Antimicrobial Chemotherapy

SIXTH EDITION

Roger Finch

Peter Davey

Mark Wilcox

William Irving

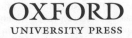

OXFORD

UNIVERSITY PRESS

OXFORD
UNIVERSITY PRESS

Great Clarendon Street, Oxford OX2 6DP

Oxford University Press is a department of the University of Oxford.
It furthers the University's objective of excellence in research, scholarship,
and education by publishing worldwide in

Oxford New York

Auckland Cape Town Dar es Salaam Hong Kong Karachi
Kuala Lumpur Madrid Melbourne Mexico City Nairobi
New Delhi Shanghai Taipei Toronto

With offices in

Argentina Austria Brazil Chile Czech Republic France Greece
Guatemala Hungary Italy Japan Poland Portugal Singapore
South Korea Switzerland Thailand Turkey Ukraine Vietnam

Oxford is a registered trade mark of Oxford University Press
in the UK and in certain other countries

Published in the United States
by Oxford University Press Inc., New York

First [edition] published by Ballière Tindall 1983
Second edition published 1989
Third edition published 1995
Fourth edition published 2000
Reprinted 2001, 2003 (twice), 2004, 2005
Fifth edition published 2007
This edition published 2012

British Library Cataloguing in Publication Data
Data available

Library of Congress Cataloging in Publication Data
Library of Congress Control Number: 2011941967

Typeset in Minion by Cenveo, Bangalore, India
Printed in Great Britain
on acid-free paper by
Ashford Colour Press Ltd, Gosport, Hampshire

ISBN 978–0–19–969765–6

10 9 8 7 6 5 4 3 2 1

Preface

Almost everyone in the developed world will receive several antibiotic courses during their lifetime. It is therefore not surprising that most clinicians and dentists will prescribe these drugs on a regular basis throughout their professional careers. Indeed, several antibiotics figure among the most frequent of all prescribed drugs.

Antibiotics are not only life-saving with regard to severe infections, such as pneumonia, meningitis, and endocarditis, but are also responsible for controlling much of the morbidity associated with non-life-threatening infectious disease; illness is abbreviated, return to normal activities is hastened, risk of infection transmission may be reduced and there is often economic benefit to the individual, as well as society, by reducing the number of working days lost. In addition, infectious complications of many commonly conducted surgical procedures are now preventable by the use of peri-operative antibiotic prophylaxis. Likewise procedures such as bone marrow and organ transplantation are also possible because of the effective control of complicating infections. These benefits are well known to healthcare professionals and to the public who no longer fear infection in the way earlier generations did. The very success of antimicrobial chemotherapy has led to a perception that such agents are generally safe and that industry will continue to generate new agents to ensure the effective control of most infectious problems.

Antibiotics have largely been derived from natural sources, mainly from environmental bacteria and fungi. Their use in clinical medicine has been one of the major successes of the past century. The term 'antibiotic' was coined by Selman A Waksman, who recognized that these 'naturally derived substances were antagonistic to the growth of other micro-organisms in high dilution.' Over the years, other agents have been developed by chemical synthesis. More recently much effort has been applied to identifying genomic research based products. The term 'antimicrobial agents' captures all such compounds which in turn have been subdivided into antibacterial, antifungal, antiparasitic (anthelminthic and antiprotozoal) and antiviral agents according to the target pathogen. However, this purist approach is often ignored in practice and the term antibiotic is somewhat loosely applied to all these agents. The reader will find all such terms in use in this book.

Antibiotics are unique among therapeutic agents in that they target invading micro-organisms rather than any pathological process arising from host cells or tissues. Furthermore, unlike other classes of drug, micro-organisms have the inherent or acquired ability to evade or inactivate antimicrobial activity of these drugs. Such resistance presents a major threat to sustaining effective treatment and prevention of infectious disease.

Indeed, controlling antibiotic resistance is one of the greatest challenges facing healthcare professionals and the public and is likely to remain so. While new drugs, vaccines and better diagnostic methods are still a requirement, the fundamental issue is to ensure that existing agents are used effectively. This can only be achieved by ensuring those doctors, dentists, and, increasingly, other healthcare professionals who use these agents in the care of their patients, pursue good prescribing practice.

Good prescribing practice is the product of sound education, with particular emphasis on the acquisition of appropriate knowledge, skills, and professional behaviour. Good science informs good practice and since the knowledge base for prescribing practice is continuously expanding, the need for life-long learning is self-evident.

Patient safety remains paramount in medicine. This is of particular importance since antibiotics are often used in the management of mild to moderate community infections and the prophylaxis of infections. The safety of antibiotics is monitored closely during drug development, at licensing and in clinical use. Since no drug is free from side effects, it is essential that the balance of risks and benefits of prescribing is understood by the prescribing practitioner. With more than 100 antimicrobial compounds currently available in the UK, this remains a particular challenge.

Setting forth the principles of rational antimicrobial chemotherapy is the whole purpose of this book. In revisiting the contents, we welcome Professor William Irving among the editors. All chapters have been revised, several rewritten and two new chapters introduced on antimicrobial stewardship and extended prescribing and also on Outpatient Parenteral Antimicrobial Therapy (OPAT), to reflect the changes that have taken place in guiding prescribing practices.

However, the basic plan of the book remains unchanged and much of the material provided by former authors has been retained attesting to its durability. As such, it reflects the vision of Professor David Greenwood, who was the inspiration for this book and who guided all previous editions so successfully.

We sincerely hope that this 6th edition of *Antimicrobial Chemotherapy* will continue to furnish students and all healthcare professionals throughout the world with the necessary framework for understanding what antimicrobial agents will and will not do, and provide a firm basis for their informed use in the treatment and control of infection.

May 2011
R.F.
P.D.
M.W.
W.I.

Contents

List of abbreviations *vii*
Historical introduction *1*

Part 1 **General properties of antimicrobial agents**

1 Inhibitors of bacterial cell wall synthesis *11*
2 Inhibitors of bacterial protein synthesis *25*
3 Synthetic antibacterial agents and miscellaneous antibiotics *40*
4 Antiviral agents *48*
5 Antiretroviral agents *61*
6 Drugs used in the treatment of viral hepatitis *68*
7 Antifungal agents *76*
8 Antiprotozoal and anthelminthic agents *82*

Part 2 **Resistance to antimicrobial agents**

9 The problem of resistance *93*
10 The genetics and mechanisms of acquired resistance *102*
11 Control of the spread of resistance and *Clostridium difficile* infection *120*

Part 3 **General principles of usage of antimicrobial agents**

12 Laboratory investigations and the treatment of infection *135*
13 General principles of the treatment of infection *146*
14 Pharmacokinetic and pharmacodynamic principles *155*
15 Prescribing in children and the elderly *164*
16 Outpatient parenteral antimicrobial therapy (OPAT) *170*
17 Adverse drug reactions *175*
18 Chemoprophylaxis and immunization *186*
19 Guidelines, formularies, and antimicrobial policies *198*
20 Antibiotic stewardship and the multi-professional antimicrobial management team *209*

Part 4 **Therapeutic use of antimicrobial agents**

21 Respiratory tract infections *223*
22 Topical use of antimicrobial agents *235*
23 Urinary infections *242*
24 Sexually transmitted infections *251*

25 Gastrointestinal infections *260*

26 Serious bloodstream infections *272*

27 Bone and joint infections *287*

28 Infections of the central nervous system *293*

29 Skin and soft tissue infections *307*

30 Tuberculosis and other mycobacterial diseases *315*

31 Infections in immunocompromised patients including HIV/AIDS *326*

32 Viral infections *334*

33 Management of HIV infection *343*

34 Treatment of chronic viral hepatitis *349*

35 Parasitic diseases *356*

36 The development and marketing of antimicrobial drugs *367*

Recommendations for further reading *379*

Index *383*

List of abbreviations

AIDS	acquired immune deficiency syndrome	HIV	human immunodeficiency virus
APA	amino-penicillanic acid	HLA	human leukocyte antigen
AZT	azidothymidine	HPV	human papilloma virus
BNF	British National Formulary	IFN	interferon
cART	combination antiretroviral therapy	IV	intravenous
CCR	chemokine receptor	MDR-TB	multidrug-resistant TB
CD	cluster of differentiation	MIC	minimum inhibitory concentrations
CDC	Centers for Disease Control	MMR	measles, mumps, and rubella (vaccination)
CMP	clinical management plan		
CMV	cytomegalovirus	MRSA	meticillin-resistant *Staph. Aureus*
CSF	cerebrospinal fluid	NANBH	non-A non-B hepatitis
CT	computed tomography	NNIS	National Nosocomial Infections Surveillance
CURB	(acronym that is a clinical prediction rule for predicting mortality in pneumonia)	NNRTI	non-nucleoside analogue reverse transcriptase inhibitors
DNA	deoxyribonucleic acid	OPAT	outpatient parenteral antimicrobial therapy
DRM	drug resistance mutation	ORF	open reading frame
EMR	electronic medical record	ORION	**O**utbreak **R**eports and **I**ntervention studies **O**f **N**osocomial (infection)
ESAC	European Surveillance of Antibiotic Consumption		
H1N1	bird influenza virus strain	PBP	penicillin binding proteins
H5N1	bird influenza virus strain	PEG	pegylated interferon
HAART	highly active antiretroviral therapy	PGD	patient group directive
HACEK group	(*Haemophilus* spp., *Actinobacillus actinomycetemcomitans, Cardiobacterium hominis, Eikenella corrodens*, and *Kingella* spp.)	PVL	Panton Vallentine Leukocydin (toxin)
		RNA	ribonucleic acid
		RTI	reverse transcriptase inhibitors
		TB	tuberculosis
HBV	hepatitis B virus	VZV	varicella-zoster virus
HBsAg	hepatitis B surface antigen	WHO	World Health Organization
HCV	hepatitis C virus	XDR-TB	extensively drug-resistant TB

Historical introduction

Although the 'antibiotic revolution' can be accurately dated to the early 1940s when Howard Florey and his colleagues in Oxford seized on Alexander Fleming's penicillin and turned it into a major therapeutic compound and Selman Waksman in the USA began his systematic pursuit of antibiotics from soil micro-organisms, the quest for chemotherapeutic agents active against pathogenic microbes began much earlier. Indeed, hopes of discovering specific antimicrobial drugs were kindled almost as soon as the microbial enemy was definitively identified by Louis Pasteur, Robert Koch, and others during the second half of the nineteenth century. By the end of that century Paul Ehrlich, often called the 'father of chemotherapy', had started the work that was to put the quest on a sound scientific footing.

Of course, the search for effective remedies is as old as mankind itself, but before the aetiological agents of infectious disease were identified and made amenable to laboratory investigation, progress had to rely entirely on the vagaries of chance and empirical observation. Not surprisingly, therefore, mankind's earliest therapeutic successes against infecting organisms came in the form of natural products such as honey that could be applied topically to infected lesions, or infusions that expelled worms visible to the naked eye. Herbal anthelminthics known since antiquity include extract of male fern (*Dryopteris filix-mas*), which is an effective vermifuge for tapeworms, and two compounds that expel intestinal roundworms: santonin (obtained from the seed-heads of *Artemisia cina*; wormseed), and oil of chenopodium (*Chenopodium ambrosioides*; American wormseed).

Observations that natural substances controlled the spectacular symptoms of certain diseases no doubt led to the initial recognition of two other ancient remedies: quinine, obtained from the bark of the cinchona tree, and emetine, an alkaloid obtained from ipecacuanha root. These compounds were introduced into Europe from South America in the seventeenth century; both are active against protozoa (the parasites of malaria and amoebic dysentery respectively), and both have survived into present-day use.

So far as antibacterial remedies were concerned, little had been achieved when Ehrlich began his work. Mercury had been used for the treatment of syphilis since the sixteenth century (giving rise to the aphorism 'one night with Venus—a lifetime with Mercury'), and chaulmoogra oil from the seeds of *Hydnocarpus* species had been used since ancient times in India for the treatment of leprosy. Otherwise the only useful antibacterial compounds were topical antiseptics that were far too toxic for systemic use. At the end of the nineteenth century hexamine, a compound that spontaneously decomposes in acid conditions to release formaldehyde, was described as being useful in urinary tract infection.

The foundations of modern chemotherapy

Oddly, in view of later developments, the foundations of twentieth century chemotherapy were built on a search for antiprotozoal agents, as it was to the newly discovered parasites of malaria and African sleeping sickness (trypanosomiasis) that Paul Ehrlich first turned his attention. He reasoned that, since these parasites could be differentiated from the tissues of infected patients by various dyes in the laboratory, such substances might display a preferential affinity for the parasites in the body as well. In a phrase, such dyes might exhibit *selective toxicity*.

Early tests of this hypothesis met with limited success, although certain aniline dyes were found to have some useful effects in trypanosomiasis of animals. Interest in dyes as chemotherapeutic agents continued, and was later to pay off in several directions, notably in helping to transform some firms in the European dyestuffs industry into large multinational pharmaceutical companies. However, Ehrlich was deflected from the study of dyes and turned to arsenicals.

Arsenicals

Arsenicals and other metallic compounds have been used in medicine at least since the time of the sixteenth century Swiss physician and alchemist, Paracelsus (Philippus Theophrastus Bombastus von Hohenheim). The explorer David Livingstone was among those who used arsenic in the treatment of nagana, a disease of ungulates, later shown by David Bruce (of *Brucella* fame) to be caused by trypanosomes. Ehrlich had also exhibited a passing interest in these compounds, and this was rekindled in 1905 by a report from the Liverpool School of Tropical Medicine that one arsenical, atoxyl, protected mice from trypanosomal infection. Ehrlich resumed research into arsenical compounds and visited the Liverpool School in 1907.

Despite its name, atoxyl was anything but atoxic and Ehrlich, together with his chemist Alfred Bertheim, set about trying to produce safer arsenical derivatives. A Japanese assistant, Sahachiro Hata, joined the team in 1909 and spirochaetes, which were thought at that time to exhibit similarities to trypanosomes, were included in the screening programme. Later that year Hata showed that arsenical compound number 606 cured rabbits infected with the spirochaetes of syphilis and, equally importantly, displayed an acceptable safety profile. Compound 606, later known as arsphenamine and marketed as Salvarsan, was the first really efficacious antibacterial agent, although its activity was restricted to spirochaetes, which are scarcely typical bacteria. An improved derivative, neoarsphenamine (Neosalvarsan), was produced in Ehrlich's laboratory in 1912.

Interest in arsenicals and other metals was also pursued elsewhere. Hopes remained of finding a drug for the treatment of African sleeping sickness, and tryparsamide and melarsoprol (Mel B) later emerged as useful compounds. Another ancient metallic remedy, tartar emetic (potassium antimony tartrate) was discovered to exhibit useful activity in two very different tropical diseases: kala azar (a protozoal disease of the reticuloendothelial system) and bilharzia (a worm infection of the blood). Tartar emetic was a familiar nostrum of Victorian medicine, and it is likely that its empirical use in previously untreatable conditions led to the discovery of its efficacy. Antimonials are still used for the treatment of kala azar, but safer drugs have been developed to treat bilharzia.

Dyes

Although Paul Ehrlich's optimistic hope of exploiting the differential affinities of dyes therapeutically came to nothing, the idea eventually bore fruit when the German dyestuffs industry started to take an interest in antimicrobial compounds. The most direct link with Ehrlich's ideas is provided by suramin (Germanin), a colourless derivative of trypan blue developed by scientists of the Bayer organization during the First World War and marketed in 1924. Like tartar emetic, suramin has proved useful in two quite unrelated parasitic diseases: trypanosomiasis and onchocerciasis (a worm disease of the skin).

Antimalarial agents

Remarkably, the very discovery of aniline dyes was sparked off by an antimalarial compound, as it was during an attempt to synthesize quinine from coal tar in 1856 that the 18 year old William Perkin, a student at the Royal College of Chemistry, stumbled on mauve purple, the first aniline dye.

The progression from dye to antimalarial was accomplished, again at Bayer, through attempts to improve the activity of Ehrlich's methylene blue. Modification of the dye produced nothing of value, but information gained on the effects of various substitutions prompted the chemists to try similar modifications on quinine-like compounds. In this way the first synthetic antimalarial drug, plasmochin (pamaquine), and the acridine derivative, atebrin (later called mepacrine or quinacrine), were produced. These compounds eventually led to the synthesis of primaquine and chloroquine, which are still in use today.

Sulphonamides

The German obsession with dyes also paid off with the discovery of the first broad-spectrum antibacterial agents, the sulphonamides. This discovery came about by another of those happy accidents with which the history of chemotherapy is littered. In 1932 Gerhard Domagk, an experimental pathologist working in the laboratories of the Bayer wing of the IG Farbenindustrie consortium, tested a number of dyes synthesized by his colleagues, Fritz Mietzsch and Josef Klarer. In one such compound, Prontosil red, a sulphonamide group had been linked to a red dye in the hope of improving the binding to bacterial cells as it was known to do with fibres. Remarkably, mice treated with Prontosil red survived an otherwise fatal infection with haemolytic streptococci, but when the compound was tested against streptococci *in vitro* it was found to have no antibacterial activity whatsoever. This paradox was explained by the Tréfouëls and their colleagues in France who showed that in the experimental animal sulphanilamide was liberated from the dye. It was this colourless compound—hitherto unsuspected of possessing any antimicrobial activity—that was responsible for the astonishing properties of Prontosil.

As a chemical, sulphanilamide had been synthesized and described as early as 1908 and Bayer were unable to protect the discovery by patent. Naturally, many other firms seized the opportunity to market the drug so that by 1940, sulphanilamide itself was available under many different trade names and a start had been made on producing the numerous sulphonamide derivatives that subsequently appeared. One proprietary version marketed in the USA, 'Elixir Sulfanilamide', was formulated in diethylene glycol and killed over 100 people. This event led to a law giving the Food and Drug Administration power to regulate the licensing of new drugs in the USA.

Such was the situation when penicillin appeared on the scene as a potential therapeutic agent in 1940.

Antibiotics

Penicillin

When Howard Florey and his team at the Sir William Dunn School of Pathology in Oxford first took an interest in penicillin in the mid-1930s, the concept of antibiosis and its therapeutic potential was not new. In fact, moulds had been used empirically in folk remedies for infected wounds for centuries and the observation that organisms, including fungi, sometimes produced substances capable of preventing the growth of others was as old as bacteriology itself. One antibiotic substance, pyocyanase, produced by the bacterium *Pseudomonas aeruginosa*, had actually been used therapeutically by instillation into wounds, at the turn of the twentieth century.

Thus, when Alexander Fleming interrupted a holiday to visit his laboratory in St Mary's Hospital in early September 1928 to make his famous observation on a contaminated culture plate of staphylococci, he was merely one in a long line of workers who had noticed similar phenomena. However, it was Fleming's observation that sparked off the events that led to the development of penicillin as the first antibiotic in the strict sense of the term.

The actual circumstances of Fleming's discovery have become interwoven with myth and legend. Attempts to reproduce the phenomenon have led to the conclusion that the lysis of staphylococci in the area surrounding a contaminant *Penicillium* colony on Fleming's original plate could have arisen only by an extraordinary concatenation of accidental events, including the vagaries of temperature of an English summer.

Early attempts to exploit penicillin foundered, partly through a failure to purify and concentrate the substance. Fleming made some attempts to use crude filtrates in superficial infections and there is documentary evidence that Cecil George Paine, a former student of Fleming's, successfully treated gonococcal ophthalmia with filtrates of *Penicillium* cultures in Sheffield as early as 1930. However, it was left to Ernst Chain, a German refugee who had been recommended to Florey as a biochemist, to obtain a stable extract of penicillin. Chain had been set the task of investigating naturally occurring antibacterial substances (including lysozyme, another of Fleming's discoveries) as a biochemical exercise. It was with his crude extracts that the first experiments were performed in mice and men. Since these extracts contained less than 1% pure penicillin, it is fortunate that problems of serious toxicity were not encountered.

Further development of penicillin was beyond the means of wartime Britain, and Florey visited the USA in 1941 with his assistant, Norman Heatley, to enlist the support of the American authorities and drug firms. Once Florey had convinced them of the potential of penicillin, progress was rapid and by the end of the Second World War bulk production of penicillin was in progress and the drug was beginning to become readily available.

Cephalosporins

The discovery of the cephalosporins (which are structurally related to the penicillins) is equally extraordinary. Between 1945 and 1948, Giuseppe Brotzu, former Rector of the University of Cagliari, Sardinia, investigated the microbial flora of a sewage outflow in the hope of discovering naturally occurring antibiotic substances. One of the organisms recovered from the sewage was a *Cephalosporium* mould that displayed striking inhibitory activity against several bacterial species—including *Salmonella typhi*, the cause of typhoid and now considered as a serotype of *S. enterica*—that were beyond the reach of penicillin at that time. Brotzu carried out some preliminary bacteriological and clinical studies, and published some encouraging results in a local house journal. However, he lacked the facilities to develop the compound further, and nothing more might have been heard of the work if he had not sent a reprint of his paper to a British acquaintance, Dr Blyth Brooke, who drew it to the attention of the Medical Research Council in London. They advised contacting Howard Florey, and Brotzu sent the mould to the Sir William Dunn School in 1948.

The first thing to be discovered by the Oxford scientists was that the mould produced two antibiotics, which they called cephalosporin P and cephalosporin N, because the former inhibited Gram-positive organisms (e.g. staphylococci and streptococci), whereas the latter was active against Gram-negative organisms (e.g. *Escherichia coli* and *S. typhi*). Neither of these substances is a cephalosporin in the sense that the term is used today: cephalosporin P proved to be an antibiotic with a steroid-like structure, and cephalosporin N turned out to be a penicillin (adicillin). The forerunner of the cephalosporins now in use, cephalosporin C, was detected later as a minor component on fractionation of cephalosporin N. Such a substance could easily have been dismissed, but it was pursued because it exhibited some attractive properties, notably stability to the enzymes produced by some strains of staphylococci that were by then threatening the effectiveness of penicillin.

Antibiotics from soil

The development of penicillin, cephalosporin C, and, subsequently, their numerous derivatives represents only one branch of the antibiotic story. The other main route came through an investigation into antimicrobial substances produced by microorganisms in soil. The chief moving spirit was Selman A. Waksman, an emigré from the Russian Ukraine, who had taken up the study of soil microbiology in the USA as a young man. In 1940, Waksman initiated a systematic search for non-toxic antibiotics produced by soil microorganisms, notably actinomycetes, a group that includes the *Streptomyces* species that were to yield many therapeutically useful compounds. Waksman was probably influenced in his decision to undertake this study by the first reports of penicillin and by the discovery by an ex-pupil, René Dubos, of the antibiotic complex tyrothricin in culture filtrates of *Bacillus brevis*.

Waksman's first discoveries were, like Dubos's tyrothricin, too toxic for systemic use, although they included actinomycin, a compound later used in cancer chemotherapy. The real breakthrough came in 1943 with the discovery by Waksman's research student, Albert Schatz, of streptomycin, the first aminoglycoside antibiotic, which was found to have a spectrum of activity that neatly complemented penicillin by inhibiting many Gram-negative bacilli and—very importantly at that time—*Mycobacterium tuberculosis*. It remained the staple treatment for tuberculosis (together with some synthetic compounds; see below) until the antibiotic rifampicin—named after the 1955 French gangster film *Rififi*—was introduced in 1968.

The success of streptomycin stimulated the pharmaceutical houses to join the chase in the years following the end of the Second World War. Soil samples by the hundred thousand from all over the world were screened for antibiotic-producing micro-organisms. Thousands of antibiotic substances were discovered and rediscovered and, although most failed preliminary toxicity tests, by the mid-1950s representatives of most of the major families of antibiotics including aminoglycosides, chloramphenicol, tetracyclines, and macrolides, had been found.

Since 1960 few truly novel antibiotics have been discovered, although a surprising number of naturally occurring molecular variations on the penicillin structure have emerged. A more fruitful approach, especially with penicillins and cephalosporins, has been to modify existing agents chemically in order to derive semi-synthetic compounds with improved properties.

Non-antibiotic antibacterial compounds

Alongside developments in naturally occurring antibiotics, chemists and microbiologists have also been successful in seeking synthetic chemicals with antibacterial activity. Most have emerged through an indefinable mixture of biochemical know-how and luck rather than the rational targeting of vulnerable processes within the microbial cell.

The first important advance came with the discovery of *para*-aminosalicylic acid and isoniazid as effective antituberculosis drugs in the early 1950s, ushering in the era of reliable triple therapy (with streptomycin) for tuberculosis. Among the rest, the nitrofurans have a long history stretching back to before the Second World War, but attracted little attention until the development of nitrofurantoin in the early 1950s. The diaminopyrimidine, trimethoprim, was first synthesized in America by George Hitchings and his colleagues in 1956.

Commercially the most successful synthetic antibacterial agents have been the quinolones. The original compound, nalidixic acid, discovered in the 1960s as a by-product of the synthesis of the antimalarial agent chloroquine, was of minor importance, but after an unpromising start quinolones began to assume a more significant role in the 1980s when derivatives such as norfloxacin and ciprofloxacin emerged that exhibited much better activity against a broader spectrum of bacteria.

Antifungal, antiparasitic, and antiviral agents

The revolution in therapy brought about by the numerous antibacterial 'wonder drugs' was not mirrored in infections caused by other microbes, but considerable progress in the treatment of non-bacterial infection was nevertheless made in the second half of the twentieth century.

Treatment of fungal infections was the first to benefit. In 1949 at the height of the search for naturally occurring antibacterial compounds, Elizabeth Hazen and Rachel Brown discovered an antibiotic with surprisingly good antifungal activity. They named it nystatin after the New York State Department of Health in whose laboratories they worked. The related polyene, amphotericin, was developed by scientists at Squibb in the 1950s. Another antifungal antibiotic, griseofulvin, had been described as early as 1939, but not used in human medicine until 1958, following the work by James Gentles in Glasgow on dermatophyte infections in experimental animals. A major step forward occurred in the 1970s with the discovery in Germany and Belgium of the unexpectedly broad-spectrum antifungal activity of certain nitroimidazole derivatives such as clotrimazole and ketoconazole (which offered the added advantage that it could be given orally) leading to the later development of the triazoles, fluconazole and itraconazole. The most recent class of antifungals, the echinocandins, are the result of screening fermentation products for novel antibiotics. These act by inhibiting fungal wall glucan synthesis and include caspofungin, used in the treatment of systemic candidiasis and aspergillosis.

Among antiprotozoal agents, most progress was made among antimalarial agents, starting with the development in America after the Second World War of a pre-war German discovery, chloroquine, and culminating in the successful testing of artemisinin, the active ingredient of an ancient Chinese herbal remedy qinghaosu in the late 1970s. Many other protozoal diseases fared less well, but patients suffering from amoebic dysentery, giardiasis, and trichomonal vaginitis (and those with infections caused by anaerobic bacteria) benefited from the development in France around 1960 of metronidazole, a synthetic compound based on the structure of a naturally-occurring antibiotic, azomycin.

Even helminthic disease treatment was to profit from the intense research activity, albeit through investigations into drugs for worm infections of farm animals. Remarkably, by the early 1980s, three anthelminthic compounds—praziquantel, albendazole, and ivermectin—were available, which between them offered safe and effective treatment for a diverse range of human worm infections.

For many years, antimicrobial agents played a very minor part in the treatment of viral infections, although prevention of a number of viral diseases through the use of vaccines was outstandingly effective. The first real breakthrough came with the nucleoside analogue aciclovir as an offshoot of anticancer research in the mid-1970s. Even this drug, the first antiviral agent to display selective toxicity, was restricted to the treatment of herpesvirus infections. Antiviral chemotherapy was not to come of age for another decade, when the emerging AIDS pandemic stimulated the pharmaceutical industry into a flurry of activity that has produced an array of drugs offering palliative if not curative therapy. The first agents to be discovered were the nucleoside reverse transcriptase inhibitors (e.g. zidovudine) which like the non-nucleoside reverse transcriptase inhibitors (e.g. efavirenz) are analogues of the naturally occurring deoxynucleotides and compete with them for incorporation in the growing viral DNA chain. Subsequent developments targeted HIV protein synthesis (protease inhibitors), entry inhibitors and inhibitors of viral integrase, which is key to viral DNA incorporation into the host chromosome.

The discovery of the first 'miracle drugs' was sanguinely declared by some to herald the virtual conquest of infection. More than 60 years of use have prompted a more sober assessment of the limitations of antimicrobial therapy. Microbes have shown amazing versatility in avoiding, with-standing, or repelling the antibiotic onslaught, while parallel medical advances have provided a large and increasing group of vulnerable patients for them to attack. Antimicrobial agents are essential tools of modern medicine, but the battle against infection is far from won. The challenge now is to preserve the remarkable achievements of the twentieth century by learning to use these powerful drugs more judiciously as well as new ways to develop new compounds.

Reference

Greenwood D (2008), *Antimicrobial Drugs: Chronicle of a twentieth century medical triumph.* Oxford: Oxford University Press.

Part 1

General properties of antimicrobial agents

Chapter 1

Inhibitors of bacterial cell wall synthesis

The essence of antimicrobial chemotherapy is selective toxicity—to kill or inhibit the microbe without harming the host (patient). In bacteria, a prime target for attack is the cell wall, since practically all bacteria (with the exception of mycoplasmas) have a cell wall, whereas mammalian cells lack this feature. Several types of antibiotics, notably β-lactam agents (penicillins, cephalosporins, and their relatives) and glycopeptides (vancomycin and teicoplanin) take advantage of this difference. Some compounds used in the treatment of tuberculosis and leprosy act on the specialized mycobacterial cell wall (p. 46).

In general bacterial cell walls conform to two basic patterns, which are distinguished by the key microbiological technique, the Gram stain. Gram-positive (staphylococci, streptococci, etc.) and Gram-negative (escherichia, pseudomonas, klebsiella, etc.) bacteria respond differently to cell wall active agents and it is helpful to understand the basis for this difference.

Cell wall construction

In both Gram-positive and Gram-negative bacteria the cell wall is formed from a cross-linked chain of alternating units of *N*-acetylglucosamine and *N*-acetylmuramic acid, known as peptidoglycan or mucopeptide. The process of synthesis is illustrated in outline in Fig. 1.1, alongside the main sites at which cell wall active antimicrobial agents act.

In Gram-positive organisms the cell wall structure is thick (about 30 nm), tightly cross-linked, and interspersed with polysugarphosphates (teichoic acids), some of which have a lipophilic tail

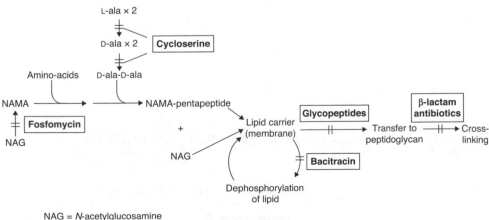

NAG = *N*-acetylglucosamine

NAMA = *N*-acetylmuramic acid

Fig. 1.1 Simplified scheme of bacterial cell wall synthesis showing site of action of cell wall-active antibiotics. Reproduced from *Medical Microbiology*, 16th edition by Greenwood D, Slack R, and Peutherer, J (2003), with permission from Elsevier.

buried in the cell membrane (lipoteichoic acids). Gram-negative bacteria, in contrast, have a relatively thin (2–3 nm), loosely cross-linked peptidoglycan layer and no teichoic acid.

External to the Gram-negative peptidoglycan is a membrane-like structure, composed chiefly of lipopolysaccharide and lipoprotein, which prevents large molecules such as glycopeptides from entering the cell. Small hydrophilic molecules enter Gram-negative bacilli through aqueous channels (porins) within the outer membrane. Differential activity among some groups of antibiotics, notably the penicillins and cephalosporins, is influenced by their ability to negotiate these porins and this, in turn, reflects the size and ionic charge of substituents carried by the individual agents.

β-lactam antibiotics

Penicillins, cephalosporins, and certain other antibiotics belong to a family of compounds, collectively known as β-lactam antibiotics, which share the structural feature of a β-lactam ring. In the penicillins the β-lactam ring is fused to a five-membered thiazolidine ring, whereas the cephalosporins display a fused β-lactam/dihydrothiazine ring structure (Fig. 1.2). The β-lactam ring is the Achilles' heel of these antibiotics because many bacteria possess enzymes (β-lactamases; see Chapter 9) that are capable of breaking open the ring and rendering the molecule antibacterially inactive.

Penicillins

The original preparations of penicillin were found on analysis to be mixtures of four closely related compounds (penicillin F, G, K, and X). Benzylpenicillin (penicillin G), often simply called 'penicillin', was chosen for further development because it exhibited the most attractive properties and because a manufacturing process was developed in which *Penicillium chrysogenum* produced benzylpenicillin almost exclusively.

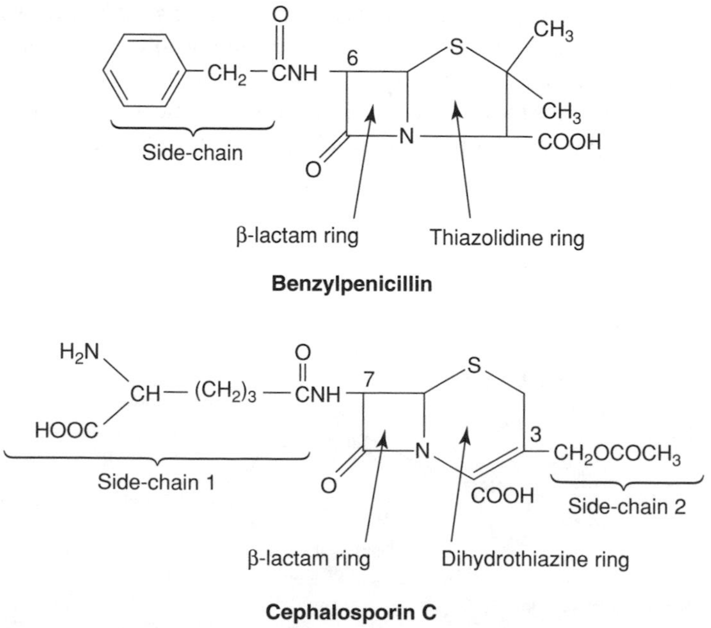

Fig. 1.2 Structures of benzylpenicillin and cephalosporin C, forerunners of the penicillin and cephalosporin groups, respectively. The fused-ring systems and the side-chains, which offer the possibility of modifications introduced in semi-synthetic derivatives, are indicated.

Early attempts to modify this structure relied on presenting the *Penicillium* mould that produced penicillin with different side-chain precursors during the manufacturing process. Later a method was discovered of removing the side chain of benzylpenicillin to liberate the penicillin nucleus, 6-amino-penicillanic acid (6-APA). Various chemical groupings could then be added to 6-APA according to the ingenuity of the chemist; a large number of compounds, collectively called semi-synthetic penicillins, have been prepared in this way.

Benzylpenicillin revolutionized the treatment of many potentially lethal bacterial infections, such as scarlet fever, puerperal sepsis, bacterial endocarditis, pneumococcal pneumonia, staphylococcal sepsis, meningococcal meningitis, gonorrhoea, syphilis (and other spirochaetal diseases), anthrax, and many anaerobic infections. The overwhelming importance of benzylpenicillin as a major breakthrough in therapy may be gauged from the fact that it remains today the treatment of choice for many of these diseases.

However, resistance has eroded the value of benzylpenicillin. Nearly all staphylococci and many strains of gonococci are now resistant. Moreover, pneumococci exhibiting reduced susceptibility to benzylpenicillin became increasingly prevalent, especially in certain geographical locales. Such strains are of two types: those for which the minimum inhibitory concentration (MIC) of benzylpenicillin is increased from the usual value of about 0.02 mg/l to 0.1–1 mg/l, and those for which the MIC exceeds 1 mg/l. The former are sufficiently sensitive to enable the antibiotic to be used successfully in high dosage, except in pneumococcal meningitis. However, penicillin is not clinically reliable in infections with strains exhibiting the higher level of resistance.

Despite its attractive properties benzylpenicillin is not the perfect antimicrobial agent:

- it exhibits a restricted antibacterial spectrum;
- it causes hypersensitivity reactions in a small proportion of persons to whom it is given;
- it is broken down by gastric acidity when administered orally;
- it is eliminated from the body at a spectacular rate by the kidneys;
- it is hydrolysed by β-lactamases produced by many bacteria, including staphylococci.

Subsequent developments have been aimed at overcoming these inherent weaknesses while retaining the attractive properties of benzylpenicillin: high intrinsic activity and lack of toxicity.

Acid stability

The first major success in improving the pharmacological properties of penicillin was achieved with phenoxymethylpenicillin (penicillin V). This compound has properties very similar to those of benzylpenicillin, but it is acid stable and thus achieves better and more reliable serum levels when given orally, at the expense of being marginally less active. Azidocillin, phenethicillin, and propicillin exhibit similar properties, but are not widely used.

Prolongation of plasma levels

Most β-lactam antibiotics are rapidly excreted, with plasma half-lives of one to three hours. Benzylpenicillin is even more rapidly eliminated and several strategies are used in order to maintain effective levels in the body. The blockbuster approach is simply to give enormous doses of this non-toxic drug. Alternatively, oral probenecid can be administered with the penicillin. Probenecid competes for sites of active tubular secretion in the kidney, slowing down the elimination of penicillin. Another solution is to use insoluble derivatives of penicillin. These are injected intramuscularly and act as depots from which penicillin is slowly liberated. Originally, mixtures of penicillin with oily or waxy excipients were used, but insoluble salts, such as procaine penicillin, were later developed. In this way an inhibitory concentration of penicillin can be maintained in the bloodstream for up to 24 h; extremely insoluble salts, such as benzathine penicillin, release penicillin even more slowly, but the concentrations achieved are, of course, correspondingly lower.

Extension of spectrum

Broadening the spectrum of benzylpenicillin to encompass Gram-negative bacilli was first achieved by adding an amino group to the side-chain to form ampicillin. Ampicillin is slightly less active than benzylpenicillin against Gram-positive cocci and is equally susceptible to staphylococcal β-lactamase. However, it displays much improved activity against some enterobacteria, including *Escherichia coli, Salmonella enterica*, and *Shigella* spp. as well as against *Haemophilus influenzae*. Oral absorption is relatively poor, but can be improved by esterifying the molecule to form so-called pro-drugs, such as pivampicillin (see p. 156). Such compounds are split by non-specific tissue esterases in the intestinal mucosa to release ampicillin during absorption. Improved absorption has also been more simply achieved by a minor modification to the molecule to produce amoxicillin.

A change of spectrum was brought about by altering the form of the linkage at the 6-position of the penicillanic acid nucleus to amidino (N–CH N) instead of acyl (CO–NH). The only penicillin of this type to become available, mecillinam (known as amdinocillin in the USA), is active against ampicillin-sensitive enterobacteria and some of the more resistant Gram-negative bacilli. However, mecillinam displays no useful activity against Gram-positive cocci. It is poorly absorbed when given orally, but a prodrug form, pivmecillinam, can be given by mouth.

Temocillin, a penicillin in which the β-lactam ring carries a methoxy group that renders it stable to most β-lactamases (as in cephamycins; see p. 18), has an unusual spectrum. It is moderately active against many Gram-negative bacilli, but has no useful activity against *Pseudomonas aeruginosa*, Gram-positive cocci, or anaerobic organisms. It was largely abandoned, but a rise in prevalence of Gram-negative bacilli that produce broad-spectrum β-lactamases has prompted its reintroduction.

Antipseudomonal penicillins

None of the agents so far mentioned has any activity against *Ps. aeruginosa*, an important opportunist pathogen, especially in burns, cystic fibrosis, and intensive care and immunocompromised patients. A simple carboxyl derivative of benzylpenicillin, carbenicillin, was found to have weak but useful activity and was used for a time in high dosage. It has been superseded by ticarcillin, the thienyl variant of carbenicillin and by a group of ureido derivatives of ampicillin, including azlocillin and piperacillin. These antipseudomonal penicillins must be administered by injection, but two esterified pro-drugs of carbenicillin, carfecillin, and carindacillin, are available in some countries.

Antistaphylococcal penicillins

By the end of the 1950s, 80% of staphylococci isolated in hospitals were resistant to benzylpenicillin because of their ability to produce penicillinase (β-lactamase). The appearance of these resistant organisms, which often gave rise to serious cross-infection problems, stimulated research into derivatives that were insusceptible to β-lactamase hydrolysis. Success was achieved with meticillin (no longer generally available), nafcillin, and a group called isoxazolylpenicillins: oxacillin, cloxacillin, dicloxacillin, and flucloxacillin. The isoxazolylpenicillins, particularly flucloxacillin, are well absorbed when given orally and are most widely used. They are highly bound to serum protein in the body (see p. 157), but this does not adversely affect their therapeutic efficacy.

Resistance to penicillinase-stable penicillins is caused not by inactivating enzymes, but by alterations to the penicillin target (p. 19). Staphylococci of this type were originally characterized by resistance to meticillin and, although this compound is no longer used in treatment, they are still known as meticillin-resistant staphylococci. Resistance extends to all β-lactam agents (or almost all—see p. 17) and often accompanies resistance to gentamicin and other antibiotics (multiresistant staphylococci). Some strains fully display the resistance phenotype only at a reduced growth temperature or in the presence of high salt concentrations. Particularly troublesome are meticillin-resistant *Staphylococcus aureus* strains (MRSA), which are an important cause of healthcare-associated infection. Some MRSA strains have a propensity to spread in healthcare institutions (e.g. EMRSA) and recently in community settings (e.g. USA 300) to give rise to mini-epidemics.

The spectrum of activity of the most important penicillins in clinical use is shown in Table 1.1.

Cephalosporins

Cephalosporins generally exhibit a somewhat broader spectrum than penicillins, though, idio-syncratically, they lack activity against enterococci. They are mostly stable to staphylococcal β-lactamase and often lack cross-allergenicity with penicillins.

The original cephalosporin, cephalosporin C, was never marketed, but has given rise to a large family of compounds that continues to expand. The extra carbon atom in the fused ring (Fig. 1.2), offers the possibility of modifications at the carbon designated C-3 (right-hand side of the molecule in Fig. 1.2). Consequently, there are many more cephalosporins than penicillins (Table 1.2). Alterations at either end of the molecule may profoundly affect antibacterial activity but, as a generalization, substituents at the C-3 position have more influence on pharmacokinetic properties. Certain cephalosporins such as cefalotin (no longer widely available) and cefotaxime have an acetoxymethyl side chain at C-3 which is slowly altered by liver enzymes. The altered cepha-losporin is usually less active than the parent antibiotic and may display altered pharmacokinetic behaviour, but there is little evidence that the clinical effectiveness is impaired. Several cepha-losporins, including cefamandole, cefotetan, cefmenoxime, cefoperazone, and the oxacephem latamoxef possess a complex side chain at the C-3 position that has been implicated in haemato-logical side effects in some patients (see p. 17).

The earliest cephalosporins, cefalotin and cefaloridine, are not absorbed when given orally. Moreover, it soon became clear that the Gram-negative organisms within their spectrum were capable of elaborating a wide variety of enzymes that exhibited potent cephalosporinase activity (see Chapter 9). As with penicillins, developments within the cephalosporin family were aimed at devising compounds with more attractive properties: oral absorption or other improved pharma-cological properties; stability to inactivating enzymes; better intrinsic activity; or a combination of these features.

Cephalosporins display diverse properties that tend to be grouped according to their relative activity against Gram-positive and Gram-negative bacteria, *P. aeruginosa*, and most recently MRSA. It is also helpful to distinguish between cephalosporins (the majority) that have to be administered parenterally and those that can be given orally (Table 1.2). Cephalosporins are com-monly described as first, second, third, fourth and, most recently, fifth generation compounds. These loose terms refer to:

- early compounds such as cefalotin and cefalexin that were available before about 1975 (first generation);
- β-lactamase stable compounds such as cefuroxime and cefoxitin (second generation);
- compounds such as cefotaxime and ceftazidime that combine β-lactamase stability with improved intrinsic activity (third generation); ceftazidime, but not cefotaxime, has good activity against *P. aeruginosa*;
- compounds such as cefepime and cefpirome that are similar to ceftazidime, i.e. with good activity against Enterobacteria and *P. aeruginosa*, but better Gram-positive activity (fourth generation);

Table 1.1 Summary of the antibacterial properties of selected penicillins

Penicillin	Staphylococci		Streptococci	Neisseria spp.	Haemophilus influenzae	Enterobacteria		Pseudomonas aeruginosa	Anaerobes
	Activity	Stability[a]				Activity	Stability[a]		
Benzylpenicillin	Very good	Poor	Very good	Very good	Fair	–	–	–	Variable
Phenoxymethylpenicillin	Very good	Poor	Very good	Good	Poor	–	–	–	Variable
Ampicillin Amoxicillin	Good	Poor	Very good	Very good	Good	Good	Poor	–	Variable
Piperacillin Ticarcillin	Good	Poor	Good	Good	Good	Variable	Variable	Good	Fair
Cloxacillin Flucloxacillin	Good	Good	Fair	Fair	Poor	–	–	–	Fair
Mecillinam	–	–	–	Fair	Poor	Good	Variable	Poor	Poor
Temocillin	–	–	–	Good	Good	Good	Very good	–	–

–, no useful activity. [a] Stability to β-lactamases of these organisms.

Table 1.2 Categorization of cephalosporins in clinical use

Parenteral compounds			Oral compounds		
Cefalotin	Cefacetrile	Ceforanide	Cefalexin[a]	Cefaloglycin	Cefroxadine
Cefaloridine	Cefapirin	Cefonicid	Cefradine[a]	Cefadroxil[a]	Cefatrizine
Cefazolin	Cefazedone	Ceftezole	Cefaclor	Cefprozil[a]	Loracarbef[b]
Cefamandole					

Compounds with improved β-lactamase stability			Compounds with improved β-lactamase stability	
Cefuroxime[a]	Cefmetazole	Cefotiam	*Non-esterified*	*Esterified*
Cefoxitin	Cefotetan	Cefminox	Cefixime[a]	Cefuroxime axetil[a]
			Ceftibuten	Cefpodoxime proxetil[a]
Compounds with improved intrinsic activity and β-lactamase stability			Cefdinir	Cefetamet pivoxil
				Cefteram pivoxil
Cefotaxime[a]	Cefmenoxime	Latamoxef[c]		Cefotiam hexetil
Ceftriaxone[a]	Ceftizoxime	Flomoxef[c]		Cefditoren pivoxil
Cefodizime	Cefuzonam			Cefcapene pivoxil

Compounds distinguished by activity against *Pseudomonas aeruginosa*		
Broad spectrum	*Medium spectrum*	*Narrow spectrum*
Ceftazidime[a]	Cefoperazone	Cefsulodin
Cefpirome[a]	Cefpimizole	
Cefepime	Cefpiramide	

Compounds distinguished by activity against MRSA
Ceftaroline

[a] Compound available in the UK (2006).

[b] Strictly a carbacephem.

[c] Strictly oxa-cephems.

- recently developed compounds, including ceftaroline and ceftobiprole (not yet licensed), are the first examples of β-lactams/cephalosporin drugs that have useful activity against MRSA, and are referred to as anti-MRSA (or fifth generation) cephalosporins.

Parenteral compounds susceptible to enterobacterial β-lactamases

Cephalosporins in this group are of limited clinical value and have been largely superseded by other derivatives; all have been abandoned in the UK. Cefazolin has the unusual property of being excreted in fairly high concentration in bile; cefamandole exhibits a modestly expanded spectrum. Others, including cefapirin, ceforanide, and cefonicid, offer no discernible advantage over earlier congeners such as cefalotin.

Parenteral compounds with improved β-lactamase stability

An important advance was achieved with the development of cephalosporins that exhibit almost complete stability to the common β-lactamases of enterobacteria such as *Esch. coli* and *Klebsiella aerogenes*. The first of these were cefuroxime and cefoxitin, the latter being one of a group of cephalosporins, collectively called cephamycins, which have a β-lactam ring modified by the addition of a stabilizing methoxy substituent. Other cephamycins available in some countries include cefotetan, cefmetazole, and cefminox. The cephamycins are unusual in displaying useful activity against anaerobes of the *Bacteroides fragilis* group.

These compounds have been overshadowed by the appearance of cephalosporins that combine almost complete stability to most β-lactamases with much improved intrinsic activity. Cefotaxime was the forerunner of this group of compounds, but several others are available: ceftizoxime and cefmenoxime are similar to cefotaxime; ceftriaxone displays a sufficiently long plasma half-life to warrant once-daily administration; cefodizime is said to possess immunomodulating properties.

Latamoxef (moxalactam), which is strictly an oxa-cephem (see below), also displays activity analogous to that of cefotaxime and its relatives, but differs in possessing useful activity against *B. fragilis* and related anaerobes. However, latamoxef has lost favour owing to toxicity problems and it is no longer widely available.

Compounds distinguished by antipseudomonal activity

Ps. aeruginosa is not susceptible to most cephalosporins and, as with penicillins, considerable efforts have been made to find derivatives that include this important opportunist pathogen in their spectrum. Ceftazidime, cefpirome, and cefepime add activity against *Ps. aeruginosa* to broad-spectrum activity comparable with that of cefotaxime and its congeners. These compounds have established a useful role in the management of *Ps. eruginosa* infections in seriously ill patients. However, the antistaphylococcal activity is suspect and cefpirome may have some advantage in this respect. Cefepime retains activity against some opportunist Gram-negative bacilli that develop resistance to cefotaxime and its relatives.

Among other antipseudomonal cephalosporins, cefoperazone, cefpimizole, and cefpiramide are not distinguished by any unusual activity against other organisms and cefsulodin is extraordinary in being virtually inactive against bacteria other than *Ps. aeruginosa*.

Oral cephalosporins

Early development of the cephalosporins yielded cefalexin, a compound of modest activity, particularly in terms of its bactericidal action against Gram-negative bacilli, but which is virtually completely absorbed when given orally. Many other oral derivatives are structurally minor variations on the cefalexin theme. Such compounds include cefradine (the properties of which are indistinguishable from those of cefalexin), cefaclor (which is more active against the important respiratory pathogen *H. influenzae*), cefadroxil (which exhibits a modestly extended plasma half-life), and cefprozil (which exhibits improved intrinsic activity). Loracarbef is a carbacephem (carbon replacing sulphur in the fused-ring structure), but is otherwise structurally identical to cefaclor. Not surprisingly, its properties closely resemble those of cefaclor.

Cefixime and ceftibuten are structurally unrelated to cefalexin. They display much improved activity against most Gram-negative bacilli, but at the expense of antistaphylococcal (and, in the case of ceftibuten, antipneumococcal) activity, which is very poor. Another compound of this type, cefdinir, appears to lack these defects.

The principle of esterification to produce pro-drugs with improved oral absorption has also been applied to cephalosporins. Two such compounds, cefuroxime axetil and cefpodoxime proxetil, are available in the UK; cefteram pivoxil, cefetamet pivoxil, cefotiam hexetil, cefditoren pivoxil, and cefcapene pivoxil are marketed elsewhere. These esters are fairly well absorbed by the oral route and deliver the parent drug into the bloodstream. Cefpodoxime, cefteram, and cefetamet are more active than the others against most organisms within the spectrum, although cefetamet has poor activity against staphylococci.

A summary of the antimicrobial spectrum of the most important cephalosporins is presented in Table 1.3.

Other β-lactam agents

In addition to penicillins and cephalosporins, various other compounds display a β-lactam ring in their structure (Fig. 1.3). Clavulanic acid, a naturally occurring substance obtained from *Streptomyces clavuligerus*, and two penicillanic acid sulphones, sulbactam and tazobactam have little useful antibacterial activity, but act as β-lactamase inhibitors. They are used in combination with β-lactamase-labile agents with a view to restoring their activity: clavulanic acid is combined with amoxicillin (co-amoxiclav) or ticarcillin; sulbactam with ampicillin; and tazobactam with piperacillin.

Structurally novel compounds that exhibit antibacterial activity in their own right include the carbapenems (imipenem, doripenem, meropenem, panipenem, and ertapenem) and aztreonam, one of a group of compounds, collectively known as monobactams, which have a β-lactam ring but no associated fused-ring system. Imipenem is readily hydrolysed by a dehydropeptidase located in the mammalian kidney and is administered together with a dehydropeptidase inhibitor, cilastatin. Aztreonam is also β-lactamase stable, but, in contrast to carbapenems, the activity is restricted to aerobic Gram-negative bacteria.

The carbapenems are stable to most bacterial β-lactamases, and exhibit the broadest spectrum of all β-lactam antibiotics, with high activity against nearly all Gram-positive and Gram-negative bacteria other than intracellular bacteria such as chlamydiae. Carbapenems are generally considered as the last line of defence in bacterial infection and tend to reserved for life-threatening infection, especially when empirical therapy is required because the causative pathogen is unknown. Given this place in the therapeutic armamentarium, a most worrying development is the recent rapid emergence of new types of carbapenemases, enzymes produced predominantly by Gram-negative bacteria, which render these valuable agents inactive.

Factors affecting β-lactam agents

Penicillins and other β-lactam antibiotics are categorized as bactericidal agents, but this is true only when bacteria are actively dividing. Moreover, the way bacteria respond to β-lactam antibiotics is affected by subtle differences in the mode of action. Several other features of the response that may sometimes have therapeutic implications have also been discovered.

Mode of action of β-lactam agents

All β-lactam antibiotics interfere with the final cross-linking reaction that gives the cell wall its strength (Fig. 1.1). However, several forms of the enzyme that performs this reaction are needed to maintain the complex molecular architecture of the cell and these are differentially inhibited by various β-lactam agents. These target enzymes belong to a group of proteins to which penicillin and other β-lactam antibiotics bind (penicillin-binding proteins; PBPs). *Esch. coli*, the best-studied species, has seven of these proteins, numbered la, lb, 2, 3, 4, 5, and 6 in order of decreasing molecular weight. PBPs 4–6 are thought to be unconnected with the antibacterial effect of β-lactam agents, since mutants lacking these proteins do not seem to be disabled in any way. Binding to the remainder has been correlated with the various morphological effects of β-lactam antibiotics on Gram-negative bacilli. Thus, cefalexin and its close congeners, as well as aztreonam, bind almost exclusively to PBP 3 and inhibit the division process, causing the bacteria to grow as long filaments. The amidinopenicillin, mecillinam, binds preferentially to PBP 2 and causes a generalized effect on the cell wall so that the bacteria gradually assume a spherical shape. Most other β-lactam antibiotics bind to PBPs 1–3 and, in sufficient concentration, induce the formation

Table 1.3 Summary of the spectrum of antibacterial activity of cephalosporins

Cephalosporin	Staphylococci	Streptococci[a]	Neisseria spp.	Haemophilus influenzae	Enterobacteria	Pseudomonas aeruginosa	Bacteroides spp.
Cefuroxime	Good	Very good	Good	Good	Good	–	–
Cefotaxime	Good	Very good	Very good	Very good	Very good	Poor	Poor
Ceftriaxone							
Ceftazidime	Fair	Good	Very good	Very good	Very good	Good	Poor
Cefpirome	Good	Very good	Very good	Very good	Very good	Good	–
Ceftaroline	Good[b]	Very good	Good	Good	Good	–	Poor
Cefalexin	Good	Good	Poor	Poor	Variable	–	–
Cefradine							
Cefadroxil							
Cefaclor	Good	Good	Fair	Good	Variable	–	–
Cefixime	Poor	Very good	Good	Good	Very good	–	–
Cefprozil	Good	Good	Very good	Very good	Very good	–	–
Cefpodoxime	Good	Very good	Very good	Good	Very good	–	–

–, no useful activity. [a]Enterococci are resistant to all cephalosporins. [b]Includes activity against MRSA.

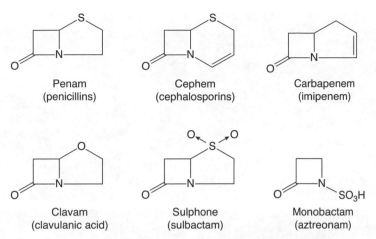

Fig. 1.3 Basic molecular structures of β-lactam antibiotics currently available (examples in parentheses).

of osmotically fragile, wall-deficient forms (called spheroplasts), which typically emerge at the cell wall growth site as the cell starts to divide. The morphological events are illustrated in Fig. 1.4. An important consequence of differences in binding is that compounds such as cefalexin, aztreonam, and mecillinam, which bind only to PBP 3 or PBP 2, are much more slowly bactericidal to Gram-negative bacilli that those that bind PBPs 1, 2, and 3. The recently developed anti-MRSA cephalosporins are active by virtue of improved affinity for the PBP that is present in MRSA strains (PBP 2a).

In Gram-negative bacilli, rupture of spheroplasts can be quantitatively prevented by raising the osmolality of the growth medium, so cell death appears to be an osmotic phenomenon. The lethal event in Gram-positive organisms, which have much thicker cell walls, appears to be autolysis triggered by the release of lipoteichoic acid following exposure to β-lactam antibiotics.

Optimal dosage effect

A further complication in Gram-positive organisms is that increasing the concentration of β-lactam antibiotics often results in a reduced bactericidal effect. The mechanism of this effect (known as the Eagle phenomenon after its discoverer) is obscure, but may be related to the multiple sites of penicillin action and the fact that cell death occurs only during active growth: saturating a relatively insusceptible penicillin-binding protein may rapidly halt growth and thereby prevent the lethal events that normally follow inhibition of another PBP by lower drug levels.

Persisters and penicillin tolerance

In both Gram-positive and Gram-negative bacteria, a proportion of the population, called persisters, survive exposure to concentrations of β-lactam antibiotics that are lethal to the rest of the culture. They remain dormant so long as the antibiotic is present and resume growth when it is removed. In addition, some strains of staphylococci and streptococci display 'tolerance' to β-lactam antibiotics in that they succumb much more slowly than usual to the lethal action of β-lactam agents. The therapeutic significance, if any, of persisters is unknown, but penicillin tolerance has been implicated in therapeutic failures in bacterial endocarditis where bactericidal activity is important for treatment success (p. 276).

Postantibiotic effect

Much has also been made of laboratory observations that the antimicrobial activity of β-lactam agents may persist for an hour or more after the drug is removed. This effect is not confined to

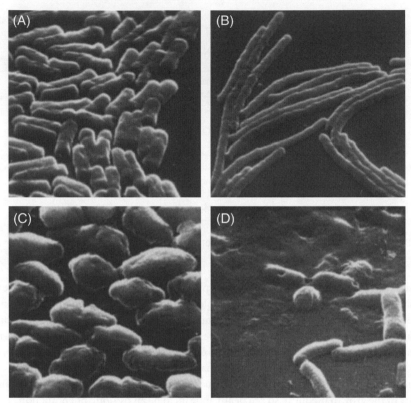

Fig. 1.4 Morphological effects of penicillins and cephalosporins on Gram-negative bacilli (scanning electron micrographs): (A) Normal *Esch. coli* cells; (B) *Esch. coli* exposed to cefalexin, 32 mg/l, for 1 h; (C) *Esch. coli* exposed to mecillinam, 10 mg/l, for 2 h; (D) *Esch. coli* exposed to ampicillin, 64 mg/l, for 1 h, showing lysed debris, central wall lesions, and a spheroplast; higher concentrations of most β-lactam antibiotics cause this effect. Reproduced from Greenwood D, O'Grady F, 'The Two Sites of Penicillin Action in Escherichia coli', *Journal of Infectious Diseases*, 1973; **128**: 791–4, by permission of Oxford University Press.

β-lactam agents and is more consistently demonstrated with Gram-positive than with Gram-negative organisms. Theoretically, knowledge of postantibiotic effects might influence the design of dosage regimens, but in practice they are too erratic to be used in this way, even if the laboratory observations could be convincingly shown to have clinical relevance, which is presently not the case.

Glycopeptides

The glycopeptides vancomycin and teicoplanin are complex heterocyclic molecules consisting of a multi-peptide backbone to which are attached various substituted sugars. These compounds bind to acyl-D-alanyl-D-alanine in peptidoglycan, thereby preventing the addition of new building blocks to the growing cell wall (Fig. 1.1). Glycopeptides are too bulky to penetrate the external membrane of Gram-negative bacteria, so the spectrum of activity is virtually restricted to Gram-positive organisms. Acquired resistance used to be uncommon, but resistant strains of enterococci are now widely prevalent and staphylococci exhibiting reduced susceptibility are causing concern. Avoparcin, a glycopeptide formerly used in animal husbandry (now banned in the European

Union), has been implicated in generating resistance in enterococci, but human use of glycopeptides is equally important. Some Gram-positive genera, including *Lactobacillus* spp., *Pediococcus* spp., and *Leuconostoc* spp. are inherently resistant to glycopeptides, but these organisms are seldom implicated in disease.

Vancomycin

This antibiotic is widely used for the treatment of infections caused by staphylococci that are resistant to meticillin and other β-lactam antibiotics, and for serious infections with Gram-positive organisms in patients who are allergic to penicillin. It is very poorly absorbed when given by mouth and must be given by injection. Oral administration is indicated in the treatment of antibiotic-associated *Clostridium difficile* infection (p. 268).

Early preparations of vancomycin contained impurities that gave the drug a reputation for toxicity. The purified formulations now available are much safer, but renal and ototoxicity still occur, particularly with high dosage. The drug is given by slow intravenous infusion (typically over 1–2 hours) to avoid 'red man syndrome' (p. 177).

Teicoplanin

This is a naturally occurring mixture of several closely related compounds with a spectrum of activity similar to that of vancomycin, although some coagulase-negative staphylococci (*Staphylococcus epidermidis* etc.) are less susceptible to teicoplanin. Some strains of enterococci that are resistant to vancomycin (those with the VanB phenotype; p. 115) retain susceptibility to teicoplanin. Unlike vancomycin, teicoplanin can be administered by intramuscular injection; it also has a much longer plasma half-life than vancomycin and a reduced propensity to cause adverse reactions.

Telavancin

Telavancin is a recently launched, once-daily, injectable, lipoglycopeptide that has increased bactericidal properties compared with vancomycin and teicoplanin. This may relate to multimodal activity, i.e. a cell membrane depolarizing effect in addition to conventional glycopeptide cell wall action.

Other cell wall active agents

Bacitracin   Topical use only

Bacitracin is a cyclic peptide antibiotic, made up of about 10 amino acids joined in a ring. It was first obtained from a strain of *Bacillus subtilis* grown from the infected wound of a 7 year old girl, Margaret Tracy, in whose honour the antibiotic was named.

The spectrum of activity of bacitracin and related cyclic peptides such as gramicidin and tyrocidine is restricted to Gram-positive organisms. They are too toxic for systemic use but are found in topical preparations. Bacitracin also finds a place in microbiology laboratories in the presumptive identification of *Streptococcus pyogenes*, which is exquisitely susceptible to its action. Bacitracin acts by preventing regeneration of the lipid carrier in the cell membrane, which is left in an unusable phosphorylated form after transporting cell wall subunits (Fig. 1.1).

Cycloserine

Cycloserine has broad-spectrum, but rather feeble, antibacterial activity. It is now used only against multiresistant *Mycobacterium tuberculosis* (p. 100). The drug bears a structural resemblance to the

D-isomer of alanine and inhibits alanine racemase. It also blocks the synthetase enzyme that links two D-ala molecules together before they are inserted into the cell wall (Fig. 1.1). Antituberculosis agents that act on special features of the mycobacterial cell wall are discussed in Chapter 3.

Fosfomycin

Fosfomycin is a naturally occurring antibiotic originally obtained from a species of *Streptomyces* isolated in Spain. It is formulated as the sodium salt for parenteral use, but this is unsuitable for oral administration. It is well tolerated, and the ready emergence of bacterial resistance that is observed *in vitro* does not appear to have been a major problem in treatment. The trometamol (tromethamine) salt, which is highly soluble, well absorbed, and excreted in high concentration in urine, is preferable to the calcium salt for oral therapy. Although fosfomycin is used for assorted purposes in some countries, it is not sufficiently reliable for serious infections. It is best reserved for uncomplicated cystitis (for which the trometamol salt is well suited), especially due to Gram-negative bacteria producing extended spectrum β-lactamases.

Fosfomycin inhibits the pyruvyl transferase enzyme that brings about the condensation of phosphoenolpyruvate and *N*-acetylglucosamine in the formation of *N*-acetylmuramic acid (Fig. 1.1). Gram-positive cocci are less susceptible than Gram-negative rods. The precise level of activity is a matter of dispute, since the in-vitro activity can be manipulated by altering the test medium. Glucose-6-phosphate potentiates the activity against many Gram-negative bacilli by inducing the active transport of fosfomycin into the bacterial cell.

Key points

Penicillins

- *Benzylpenicillin (penicillin G)* is the original penicillin and still best against streptococci and spirochaetes.
- *Amoxicillin (oral)/ampicillin (injection)* is used if broader spectrum is needed.
- *Flucloxacillin* is best for staphylococci, except MRSA.
- *Piperacillin/ticarcillin* are usually given with a β-lactamase inhibitor (tazobactam/clavulanic acid) for serious infection, especially if a risk of pseudomonas.

Cephalosporins

- *Cefuroxime* is a good broad-spectrum, intravenous work-horse antibiotic.
- *Cefotaxime/ceftriaxone* are more active than cefuroxime and used for serious infections.
- *Ceftazidime* is reserved for serious infection, especially if a risk of pseudomonas.
- *Cefalexin/cefradine/cefaclor* oral absorption is their chief virtue.
- All cephalosporins are associated with the risk of inducing *C. difficile* infection.

Further reading

Finch RG, Greenwood D, Norrby SR, Whitley RJ (2010), *Antibiotic Chemotherapy* (9th edn) London: Elsevier.

Chapter 2

Inhibitors of bacterial protein synthesis

The remarkable process by which proteins are manufactured on the ribosomal conveyor belt according to a blueprint provided by the cell nucleus is of fundamental importance to cell life. Although the general mechanism is thought to be universal, the process as it occurs in bacterial cells is sufficiently different from mammalian protein synthesis to offer scope for the selective toxicity required of therapeutically useful antimicrobial agents. The chief difference involves the actual structure of the protein and RNA components of the ribosomal workshop.

In order to understand how the various inhibitors of protein synthesis work it is helpful to be aware of the main features of the process. The first step is the formation of an initiation complex, consisting of messenger RNA (mRNA), transcribed from the appropriate area of a DNA strand; the two ribosomal subunits; and methionyl transfer RNA (tRNA) (N-formylated in bacteria) which occupies the 'peptidyl donor' site (P site) on the larger ribosomal subunit. Aminoacyl tRNA appropriate to the next codon to be read slots into place in the aminoacyl 'acceptor' site (A-site), and an enzyme called peptidyl transferase attaches the methionine to the new amino acid with the formation of a peptide bond. The mRNA and the ribosome now move with respect to one another so that the dipeptide is translocated from the A- to the P-site and the next codon of the mRNA is aligned with the A-site in readiness for the next aminoacyl tRNA. The process continues to accumulate amino acids in the nascent peptide chain according to the order dictated by mRNA until a 'nonsense' codon is encountered, which signals chain termination.

The selective activity of therapeutically useful inhibitors of protein synthesis is far from absolute. Some, such as tetracyclines and clindamycin, have sufficient activity against eukaryotic ribosomes to be of value against certain protozoa. Moreover, the mitochondria of mammalian and other eukaryotic cells (which may have been derived from endosymbiotic bacteria during the course of evolution) carry out protein synthesis that is susceptible to some antibiotics used in therapy. The selectivity of these antibiotics is, therefore, due not only to structural differences in the ribosomal targets, but also access to, and affinity for, those targets.

Inhibitors of bacterial protein synthesis with sufficient selectivity to be useful in human therapy include aminoglycosides, chloramphenicol, tetracyclines, fusidic acid, macrolides, lincosamides, streptogramins, oxazolidinones, and mupirocin.

Aminoglycosides

Classification

The first aminoglycoside, streptomycin, discovered in 1943 (see Historical introduction), was later found to be just one of a large family of related antibiotics produced by various species of *Streptomyces* and *Micromonospora*. Aminoglycosides derived from the latter genus, such as gentamicin, are distinguished in their spelling by an 'i' rather than a 'y' in the 'mycin' suffix.

Structurally, most aminoglycosides consist of a linked ring system composed of aminosugars and an aminosubstituted cyclic polyalcohol (aminocyclitol). One antibiotic usually included with the group, spectinomycin, contains no aminoglycoside substituent and is properly regarded as a pure aminocyclitol.

The aminocyclitol moiety of most aminoglycosides consists of one of two derivatives of streptamine: streptidine (present in streptomycin and its relatives) or deoxystreptamine (present in most other therapeutically useful aminoglycosides) (Fig. 2.1). Deoxystreptamine-containing aminoglycosides can, in their turn, be subdivided into two major groups: the neomycin group and the kanamycin group. The aminoglycosides most commonly used in medicine, including gentamicin and tobramycin, belong to the kanamycin group. The designation 'kanamycin', 'gentamicin', or 'neomycin' indicates a family of closely related compounds and commercial preparations usually contain a mixture of these. For example, gentamicin, as used therapeutically, is a mixture of several structural variants of the gentamicin C complex (Fig. 2.2).

General properties

The aminoglycosides are potent, broad-spectrum bactericidal agents that are very poorly absorbed when given orally and are therefore administered by injection. The spectrum includes most Gram-negative bacilli and staphylococci. They lack useful activity against streptococci and anaerobes, but the activity against streptococci can often be improved by using them in conjunction with penicillins, with which they interact synergistically. Aminoglycosides penetrate poorly into mammalian cells and thus are of limited value in infections caused by intracellular bacteria. Some members of the group display important activity against *Mycobacterium tuberculosis* or *Pseudomonas aeruginosa*. All of them display considerable toxicity affecting both the ear and the kidney (Table 2.1).

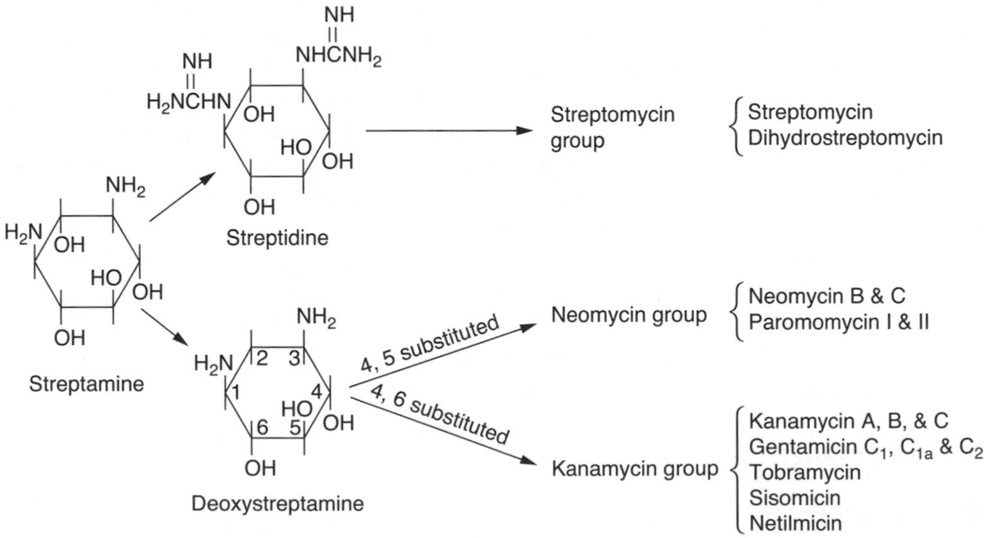

Fig. 2.1 Grouping of therapeutically useful aminoglycosides according to characteristics of the aminocyclitol ring. In most aminoglycosides the aminocyclitol moiety is either streptidine or deoxystreptamine, both derivatives of streptamine. The deoxystreptamine group can be subdivided into those in which sugar substituents are linked at the 4- and 5-hydroxyls, and those substituted at the 4- and 6-hydroxyl positions.

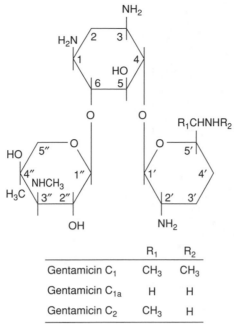

	R_1	R_2
Gentamicin C_1	CH_3	CH_3
Gentamicin C_{1a}	H	H
Gentamicin C_2	CH_3	H

Fig. 2.2 Structure of the gentamicin C complex, showing the ring numbering system and variations in structure of the different gentamicins.

Aminoglycoside assay

Because of their toxicity, use of aminoglycosides requires careful laboratory monitoring to make sure that plasma concentrations are adequate, but not so high that toxic levels are reached. Assays should be performed if treatment is for longer than 48 h, particularly if there is any renal impairment, and always in older patients. Indeed it might be considered negligent if a patient developed side effects attributable to aminoglycoside therapy and the drug concentration(s) had not been monitored.

The therapeutic range of concentrations of aminoglycosides such as gentamicin in plasma was originally thought to be 2–10 mg/l, but it is far from certain that single high peak concentrations correlate simply with adverse effects. Indeed, it is now common to use once-daily aminoglycoside therapy, which requires a dosage that achieves relatively high peak concentrations and low trough levels (<1 mg/l) before the next dose is administered. Such regimens have been shown to be as safe as conventional multi-dose therapy.

Mode of action

Streptomycin binds to a particular ribosomal protein and a single amino acid change in this protein results in streptomycin resistance. Aminoglycosides of the kanamycin and neomycin groups bind at a different site and are generally unaffected. Several effects of the binding of streptomycin and other aminoglycosides have been noted, including a tendency to cause misreading of certain codons of mRNA resulting in the production of defective proteins, some of which may affect membrane integrity. Other evidence suggests that the primary site of action is the formation of non-functioning initiation complexes, or inhibition of the translocation step in polypeptide synthesis. None of these hypotheses fully explains the potent bactericidal activity of aminoglycosides

Table 2.1 Summary of the antibacterial spectrum and toxicity of some aminoglycosides

Aminoglycoside	Activity against:						Relative degrees of:	
	Staphylococci	Streptococci	Enterobacteria	Pseudomonas aeruginosa	Mycobacterium tuberculosis		Ototoxicity	Nephrotoxicity
Streptomycin	Good	Poor	Good	Poor	Good		+++	+
Kanamycin	Good	Poor	Good	Poor	Good		++	++
Gentamicin	Good	Fair	Good	Good	Poor		++	++
Tobramycin	Good	Poor	Good	Good	Poor		++	++
Netilmicin	Good	Poor	Good	Good	Poor		+	+
Amikacin	Good	Poor	Good	Good	Good		++	+
Neomycin	Good	Poor	Good	Poor	Fair		+++	+++

Streptomycin: mainly tuberculosis.

compared with other inhibitors of protein synthesis. Aminoglycosides enter bacteria by an active transport process involving respiratory quinones. These are absent in streptococci and anaerobes which are consequently resistant.

Streptomycin

The use of streptomycin has declined with the appearance of other aminoglycosides, although it is still a component of several antituberculosis regimens recommended by the World Health Organization (see Chapter 25). It is also used in the treatment of some rarer conditions, including plague, brucellosis, bartonellosis, and tularaemia, possibly for want of adequate evidence that more modern agents might be effective.

Neomycin group

Neomycin is the most ototoxic of the aminoglycosides and it is now little used, except in topical preparations; even this use is discouraged because of the risk of promoting the emergence of aminoglycoside resistance. It has also been given orally together with other agents to sterilize the gut (for example, before abdominal surgery or in patients in intensive care units), but the inactivity of aminoglycosides against anaerobes ensures that most of the gut flora escapes, and the procedure is not without risk of systemic toxicity. Framycetin, a common component of topical preparations, is identical to neomycin B.

One aminoglycoside of the neomycin group, paromomycin, is unusual in being active against the protozoa causing amoebic dysentery and leishmaniasis as well as some tapeworms. However, other drugs are preferred in the treatment of these parasitic diseases (see Chapter 5).

Kanamycin group

Important members of this large group include kanamycin itself, gentamicin, tobramycin, netilmicin, and a semi-synthetic derivative of kanamycin A, amikacin.

In its naturally occurring form, kanamycin is a mixture of three closely related compounds, kanamycin A, B, and C. Pharmaceutical preparations consist almost exclusively of kanamycin A, although kanamycin B (bekanamycin) is available in some countries. The spectrum of activity is similar to that of streptomycin (and includes *M. tuberculosis*), but it retains activity against streptomycin-resistant strains and is less likely to cause vestibular damage.

Kanamycin has largely been superseded by gentamicin and tobramycin (deoxykanamycin B), which are more active against many enterobacteria and, more importantly, *Ps. aeruginosa*. This has been a major factor in the popularity of these agents for the 'blind' therapy of serious infection before the results of laboratory tests are known. The relative merits of gentamicin and tobramycin have been the subject of much debate. Tobramycin appears to be marginally less toxic and slightly more active against *Ps. aeruginosa*; against other susceptible bacteria, gentamicin probably has the edge. Netilmicin (*N*-acetyl sisomicin) is said to be somewhat less toxic than its predecessors.

Other members of the kanamycin group are available in some countries. They include sisomicin, dibekacin, micronomicin (gentamicin C_{2B}), ribostamycin, and astromicin. They offer little advantage over gentamicin or tobramycin, although some have different patterns of stability to aminoglycoside-modifying enzymes (see p. 111).

Amikacin and arbekacin are semi-synthetic derivatives of kanamycin A and dibekacin respectively, in which an α-aminobutyric acid substituent has been added to an amino group on the deoxystreptamine ring. These compounds were specifically developed to resist most aminoglycoside-modifying enzymes, although they have lower intrinsic activity than gentamicin or tobramycin.

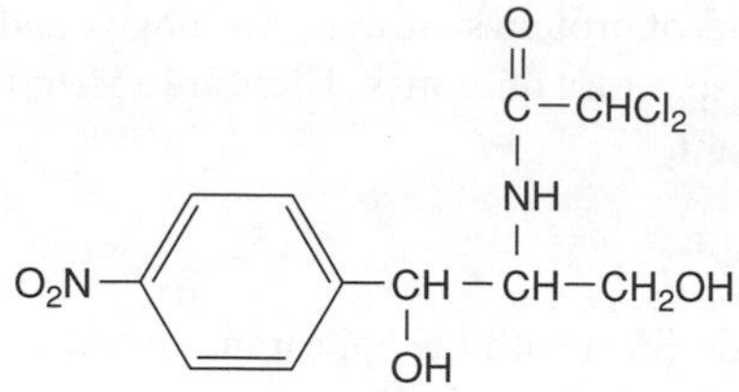

Fig. 2.3 Structure of chloramphenicol.

Amikacin is most widely used and is popular in units troubled by gentamicin resistance. Strains of bacteria that are resistant to gentamicin by non-enzymic mechanisms are cross-resistant to amikacin and other aminoglycosides.

Spectinomycin

Spectinomycin exhibits properties that separate it from the true aminoglycosides. It displays inferior antibacterial activity against most species and generally achieves a bacteristatic rather than a bactericidal effect. Its sole use is in the treatment of gonorrhoea in patients who are either hypersensitive to penicillin, or infected with gonococci that are resistant to penicillin and other options (see p. 253).

Chloramphenicol

Chloramphenicol was one of the first therapeutically useful antibiotics to appear from systematic screening of *Streptomyces* strains in the wake of the discovery of streptomycin in the 1940s. Although it is a naturally occurring compound, it is a relatively simple molecule (Fig. 2.3) and can readily be synthesized. Attempts to modify the structure have generally resulted in a marked loss of activity, but thiamphenicol, a compound in which a sulphomethyl group replaces the nitro group of chloramphenicol, displays antibacterial activity comparable with that of chloramphenicol itself.

Pure chloramphenicol is very insoluble in water and tastes extremely bitter. These problems have been overcome by pro-drug forms of the antibiotic: chloramphenicol palmitate and stearate to improve palatability and chloramphenicol succinate to improve solubility for injection. These pro-drugs lack antibacterial activity, but serve to release chloramphenicol in the body; they should not be used for laboratory tests of bacterial sensitivity.

Chloramphenicol acts by inhibiting the peptidyl transferase reaction—the step at which the peptide bond is formed—on bacterial ribosomes. The spectrum of activity embraces most Gram-positive and Gram-negative bacteria, and also extends to chlamydiae and rickettsiae, strictly intracellular bacteria that cause a variety of infections, including trachoma, psittacosis, and typhus (Table 2.2). Resistance is usually due to bacterial enzymes that acetylate the two hydroxyl groups.

The action of chloramphenicol against enterobacteria is largely bacteristatic, but against some bacteria, including the Gram-positive cocci, it may display quite potent bactericidal activity. The drug also possesses the important properties of diffusing well into cerebrospinal fluid and of penetrating into cells—a very useful feature in the treatment of diseases such as typhoid, typhus, and other conditions where intracellular bacteria are involved. Resistance to chloramphenicol is generally uncommon, although resistant strains of the typhoid bacillus, *Salmonella enterica*, serotype Typhi, cause serious problems in areas of the world where the disease is endemic.

Table 2.2 Summary of the antibacterial spectrum of inhibitors of protein synthesis in common use

Antibiotic	Staphylococci	Streptococci	Neisseria spp.	Haemophilus influenzae	Entero-bacteria	Pseudomonas aeruginosa	Anaerobes	Rickettsiae and chlamydiae	Mycoplasmas
Aminoglycosides	Good	Poor	Fair	Fair	Good	Variable	–	–	Fair
Chloramphenicol	Good	Good	Good	Good	Good	Poor	Good	Good	Fair
Clindamycin	Very good	Good	–	–	–	–	Good	Fair	Variable
Fusidic acid	Very good	Fair	Good	–	–	–	Fair	–	–
Macrolides	Very good	Very good	Good	Good	–	–	Fair	Good	Variable
Mupirocin	Very good	Very good	Good	Good	–	–	–	–	–
Linezolid	Very good	Very good	Poor	Poor	–	–	Poor	. . .	. . .
Streptogramins	Very good	Very good	Good	Good	–	–	Fair	. . .	. . .
Tetracyclines	Good	Good	Good	Good	Good[a]	Poor	Fair	Good	Good
Tigecycline	Very good	Very good	Good	Good	Good[ab]	Poor	Good		

–, no useful activity; . . ., no information.

N.B: Individual strains of susceptible species may be resistant to any of these agents.

[a] Poor activity against *Proteus* spp., *Providentia* spp., and *Morganella* spp.

[b] Generally better anti-Gram-negative activity compared with other tetracyclines.

Therapeutic use

Given its attractive qualities it is a great pity that chloramphenicol displays one grave drawback: potentially fatal aplastic anaemia (p. 183). This rare side effect has generally relegated chloramphenicol to the role of a reserve drug for use in life-threatening infections caused by bacteria resistant to safer compounds. It was once popular for the treatment of meningitis, including neonatal meningitis when, however, another potentially fatal side effect of the antibiotic ('grey baby syndrome'; p. 166) may follow if the dosage is not properly adjusted. Because it is effective and cheap chloramphenicol is still widely used in the developing world, especially for typhoid fever and meningitis. It is also commonly used as a topical agent for the treatment of bacterial conjunctivitis.

Tetracyclines

The first tetracycline, chlortetracycline (Fig. 2.4), was described in 1948 as a product of *Streptomyces aureofaciens*. Oxytetracycline and tetracyline itself (so called because it lacks both the chlorine of chlortetracycline and the hydroxyl of oxytetracycline) quickly followed. These, and other members of the group including demeclocycline, doxycycline, lymecycline, methacycline, and minocycline, are closely related structural variants of the same tetracyclic molecule. Tigecycline is a relatively new glycylcycline; it is a synthetic derivative of minocycline.

The tetracyclines exhibit a very broad spectrum, displaying good activity against most Gram-positive and Gram-negative bacteria (excluding *Proteus* spp. *Providentia* spp., *Morganella* spp., and *Pseudomonas aeruginosa*), rickettsiae, chlamydiae, mycoplasmas, and spirochaetes (Table 2.2). They generally have similar antibacterial activity and are distinguished more by their pharmacokinetic behaviour. Of the older tetracyclines, doxycycline and minocycline are the most widely used. These derivatives are more completely absorbed when given orally and, unlike the others, they do not aggravate renal failure so that they can be used in patients suffering renal impairment; they also exhibit marginally better antibacterial activity, and they display sufficiently long serum half-lives to allow them to be given only once or twice daily. Tetracyclines should not be given to young children (see p. 180).

Susceptible bacteria concentrate tetracyclines by an active transport process. In the cell they interfere with the binding of aminoacyl tRNA to the A-site on the ribosome. Like chloramphenicol, the tetracyclines are predominantly bacteristatic. The mechanism of the most common form of resistance is unusual in that a new protein is produced which appears to prevent uptake of the drug (p. 117). There is almost complete cross-resistance between tetracyclines, although minocycline may retain activity against some tetracycline-resistant strains.

Tigecycline is additionally active against some multiply resistant Gram-negative bacteria (for example, *Acinetobacter* spp.), MRSA, anaerobes, and strains that are resistant to earlier compounds. It is only available as an intravenous formulation, but achieves very modest blood concentrations largely because of its widespread penetration throughout the body (often referred to as a high volume of distribution) (see Chapter 14).

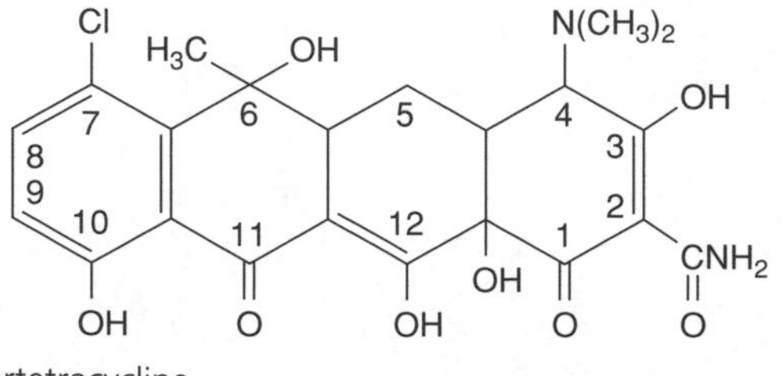

Fig. 2.4 Structure of chlortetracycline.

The bacterial ribosome is the target for the tetracyclines. Binding to the 30S ribosomal subunit at the A-site blocks entry of amino-acyl transfer RNA molecules into the ribosome, preventing incorporation of amino acid residues into elongating peptide chains. Tigecycline binds to the 30S ribosomal subunit with higher affinity than the tetracyclines, and interacts with another region of the A-site in an unusual way. These methods of action likely explain why tigecycline is active against strains with either of the two main mechanism of tetracycline resistance—ribosomal protection and drug efflux.

Therapeutic use

The therapeutic importance of tetracyclines has declined over the years with the upsurge of resistant strains, particularly among enterobacteria and streptococci. They are still widely used for the treatment of respiratory infections, particularly chronic bronchitis and mycoplasma pneumonia, and in selected skin infections. Traditionally, they are the drugs of choice for rickettsial and chlamydial infections of all types, although use for the latter indication has been eroded by the newer macrolides (see below). Tigecycline is used as a second- or third-line antibiotic to treat more difficult skin and soft tissue or intra-abdominal infections, typically where broad spectrum coverage is needed (but pseudomonas infection is not suspected).

Tetracyclines are active against malaria parasites and some other protozoa. Doxycycline is sometimes used for antimalarial prophylaxis and in combination with quinine in the treatment of *Plasmodium falciparum* infections.

Fusidic acid

Fusidic acid is the only therapeutically useful member of a group of naturally occurring antibiotics that display a steroid-like structure (Fig. 2.5). The antibiotic acts to prevent the translocation step in bacterial protein synthesis by inhibiting one of the substances (factor G) essential for this reaction.

Fusidic acid is active *in vitro* against Gram-positive and Gram-negative cocci, *M. tuberculosis*, *Nocardia asteroides*, and many anaerobes; the ribosomes of Gram-negative bacilli are susceptible to the action of the drug, but access is denied by the Gram-negative cell wall.

Staphylococcus aureus is particularly susceptible to fusidic acid and the compound is usually regarded simply as an antistaphylococcal agent. It penetrates well into infected tissues, including bone, and it is favoured by some authorities for the treatment of staphylococcal osteomyelitis.

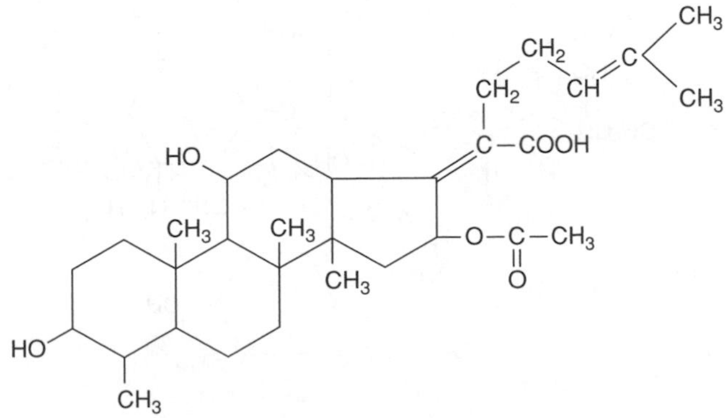

Fig. 2.5 Structure of fusidic acid.

A potential drawback is the presence in any large staphylococcal population of a small number of fusidic acid resistant variants that can proliferate during therapy. For this reason, fusidic acid is almost always administered together with another antibiotic (when given systemically), often a penicillin.

Fusidic acid is usually free from side effects when given orally. Intravenous administration of the diethanolamine salt is sometimes accompanied by a reversible jaundice. Topical preparations are available (for example to treat superficial skin infections), but their use risks encouraging the emergence of resistance.

Macrolides

The earliest macrolide, erythromycin, was discovered in 1952 as a product of *Streptomyces erythreus*. This and related antibiotics share a similar molecular structure characterized by a 14-, 15-, or 16-membered macrocyclic lactone ring substituted with some unusual sugars (Fig. 2.6). All members of the group are thought to act by causing the growing peptide chain to dissociate from the ribosome during the translocation step in bacterial protein synthesis.

Macrolides are most notable for their antistaphylococcal and antistreptococcal activity, though the spectrum encompasses other important pathogens, including chlamydiae, *Mycoplasma pneumoniae*, legionellae, and some mycobacteria; they lack useful activity against enterobacteria and *Ps. aeruginosa* (Table 2.2). Resistance is common among staphylococci, but less so in streptococci. However, resistant *Streptococcus pyogenes* strains are increasing in prevalence.

Macrolides have many attractive properties as well-tolerated oral compounds that display good tissue penetration. Their spectrum of activity makes them particularly suitable for the treatment of respiratory and soft-tissue disease and for infections caused by susceptible intracellular bacteria. They are also used in campylobacter enteritis if the severity of infection warrants antimicrobial treatment, and in *Legionella pneumophila* pneumonia.

Erythromycin

Erythromycin, the oldest and most widely used macrolide antibiotic, was discovered at a time when resistance of staphylococci to penicillin was first becoming a serious problem. In the fear that its

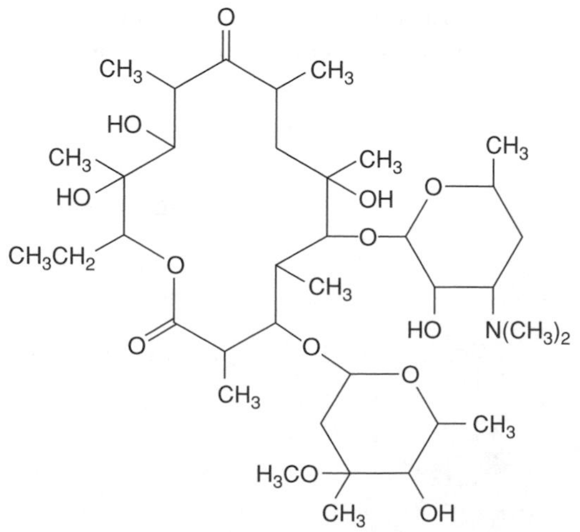

Fig. 2.6 Structure of erythromycin.

usefulness might be similarly compromised, it was at first used as a reserve antistaphylococcal agent or for streptococcal infections in patients allergic to penicillin.

Erythromycin base is broken down in the acid conditions of the stomach and it is administered in the form of enteric-coated tablets that protect the antibiotic until it reaches the absorption site in the duodenum. Alternatively, the stearate salt or esterified pro-drug forms are used for oral administration. Two ester formulations are in general use: the ethylsuccinate and the estolate. Erythromycin lactobionate and erythromycin gluceptate are available for intravenous use. The estolate is generally regarded as the most toxic formulation because of its propensity to cause reversible cholestatic jaundice. However, this uncommon complication can arise with any of the preparations. Erythromycin is liable to cause nausea and abdominal cramps and this has diminished its popularity. Indeed, this side effect is used to an advantage in some patients in intensive care units to stimulate the bowel, and thus to help excrete gut contents that would otherwise be retained by individuals who are paralyzed and sedated.

Erythromycin derivatives

Efforts to modify the properties of erythromycin have been more successful in generating compounds with improved pharmacological features rather than enhanced antibacterial activity. Much interest has centred on altering the molecule in such a way that the reactive groups responsible for the acid lability are modified. Such changes increase the bioavailability and often extend the plasma half-life. Any improvement in antibacterial activity is generally modest, but enhanced tissue penetration may render these compounds more effective. Acid-stable derivatives of erythromycin also appear to be less prone to cause gastrointestinal upset. Macrolides of this type include azithromycin, clarithromycin, dirithromycin, and roxithromycin.

Azithromycin

In this semi-synthetic macrolide, a nitrogen atom has been inserted into the lactone ring of erythromycin to produce a 15-membered ring structure that is described as an azalide. Azithromycin has a considerably improved bioavailability and a much extended plasma half-life compared with erythromycin. The antibacterial spectrum is similar to that of erythromycin, although it is somewhat more active against some important respiratory pathogens such as *H. influenzae* and *L. pneumophila*; there is also some improvement in activity against enteric Gram-negative bacilli, but this is unlikely to be of therapeutic benefit.

The most important property of azithromycin is the long terminal half-life, which enables it to be administered once a day. A single dose is effective in chlamydial and gonococcal infections of the genital tract.

Clarithromycin

This derivative of erythromycin is altered in the body to yield a metabolite that retains antibacterial activity, but has altered pharmacokinetic properties. The activities of clarithromycin and its metabolite are similar to that of erythromycin, although concentrations required to inhibit legionellae and chlamydiae are generally lower.

There have been claims of much enhanced penetration into pulmonary sites, beneficial interactions between the parent compound and the metabolite, and other minor advantages. It is doubtful whether these translate into significantly improved therapeutic efficacy, but clarithromycin is better absorbed and less prone to cause abdominal discomfort than earlier macrolides. It has been successfully used in combination regimens for the treatment of infections with *Helicobacter pylori* and some mycobacteria, notably those of the *M. avium* group.

Dirithromycin

Dirithromycin is slightly less active than erythromycin against most organisms within the spectrum, but it has a much extended plasma half-life and has been successfully used for once-daily treatment of respiratory tract, skin, and soft tissue infections.

Roxithromycin

Roxithromycin is another erythromycin derivative and, not surprisingly, exhibits activity very similar to the older drug. It differs, however, in having an extended plasma half-life, a feature that may be related to extensive binding to plasma proteins.

Ketolides

A new class of erythromycin derivatives, the ketolides, has been obtained by introducing a keto function into the macrolactone ring of erythromycin after removal of one of the sugars. These compounds share the Gram-positive spectrum of the earlier macrolides, but retain activity against macrolide-resistant strains.

The only compound of this type presently available is telithromycin. However, its use has been restricted because of rare but serious reports of acute liver failure. Also, telithromycin may cause worsening of symptoms, including breathing problems, when taken by people with myasthenia gravis (a disease that causes muscle weakness).

Other macrolides

Other macrolides that have been used in various parts of the world include oleandomycin (or its better absorbed derivative triacetyloleandomycin) and a series of compounds with a 16-membered ring, including spiramycin, josamycin, midecamycin, kitasamycin, and rokitamycin. None of them seems to offer much therapeutic advantage over erythromycin. Spiramycin is sometimes used as an alternative to pyrimethamine in infections caused by the protozoan parasite, *Toxoplasma gondii*.

Lincosamides

The original lincosamide, lincomycin, a naturally occurring product of *Streptomyces lincolnensis*, has been superseded by clindamycin (7-chloro-7-deoxylincomycin; Fig. 2.7), which exhibits improved antibacterial activity.

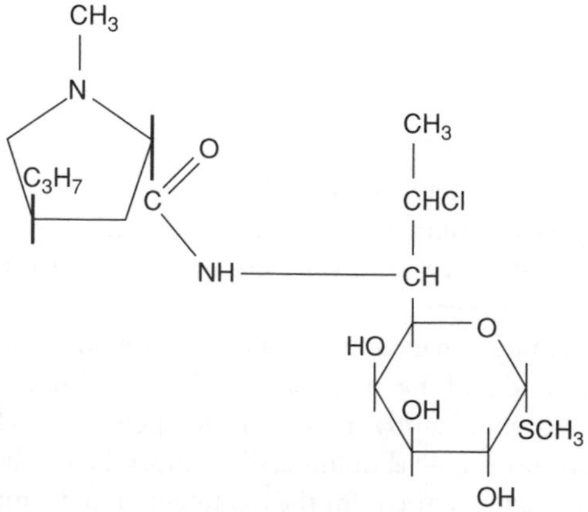

Fig. 2.7 Structure of clindamycin.

Lincosamides interfere with the process of peptide elongation in a way that has not been precisely defined. The ribosomal binding site is probably similar to that of erythromycin, since resistance to erythromycin caused by methylation of the ribosomal binding site affects lincosamides as well.

Lincomycin and clindamycin possess good antistaphylococcal and antistreptococcal activity, and *in vitro* studies demonstrate reduced toxin release by producer strains even in the presence of low concentrations of clindamycin. This attribute has led to a niche use for this antibiotic, usually in combination, in life-threatening staphylococcal and streptococcal infections thought to be mediated by toxin release (for example, necrotizing fasciitis). Clindamycin has also proved therapeutically useful in the treatment of infections due to *Bacteroides fragilis* and some other anaerobes. Enterobacteria and *Ps. aeruginosa* lie outside the spectrum of activity (Table 2.2). Clindamycin exhibits some activity against parasitic protozoa and has been used in toxoplasmosis, malaria, and babesiosis.

Clindamycin hydrochloride, like chloramphenicol, is extremely bitter. For oral administration the drug is formulated in capsules or as the biologically inactive palmitate, which liberates the parent compound *in vivo*. Clindamycin phosphate, the soluble form used for intravenous administration, is similarly inactive in the test-tube, but is hydrolyzed to the active drug in the body.

Patients treated with clindamycin (or lincomycin) sometimes experience diarrhoea caused by a clostridial toxin, which occasionally develops into a potentially fatal pseudomembranous colitis (see p. 268). Other antibiotics, notably ampicillin and broad-spectrum cephalosporins, may also cause this side effect.

Streptogramins

Each member of the streptogramin family is not one antibiotic, but two: they are produced as synergistic mixtures by various species of *Streptomyces*. One of these compounds, virginiamycin, has been extensively used as a growth promoter in animal husbandry. Another streptogramin, pristinamycin, is sometimes used as an antistaphylococcal agent in continental Europe, but plasma concentrations after oral administration do not greatly exceed inhibitory levels and solubility problems have militated against parenteral use. A formulation consisting of the water-soluble derivatives, quinupristin and dalfopristin, is, however, suitable for infusion and is now preferred for human therapy.

The two components of streptogramin antibiotics are structurally different. Alone they exhibit feeble bacteristatic activity, but in combination the effect is bactericidal. Component A causes distortion of the aminoacyl-tRNA binding site, hindering further growth of the peptide chain. It is thought that component B binds to an adjacent site and that the combined effect is to constrict the channel through which the nascent peptide is extruded from the ribosome. Protein synthesis is completely blocked and the consequences are lethal to the bacterial cell.

The activity of streptogramins is virtually restricted to Gram-positive organisms. Their major claim to attention is that they retain activity against multiresistant staphylococci and some enterococci, notably *Enterococcus faecium*. Unfortunately, *E. faecalis*, which is more commonly encountered, is often resistant.

Mupirocin

Mupirocin (formerly known as pseudomonic acid) is a component of the antibiotic complex produced by the bacterium *Ps. fluorescens*. The novel structure consists of monic acid with a short fatty acid side chain (Fig. 2.8). The terminal portion of the molecule distal to the fatty acid resembles isoleucine, and mupirocin inhibits protein synthesis by blocking incorporation of the amino acid into polypeptides. The analogous process in mammalian cells is unaffected.

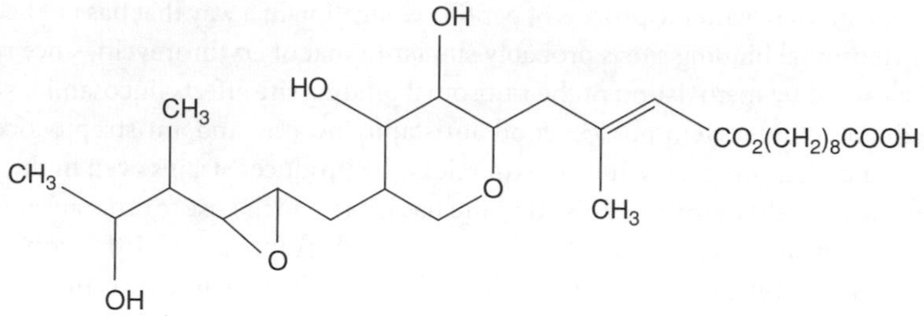

Fig. 2.8 Structure of mupirocin.

The spectrum of activity embraces staphylococci and streptococci, but excludes most enteric Gram-negative bacilli (Table 2.2). Hopes that mupirocin might be useful in systemic therapy were thwarted by the realization that the compound is inactivated in the body. Consequently, its use is restricted to topical preparations. Mupirocin has proved particularly useful in the eradication or suppression of staphylococci (typically MRSA) from nasal carriage sites. However, resistance emergence occurs if the drug is used frequently, and especially if used on multiple occasions or for prolonged periods in patients with long-term colonization by MRSA.

Oxazolidinones

Several oxazolidinones have attracted attention over the years owing to their activity against Gram-positive organisms, including staphylococci, pneumococci, and enterococci. They are well absorbed by the oral route and exhibit bacteristatic activity. They act at an early stage in protein synthesis by blocking the formation of the 70 S initiation complex. A principal attraction of these compounds is that they do not show cross-resistance to other classes of drugs.

The most widely investigated member of the family, linezolid, has been available for several years. It is a available in both oral and intravenous formulations, and is an effective and useful agent in patients infected with multiresistant strains of staphylococci or other Gram-positive cocci. The drug is active against *M. tuberculosis* and there is some evidence that it might be useful in infections with drug-resistant strains. The chief limitation of linezolid is an effect on bone marrow cells that largely limits the length of treatment to two weeks. Rare instances of peripheral or optic neuropathy have also been reported, typically associated with use longer that two to four weeks.

Resistance to linezolid has been slow to emerge, and was limited to very occasional staphylococcal strains with ribosomal mutations. However, a worrying recent development has been reports of linezolid resistance in *S. aureus* strains that is mediated by the *cfr* gene, so named because it was originally noted to cause resistance to chloramphenicol and florfenicol (formerly in bacteria recovered from animals). Actually, the *cfr* gene encodes a RNA methyltransferase that affects the binding of at least five chemically unrelated antimicrobial classes: phenicols, lincosamides, oxazolidinones, pleuromutilins, and streptogramin *A* antibiotics. The *cfr* gene can be transferred on plasmids and thus there is a risk or more widespread dissemination of this mode of resistance.

Key points

- Gentamicin is a good all-purpose aminoglycoside for serious infections, but streptococci, anaerobes, and intracellular organisms are not covered; need to monitor plasma levels.
- Tetracyclines still have a role in selected community-acquired respiratory tract and skin infections, but must not be given to children because of teeth staining.
- Chloramphenicol is still widely used in the developing world given its low cost, but has serious albeit rare side effects.
- Azithromycin is increasingly used as a single dose treatment for chlamydial infections to ensure compliance.
- Linezolid is used as an oral (or IV) alternative to glycopeptides, particularly for the treatment of MRSA infection.

Further reading

Finch RG, Greenwood D, Norrby SR, Whitley RJ (2010), *Antibiotic Chemotherapy* (9th edn) London: Elsevier.

Chapter 3

Synthetic antibacterial agents and miscellaneous antibiotics

Various targets other than the cell wall and ribosome are open to attack by chemotherapeutic agents. This chapter describes the properties of inhibitors of bacterial nucleic acid synthesis, compounds that act on the bacterial cell membrane, and agents used solely for the treatment of mycobacterial disease. Many of these compounds are synthetic chemicals rather than antibiotics in the strict sense.

Inhibitors of nucleic acid synthesis

Given the universality of nucleic acid as the basis of life, it is surprising that so many antimicrobial agents have been discovered that selectively interfere with the functions of DNA and RNA. Some, like the sulphonamides and diaminopyrimidines, achieve their effect indirectly by interrupting metabolic pathways that lead to the manufacture of nucleic acids; others, of which the quinolones and nitroimidazoles are prime examples, exert a more direct action.

Sulphonamides

The discovery of Prontosil in the 1930s was a major breakthrough in the chemotherapy of bacterial infections (see Historical introduction). However, the emergence of resistant strains and the appearance of safer and more potent agents have relegated the sulphonamides to a minor place in therapy. Even in their traditional role—uncomplicated urinary infection—they are now seldom used. They are still found in combination products with trimethoprim, pyrimethamine, and other diaminopyrimidines (see below).

The antibacterial activity of the Prontosil dye is due to the liberation in the body of sulphanilamide, an analogue of *para*-aminobenzoic acid (Fig. 3.1), which is essential for bacterial folate synthesis. Most bacteria synthesize folic acid and cannot take it up preformed from the environment. Mammalian cells, in contrast, use preformed folate and cannot make their own. Sulphonamides block an early stage in folate synthesis leading to various effects, including a failure to synthesize purine nucleotides and thymidine. Chemical modification of the sulphanilamide molecule has resulted in the production of hundreds of different sulphonamides, which differ chiefly in their pharmacological properties.

Sulphonamides have a broad antibacterial spectrum, though the activity against enterococci, *Pseudomonas aeruginosa*, and anaerobes is poor. They are predominantly bacteristatic, and relatively slow to act: several generations of bacterial growth are needed to deplete the folate pool before inhibition of growth occurs. Resistance emerges readily, and bacteria resistant to one sulphonamide are cross-resistant to the others. Sensitivity tests present problems in the laboratory since results depend critically on the composition of the culture medium and the inoculum size.

Diaminopyrimidines

Diaminopyrimidines inhibit dihydrofolate reductase, the enzyme that generates tetrahydrofolate (the active form of the vitamin) from metabolically inactive dihydrofolate. Trimethoprim (Fig. 3.2),

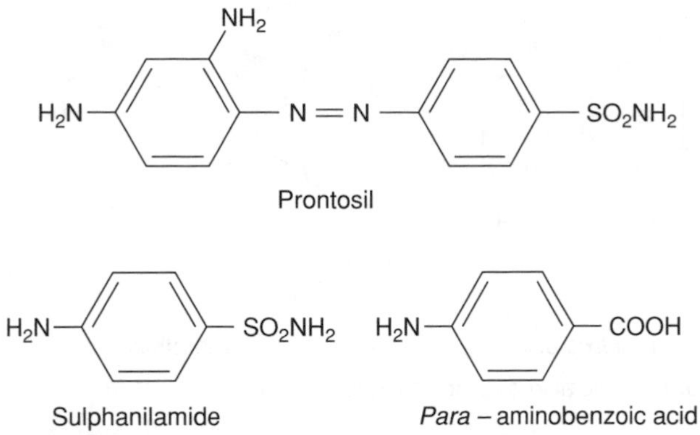

Fig. 3.1 Structures of prontosil, sulphanilimide, and p-aminobenzoic acid.

the most important antibacterial agent of this type, exhibits far greater affinity for the dihydro-folate reductase of bacteria than for the corresponding mammalian enzyme; this is the basis of the selective toxicity of the compound.

Since sulphonamides and trimethoprim act at different points in the same metabolic pathway they interact synergistically: bacteria are inhibited by much lower concentrations of the combination than by either agent alone. For this reason trimethoprim and sulphonamides are often combined in therapeutic formulations, although trimethoprim alone is probably as effective and less toxic. The most commonly used combination is trimethoprim and sulfamethoxazole (co-trimoxazole), but combinations of trimethoprim with sulfadiazine (co-trimazine) and sulfamoxole (co-trifamole) are also available in some countries.

Trimethoprim is active in low concentration against many common pathogenic bacteria, although *Ps. aeruginosa* is a notable exception. Resistance is on the increase and the prevalence varies considerably between countries (see Fig. 20.2). The drug is rapidly absorbed from the gut and excreted almost exclusively by the kidneys with a plasma half-life of about 10 h.

The chief use for trimethoprim is in urinary tract infection. In the UK the use of the combination with sulfamethoxazole (co-trimoxazole) declined greatly during the 1980s because of concern about life threatening adverse effects (agranulocytosis and Stevens Johnson syndrome, see Chapter 15). In the 1990s co-trimoxazole was principally used in pneumonia caused by the fungus, *Pneumocystis carinii* (*P. jiroveci*; see p. 80 and Chapters 7, 31, and 33). However, co-trimoxazole has a relatively low risk of causing *C. difficile* infection (see p. 268) and is available in both IV and oral formula-tions. In the past ten years co-trimoxazole has been increasingly used in UK hospitals as an alterna-tive to ciprofloxacin and broad spectrum beta-lactam antibiotics. .

Analogues of trimethoprim, including tetroxoprim and brodimoprim, are marketed in combination with sulphonamides in some countries, but offer few, if any advantages. Other diaminopyrimidines

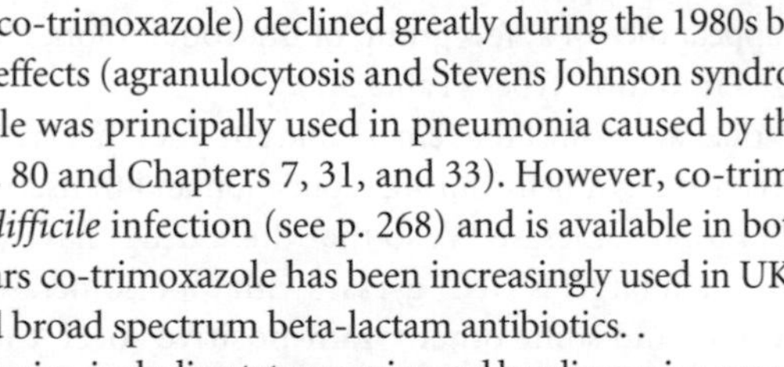

Fig. 3.2 Structure of trimethoprim.

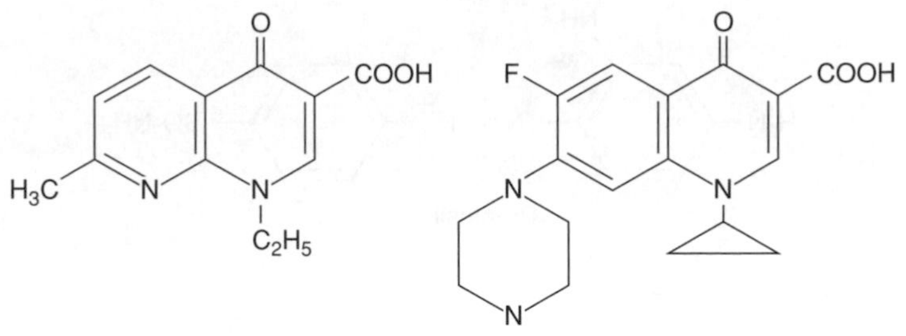

Fig. 3.3 Structures of nalidixic acid and ciprofloxacin.

include the antimalarial agents pyrimethamine and proguanil (Chapter 5); the anti-pneumocystis agent trimetrexate; and the antineoplastic agent methotrexate.

Quinolones

Nalidixic acid (Fig. 3.3) was the first representative to appear of a family of compounds that share close similarities of structure. These agents are generically known as quinolones, although they embrace a variety of molecular types, depending on the arrangement of nitrogen atoms within the heterocyclic structure.

Among the earlier quinolones are two with modestly improved antibacterial activity: flumequine (which bears a fluorine atom at the C-6 position) and pipemidic acid (with a piperazine substituent at C-7). During the 1980s a new series of quinolones were synthesized in which these two features were combined. These compounds, of which ciprofloxacin (Fig. 3.3) is a typical example, exhibit considerably enhanced activity. In some subsequent derivatives, piperazine was replaced by other substituents, and members of this family of compounds are now generally referred to as fluoroquinolones. Although flumequine is strictly a fluoroquinolone, the term is usually restricted to compounds that exhibit superior intrinsic activity.

Further attempts to improve the pharmacological and antimicrobial properties of these compounds have led to the appearance of a new group of fluoroquinolones, so that these agents can now be loosely categorized into three types (Table 3.1).

All antibacterial quinolones act against the remarkable enzymes that are involved in maintaining the integrity of the supercoiled DNA helix during replication and transcription. Two enzymes are affected, DNA gyrase and topoisomerase IV, so that these drugs have a dual site of action. In Gram-negative bacilli the main target is DNA gyrase, with topoisomerase IV as a secondary site, but in *Staphylococcus aureus* and some other Gram-positive cocci, the situation is reversed. Relative affinity for the two sites has led to claims of differential activity, especially among some of the newer quinolone derivatives.

Quinolones are generally well tolerated, but rashes and gastrointestinal disturbances may occur; photophobia and various non-specific neurological complaints are also sometimes encountered. These compounds affect the deposition of cartilage in experimental animals, and licensing authorities have cautioned against their use in children and pregnant women. Several promising fluoroquinolones have had to be withdrawn or have had their use restricted because of unexpected toxicity.

Nalidixic acid and its early congeners

Several quinolone derivatives, including cinoxacin, oxolinic acid, and pipemidic acid, were introduced into clinical use in various countries following the marketing of nalidixic acid in the 1960s. They are all well absorbed when taken by mouth and are more or less extensively metabolized in the body before being excreted into the urine. Most Gram-negative bacteria, with the exception

Table 3.1 Summary of spectrum of activity of quinolones available in the UK (2011)

Quinolone	Enterobacteria	*Pseudomonas aeruginosa*	Staphylococci	Streptococci	*Bacteroides fragilis*	Chlamydiae
Narrow spectrum quinolones						
Nalidixic acid	Good	Poor	Poor	Poor	Poor	Poor
Norfloxacin	Very good	Good	Fair	Poor	Poor	Poor
Fluoroquinolones						
Ciprofloxacin	Very good	Good	Fair	Fair	Poor	Poor
Levofloxacin	Very good	Good	Fair	Fair	Fair	Good
Moxifloxacin	Very good	Poor	Good	Good	Fair	Good
Ofloxacin	Very good	Good	Fair	Fair	Poor	Fair

of *Ps. aeruginosa*, are susceptible to nalidixic acid and its early congeners, but Gram-positive organisms are usually resistant (Table 3.1). Susceptible bacteria readily develop resistance in the laboratory and the emergence of resistance sometimes occurs during treatment so these drugs are now rarely used in clinical practice.

Fluoroquinolones

After the appearance, over a 20 year period, of a series of compounds that offered little improvement over nalidixic acid, the discovery of a family of quinolones that exhibited greatly improved properties came as a surprise. These compounds are much more active than earlier derivatives against enterobacteria, *Ps. aeruginosa*, and many Gram-positive cocci (Table 3.1), though the activity is somewhat reduced in acidic conditions and in the presence of divalent cations such as magnesium. The spectrum also includes certain problem organisms such as chlamydiae, legionellae, and some mycobacteria. Similar compounds, including enrofloxacin, danofloxacin, and sarafloxacin, have been introduced into veterinary practice and there has been considerable debate about the impact this may have had on the development of resistance.

The success of the first fluoroquinolones led to an intensive search for derivatives with further improved properties and this has borne fruit with several new agents now on the world market, or at an advanced stage of development. These compounds are characterized by enhanced activity against Gram-positive cocci, including *Staph. aureus* and *Streptococcus pneumoniae* as well as chlamydiae and mycoplasmas; clinafloxacin, gatifloxacin, moxifloxacin, and trovafloxacin also have sufficient activity against anaerobes of the *Bacteroides fragilis* group to make treatment of infections with those organisms feasible. They are not reliably active against *Ps. aeruginosa*.

Fluoroquinolones are usually administered orally, although some, including ciprofloxacin, ofloxacin, and levofloxacin (the L-isomer of ofloxacin), can also be given by injection. Therapeutic dosages achieve relatively low concentrations in plasma, but the compounds are well distributed in tissues and are concentrated within mammalian cells. The major route of excretion is usually renal, in the form of native compound or glucuronide and other metabolites, some of which retain antibacterial activity. Some fluoroquinolones, notably moxifloxacin, exhibit long terminal half-lives; these compounds are partly excreted by the biliary route and this may help to explain the long half-life.

Ciprofloxacin is the most widely used fluoroquinolone; among other indications, it is now the drug of choice for typhoid fever and other serious enteric diseases. The newer derivatives were targeted at the treatment of respiratory infections in the community and, although they are undoubtedly effective, there is no convincing evidence that they are more effective than other antibiotics. In contrast there is growing evidence that use of fluoroquinolones in hospitals is associated with increased prevalence of *C. difficile* infection and MRSA infections. In addition fluoroquinolone resistance is increasing rapidly in *Esch. coli* in the community and in hospitals. Consequently many hospital antibiotic policies now restrict the use of fluoroquinolones. In primary care ESAC (European Surveillance of Antimicrobial Consumption) has proposed that seasonal variation in fluoroquinlone use should be a quality indicator. The rationale for this is that fluoroquinolones should not be used for respiratory infections in primary care, consequently winter use should be no greater than summer use.

Nitroimidazoles

As a group, the imidazoles are remarkable in that derivatives are known, which between them cover bacteria, fungi, viruses, protozoa, and helminths—in fact, the whole antimicrobial spectrum. Outside the antimicrobial field certain imidazoles have been shown to exhibit radio-sensitizing properties and have attracted attention as adjuncts to radiation therapy for some tumours.

The members of this family of compounds used as antibacterial agents are 5-nitroimidazoles, of which metronidazole is best known. Related 5-nitroimidazoles include tinidazole, ornidazole, secnidazole, and nimorazole; they share the properties of metronidazole but have longer plasma half-lives.

Metronidazole was originally used for the treatment of trichomoniasis, and subsequently for two other protozoal infections—amoebiasis and giardiasis. The antibacterial activity of the compound was first recognized when a patient suffering from acute ulcerative gingivitis responded spontaneously while receiving metronidazole for a *Trichomonas vaginalis* infection. Anaerobic bacteria are commonly incriminated in gingivitis, and it was subsequently shown that metronidazole possesses potent antibacterial activity against strict anaerobes and also some micro-aerophilic bacteria, including *Gardnerella vaginalis* and *Helicobacter pylori*.

Metronidazole is so effective against anaerobic bacteria and resistance is so uncommon that it is now the drug of choice for the treatment of anaerobic infections. It is also commonly used for prophylaxis in some surgical procedures in which post-operative anaerobic infection is a frequent complication. It is an alternative to vancomycin in the treatment of non-severe antibiotic-associated colitis caused by *Clostridium difficile* toxins (p. 268) (see Fig. 25.2).

The basis of the selective activity against anaerobes resides in the fact that a reduction product is produced intracellularly at the low redox values attainable by anaerobes, but not by aerobes. The reduced form of metronidazole is thought to induce strand breakage in DNA by a mechanism that has not been precisely determined.

The 5-nitroimidazoles are generally free from serious side effects, though gastrointestinal upset is common and ingestion of alcohol induces a disulfiram-like reaction. Since these drugs act on DNA they are potentially genotoxic and tumorigenic, but there is no evidence that these problems have arisen despite widespread clinical use. None the less, these compounds are best avoided in pregnancy.

Nitrofurans (nitrofurantoin)

A number of nitrofuran derivatives have attracted attention over the years, among which nitrofurantoin is much the most important. Others have very limited role, for example nifurtimox is only used in Chagas' disease; (see p. 361).

Nitrofurantoin is the only nitrofuran derivative available in the UK. Its use is restricted to the treatment of urinary infection since it is rapidly excreted into urine after oral absorption and the small amount that finds its way into tissues is inactivated there. It is active against most urinary tract pathogens, but *Proteus* spp. and *Ps. aeruginosa* are usually resistant. The occurrence of resistant strains among susceptible species is uncommon. The activity is affected by pH, being favoured by acid conditions.

The mode of action of nitrofurantoin (or other nitrofurans) has not been precisely elucidated and is probably complex. The nitro group is reduced intracellularly in susceptible bacteria and it is likely that one effect, as with metronidazole, is the interaction of a reduction product with DNA.

Rifamycins (rifampicin)

The clinically useful rifamycins, of which rifampicin (known in the USA as rifampin) is the most important, are semi-synthetic derivatives of rifamycin B, one of a group of structurally complex antibiotics produced by *Streptomyces mediterranei*. These compounds interfere with mRNA formation by binding to the β-subunit of DNA-dependent RNA polymerase. Resistance readily arises by mutations in the subunit. For this reason, the drugs are normally used in combination with other agents.

Rifampicin

Rifampicin is one of the most effective weapons against two major mycobacterial scourges of mankind: tuberculosis and leprosy. It also exhibits potent bactericidal activity against a range of other bacteria, notably staphylococci and legionellae. Rifampicin is now often used in combination with other drugs in Legionnaires' disease and staphylococcal prosthetic device infections. It is also used as a single agent to eliminate meningococci from the throats of carriers and for the protection of close contacts of meningococcal and *Haemophilus influenzae* type b disease.

Rifampicin is well absorbed by the oral route, although it may also be given by intravenous infusion. Serious side effects are relatively uncommon, but can be more troublesome when the drug is used intermittently, as it may be in antituberculosis regimens. Hepatotoxicity is well recognized and the antibiotic induces hepatic enzymes, leading to self-potentiation of excretion and antagonism of some other drugs handled by the liver, including oral contraceptives. A potentially alarming side effect arising from the fact that rifampicin is strongly pigmented is the production of red urine and other bodily secretions; contact lenses may become discoloured. Patients should be warned of these potential problems.

Two other rifamycin derivatives (rifabutin and rifapentine) have a limited role in the treatment of infections caused by organisms of the *Mycobacterium avium* complex, which often cause disseminated disease in patients with cancer or acquired immune deficiency syndrome (AIDS). Rifaximin is a non-absorbed oral rifamycin which is used in some countries for the treatment of travellers' diarrhoea, and *C. difficile* infection (see p. 268), and the prevention of hepatic encephalopathy.

Fidaxomicin

Fidaxomicin (previously known as OPT-80) is a macrocyclic antibiotic that inhibits bacterial RNA polymerase, but at a different site to rifamycins and so there is no cross resistance with the latter. Fidaxomicin is poorly absorbed from the gut following oral administration, and compared with vancomycin significantly reduces the rate of recurrence following resolution of *Clostridium difficile* infection (p. 268). It has been launched in the US in 2011 and European marketing is anticipated in 2012.

Agents affecting membrane function

Polymyxins

The polymyxins are a family of compounds produced by *Bacillus polymyxa* and related bacteria. Only polymyxins B and E are used therapeutically. Polymyxin E is usually known by its alternative name, colistin. Structurally, the polymyxins are cyclic polypeptides with a long hydrophobic tail. They act like cationic detergents by binding to the cell membrane and causing the leakage of essential cytoplasmic contents. The effect is not entirely selective, and both polymyxin B and colistin exhibit considerable toxicity so are not used for systemic therapy. They have a limited role in topical therapy such as in selective decontamination regimens (See Chapters 18 and 31) and in cystic fibrosis by instillation into the lungs of those suffering exacerbation of pseudomonal infection.

Other membrane-active agents

Daptomycin, a semi-synthetic lipopeptide antibiotic not unlike the polymyxins in structure, has various effects on bacteria, but the primary mode of action is thought to lie in disruption of the cell membrane. Development of the compound in the 1980s was stopped because of fears of toxicity, but the rise to prominence of multiresistant Gram-positive cocci revived commercial interest and it is now marketed for serious infections of the skin and soft tissues that are unresponsive to other agents, especially those caused by multiresistant staphylococci. Activity is restricted to Gram-positive cocci and is greatly enhanced *in vitro* by the presence of magnesium ions.

Antibiotics of the tyrothricin complex (gramicidin and tyrocidine), which are used in some topical preparations, are cyclic peptides that bind to the cell membrane and interfere with its function. These agents possess good activity against Gram-positive organisms, but they also bind to mammalian cell membranes and are far too toxic to be used systemically in humans.

Toxicity also precludes the systemic use of the many disinfectants, including phenols, quaternary ammonium compounds, biguanides, and others, that achieve their antibacterial effect wholly or in part by interfering with the integrity of the cell membrane.

Antimycobacterial agents

Compared with the number of agents at the disposal of the prescriber for the therapy of most bacterial infections, the resources available to treat mycobacterial disease are precariously meagre. Part of the reason is that mycobacteria are unusual organisms with a relatively impermeable waxy coat, but the fact that they are very slow growing and are able to survive and multiply within macrophages and necrotic tissue also makes them difficult targets.

In general, the development of drugs for the treatment of tuberculosis and leprosy has evolved along specialized lines, but some important antimycobacterial agents, such as rifampicin (see above) and certain aminoglycosides (Chapter 2), have wider uses. Agents specifically used for the treatment of tuberculosis include isoniazid (isonicotinic acid hydrazide), pyrazinamide, ethambutol, and thiacetazone (thioacetazone). *Para*-aminosalicylic acid, which was formerly much used in antituberculosis regimens, is no longer recommended, but this and other compounds with activity against *Mycobacterium tuberculosis*, such as capreomycin, cycloserine, and viomycin, may be considered if first-line treatment fails. In leprosy, the most important agents (apart from rifampicin) are dapsone (or its pro-drug, acedapsone) and clofazimine. The thioamides ethionamide and protionamide (prothionamide) are sometimes used, but are hepatotoxic.

Some fluoroquinolones and macrolides display quite good activity against mycobacteria, including *M. leprae* and organisms of the *M. avium* complex, and these agents widen the options for treating mycobacterial disease at a time when resistance is emerging as a serious problem.

Because of the difficulties in studying mycobacteria in the laboratory, less is known about the mode of action of antimycobacterial drugs than about other antibacterial agents. Various theories have been put forward to explain the action of isoniazid. The most widely held view is that an oxidized product inhibits the formation of the mycolic acids that are peculiar to the cell walls of acid-fast bacilli. Other derivatives of nicotinic acid, including pyrazinamide, ethionamide, and protionamide, may act in the same way. Ethambutol probably inhibits the formation of arabinogalactan, a polysaccharide component of the mycobacterial cell wall. Dapsone (diaminodiphenyl sulphone) and *para*-aminosalicylic acid are related to the sulphonamides and have been assumed to share the same mode of action, but this is by no means certain. The mode of action of the antileprosy agent clofazimine has not been determined, but it may, like rifampicin, inhibit DNA-dependent RNA polymerase. Some puzzling aspects of the idiosyncratic spectrum of antimycobacterial agents may be explained by differences in uptake into susceptible cells.

Further information on these agents is given in the context of their use in Chapter 30.

Key points

Miscellaneous antibacterial agents

♦ *Trimethoprim*: use alone for uncomplicated cystitis.

♦ *Co-trimoxazole*: use is increasing in hospitals because of relatively low risk of causing *C. difficile* infection.

♦ *Ciprofloxacin*: use is decreasing in hospitals and primary care because of concerns about growing resistance and association with *C. difficile* infection. Should not be used for community-acquired respiratory infections.

♦ *Metronidazole*: drug of choice for anaerobic infections.

♦ *Nitrofurantoin*: useful for uncomplicated cystitis and prophylaxis against recurrent cystitis.

♦ *Rifampicin*: essential component of regimens for treatment of tuberculosis and leprosy and also has a role in treatment of staphylococcal infections.

Chapter 4

Antiviral agents

Viruses are almost as versatile as bacteria in the range of diseases they can cause. Vertebrates, insects, plants, and even bacteria are all open to attack. Some viruses of vertebrates (arboviruses) develop in and are transmitted by mosquitoes or other arthropods; others—rabies is a good example—can infect a wide range of mammalian hosts. In general, however, viruses are highly specific in their host range.

All viruses are obligate intracellular parasites; that is, they replicate only within living cells and cannot usually survive for long outside the host cell. Selectivity usually extends not only to the host, but also to the type of cell within the host, as viruses only infect cells that express appropriate receptors on their surface. The preference of a virus for certain types of cell is known as the tropism of the virus, and this often accounts for the characteristic clinical manifestations of particular viral infections. For example, some viruses preferentially infect liver cells, thereby giving rise to hepatitis.

Most viruses that infect man gain entry to the body by adsorption to superficial cells of the mucous membranes of the respiratory, intestinal, and genital tracts, or of the conjunctivae. Others may be swallowed in contaminated food or water, and gain entry through the gastrointestinal tract, or find their way in through damaged skin, insect bites, or direct inoculation. Intact skin is normally impermeable to viruses, although wart virus is an exception.

The principal types of virus causing human disease are listed in Table 4.1.

Properties of viruses

Viruses are deceptively simple. Sizes range from about 20 nm (parvovirus) to 300 nm (poxvirus); consequently, even the biggest viruses fall barely within the limits of resolution of conventional light microscopy and the electron microscope must be used to visualize them.

Complete virus particles (virions) consist of a nucleic acid core (the viral genome), surrounded by a few proteins, and possibly a lipid envelope. The nucleic acid may be DNA or RNA (never both), single or double stranded, circular or linear, continuous or segmented. This provides all the information needed for viral replication once it is released within the host cell. The proteins serve a number of functions. The capsid, or protein coat surrounding the nucleic acid consists of repeating structural units made up of one to three different protein molecules that are generally arranged in helical or icosahedral symmetry. The nucleic acid surrounded by its capsid is referred to as the nucleocapsid of the virus. Many viral proteins have enzymatic properties. These include polymerases and proteases that are necessary for replication and assembly of viral particles. Proteins protruding from the surface coat of the virus act as ligands that will bind to cellular receptors during the first stage of infection of a cell. The lipid envelope possessed by some viruses is derived from membranes of the host cell.

Targets for antiviral drugs

Virus infection of and replication within cells proceeds via a number of distinct steps, each of which, theoretically, provides a possible target for attack (Fig. 4.1). Although the exact details of these steps vary between different viruses, they can be broadly summarized as follows:

◆ *Attachment to the cell surface.* This involves a specific interaction between proteins (ligands) on the surface of the virus, with receptors on the surface of the cell. The nature of the viral

Table 4.1 Principal types of virus causing human disease

Family	Examples	Diseases	Mode of transmission
RNA Viruses			
Orthomyxoviruses	Influenza A and B viruses	Influenza	Respiratory
Paramyxoviruses	Mumps virus	Mumps	Respiratory
	Measles virus	Measles	
	Respiratory syncytial virus	Bronchiolitis (especially babies)	
	Human metapneumovirus	Bronchiolitis (especially babies)	
	Parainfluenza viruses	Croup; bronchiolitis (especially babies)	
Rhabdoviruses	Rabies virus	Rabies	Bite of rabid animal
Arenaviruses	Lassa virus	Lassa fever	Respiratory/rodent reservoir
Filoviruses	Ebola, Marburg	Acute haemorrhagic fever	Direct contact
Togaviruses	Rubella virus	German measles (rubella)	Respiratory/congenital
Flaviviruses	Many arboviruses	Yellow fever	Arthropod vectors
	Hepatitis C virus	Hepatitis	Inoculation
Picornaviruses	Enteroviruses:	Meningitis; Paralysis	Faecal–oral
	Polio		
	Echo		
	Coxsackie A and B		
	Hepatitis A virus	Hepatitis	
	Rhinoviruses	Colds	Respiratory
Hepeviruses	Hepatitis E	Hepatitis	Faecal–oral
Retroviruses	Human immunodeficiency Viruses	AIDS	Sexual/inoculation/vertical
	Human T-cell lymphotropic viruses	T-cell leukaemia; lymphoma	Inoculation/sexual/vertical
Reoviruses	Rotavirus	Infantile diarrhoea	Faecal–oral
Caliciviruses	Norovirus (Norwalk virus)	Gastroenteritis	Faecal–oral
Coronaviruses	Human coronavirus	Colds	Respiratory
		Severe acute respiratory syndrome (SARS)	
DNA Viruses			
Poxviruses	Variola	Smallpox (now eradicated)	Mainly respiratory
	Vaccinia	Smallpox vaccine	Vaccination
	Molluscum contagiosum	Skin disease	Contact
	Orf	Skin disease	Contact with sheep

Table 4.1 (continued)

Family	Examples	Diseases	Mode of transmission
Herpesviruses	Herpes simplex virus types 1 and 2	Cold sores; genital herpes	Saliva/contact/sexual
	Varicella zoster	Chickenpox; shingles	Respiratory
	Cytomegalovirus	Non-specific illness	Close contact/kissing
	Epstein–Barr virus	Glandular fever	Saliva, e.g. kissing
	Human herpesvirus type 6	Roseola infantum (sixth disease)	Saliva
	Human herpesvirus type 7	Not known	Saliva
	Human herpesvirus type 8	Kaposi's sarcoma	Sexual
Adenoviruses	Many serotypes	Conjunctivitis; pharyngitis; infantile diarrhoea	Respiratory
Papillomaviruses	Human papillomaviruses (HPV)	Cervical cancer; Warts	Contact
Polyomaviruses	JC, BK viruses	Progressive Multifocal Leukoencephalopathy; BK nephropathy	Faecal–oral; respiratory
Hepadnaviruses	Hepatitis B virus	Hepatitis	Inoculation/sexual/vertical
Parvoviruses	Parvovirus B 19	Erythema infectiosum (fifth disease)	Respiratory

ligands and cellular receptors is known in great detail for some viruses (e.g. the gp120 of human immunodeficiency virus (HIV) and the CD4 molecule on T lymphocytes), but not at all for others;

◆ *Entry into the host cell*. Some viruses can enter cells by fusion of their own outer lipid membrane with the plasma membrane of the cell, resulting in release of viral nucleocapsid into the cell cytoplasm. In other cases, the process of translocation of the viral particle from the outside of the cell to the inside is very poorly understood;

◆ *Uncoating of the viral genome*. The viral nucleic acid must be released from its capsid before replication. This process may be mediated by cellular lysosomal enzymes.

◆ *Macromolecular synthesis*. Within the cell, multiple copies of the viral genome are made, and mRNA derived from the virus is translated into multiple copies of the proteins encoded by the viral genome. Many viruses use enzymes present within the host cell to perform these activities, but some carry their own enzymes for certain synthetic processes that are not present within the host cell. A good example is HIV, which copies its RNA genome into a DNA intermediate. Since host cells are not able to convert RNA into DNA, the necessary reverse transcriptase must be encoded by the HIV genome itself, and the enzyme carried into the cell within the viral particle;

◆ *Assembly*. Before final assembly into new viral particles, viral polyproteins may be digested by viral protease enzymes, and individual proteins may be modified by host cell processes such as glycosylation or phosphorylation;

◆ *Release*. The infected cell has by now become little more than a viral factory and complete viral particles may be released by destruction of the cell, or by continuous export through the cell membrane.

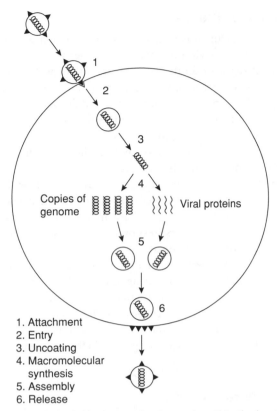

1. Attachment
2. Entry
3. Uncoating
4. Macromolecular
   synthesis
5. Assembly
6. Release

Fig. 4.1 Schematic representation of the virus replication cycle within the host cell, showing the stages that are theoretically open to inhibition by antiviral agents.

Virus–cell interactions

The viral replication cycle described above is representative of an acute viral infection: virus enters the cell, replicates, disrupts normal cellular function, and is released, often resulting in cell death. However, viruses may interact with cells in other ways. Some viruses can undergo latency within cells: the viral genome is present within the cell, usually as an episome within the cell nucleus, but no replication of the genome occurs, and few, if any, viral proteins are synthesized. The latent virus may cause the cell no harm, but it has the propensity, under certain conditions, to become reactivated, with consequent viral replication and damage to the cell. All herpesviruses undergo latency, one consequence of which is that once individuals becomes infected with a herpesvirus, they remain infected for their lifetime.

Another form of virus–cell interaction is chronic or persistent infection. In this, there is a steady production and release of virus, but the host cell is able to survive. However, host cell function may be impaired, and the expression of viral antigens on the cell surface can lead to a chronic inflammatory state as in chronic infection of hepatocytes with hepatitis B or C viruses leading to chronic hepatitis.

A further potential consequence of virus–cell interaction is transformation, whereby virus infection leads to uncontrolled cell division, resulting in an immortal cell line. For example, Epstein–Barr virus infection of B lymphocytes in vitro results in stimulation of cell division, and the establishment of a continuous lymphoblastoid cell line. The molecular mechanisms underlying this process, and possible means of interfering with them, are of great interest, since several viruses, including Epstein–Barr virus, have been implicated in initiating malignant change *in vivo*.

Limitations of antiviral therapy

Although all stages of the cycle of virus replication are potential targets for antiviral drugs, the intimate relationship between the virus and its host cell means that the design or discovery of compounds that are selectively toxic for the virus is beset with considerable problems. Moreover, antiviral therapy may be at a disadvantage for quite a different reason: in many viral diseases, initial infection and spread is commonly asymptomatic and the onset of illness, often at the peak of viral multiplication, occurs when the host defences have been fully mobilized. Unless the patient is immunodeficient in some way, these defences are usually quite able to deal with the infection unassisted. Consequently, initiation of antiviral therapy at the onset of symptoms may have little influence on the course of the disease.

Viruses that undergo latency pose a further problem. Unless the latently infected cells can be killed or removed, the virus cannot be eliminated from the patient. Achieving such elimination by therapeutic intervention is a daunting task, as there are no virus-specific metabolic processes occurring in those cells, and there is no expression of viral antigens on the cell surface against which an immune response could be mounted.

Despite these discouraging considerations, significant progress has been achieved in the development of antiviral compounds and an increasing number of antiviral agents is now in regular use (Table 4.2). Many are nucleoside analogues that interfere with viral replication, but other targets have been successfully exploited. Much research emphasis has been concentrated on agents that act to inhibit the replication of HIV, and on development of effective therapies for the treatment of chronic viral hepatitis. Antiviral drugs used in the treatment of these two conditions are discussed in Chapters 5 and 6 respectively.

Properties of antiviral agents

Aciclovir

Aciclovir was the first antiviral drug with selective toxicity: it inhibits the replication of certain viruses while exhibiting virtually no toxic side effects on host cells. Structurally, it is acycloguanosine (Fig. 4.2), an analogue of the purine nucleoside, guanosine, in which the deoxyribose moiety has lost its cyclic configuration. Aciclovir itself is inactive; in order to achieve its antiviral effect, it must first be phosphorylated to the triphosphate form within the infected cell. Although the second and third phosphate groups are added by cellular enzymes, the initial phosphorylation step is accomplished by a viral thymidine kinase, specified by herpes simplex and varicella zoster viruses; the cellular form of this enzyme is much less efficient in producing aciclovir monophosphate. This unique feature contributes significantly to the selective toxicity of aciclovir, for two reasons: first, it means that the active form of the drug is produced only in virally infected cells; secondly, by the law of mass action, once the equilibrium

aciclovir ↔ aciclovir monophosphate

is shifted to the right within an infected cell, more free aciclovir will enter the cell from the extracellular space, thus resulting in concentration of the drug precisely where it is needed: in the infected cell.

Mode of action

As an analogue of guanosine triphosphate, aciclovir triphosphate will compete with GTP for incorporation into a growing DNA chain. Incorporation results in chain termination, since it lacks the 3′-hydroxyl group necessary to form the 5′-3′ phosphodiester linkage with the next base.

Table 4.2 Principal antiviral agents* in present use

Compound	Indication	Mode of action	Route of administration
Aciclovir	Herpes simplex; Varicella–zoster	Nucleoside analogue	Oral; topical; intravenous
Amantadine	Influenza A	Uncoating of virus	Oral
Cidofovir	Cytomegalovirus	Nucleotide analogue	Intravenous
Famciclovir	Herpes simplex; Varicella–zoster	Nucleoside analogue[a]	Oral
Fomivirsen	Cytomegalovirus	Anti-sense oligonucleoside	Intra-ocular
Foscarnet	Cytomegalovirus	DNA polymerase inhibitor	Intravenous
Ganciclovir	Cytomegalovirus	Nucleoside analogue	Intravenous
Ribavirin	Respiratory syncytial virus	Nucleoside analogue	Nebulizer
	Chronic hepatitis		Oral
Valaciclovir	Herpes simplex; Varicella–zoster	Nucleoside analogue[a]	Oral
Valganciclovir	Cytomegalovirus	Nucleoside analogue[a]	Oral
Oseltamivir	Influenza	Neuraminidase inhibitor	Oral
Zanamivir	Influenza	Neuraminidase inhibitor	Inhalation

* other than anti-HIV agents, see Chapter 5, and agents used in the treatment of viral hepatitis, see Chapter 6.
[a] Prodrug formulation.

Viral DNA polymerase enzymes bind aciclovir triphosphate with a much greater affinity than do the corresponding cellular enzymes. This preferential binding creates a third level of antiviral selectivity, as aciclovir triphosphate acts as a direct inhibitor of viral DNA polymerase.

Resistance

It is theoretically possible for a virus to become resistant to aciclovir in several ways:

◆ Strains of virus that lack the thymidine kinase enzyme, known as TK⁻ variants, are inherently resistant to the drug, as they cannot generate the active form;

◆ Mutations in the *TK* gene may alter the thymidine kinase molecule, such that it becomes unable to perform the first phosphorylation step;

◆ Alterations in viral DNA polymerase may reduce the ability of the enzyme to bind aciclovir triphosphate, and thereby to escape the inhibitory properties of the drug.

All these mechanisms occur in the laboratory and in nature. However, TK⁻ strains, and those with altered thymidine kinases exhibit reduced virulence, and DNA polymerase mutants are the ones that cause most clinical difficulties. These emerge particularly in immunocompromised patients including those with HIV infection, in whom recurrent herpes simplex virus infections cause frequent and extensive disease necessitating prolonged treatment with aciclovir.

Aciclovir represents a prime example of what a good antiviral drug should be. It has potent antiviral activity, but is virtually free of toxic side effects. It can be life-saving in certain infections, and in others can significantly decrease morbidity (see Chapter 32). However, it is relatively poorly absorbed when given orally, and in life-threatening infection it must be given intravenously.

Analogues of aciclovir

Several structural analogues of aciclovir have been developed. Valaciclovir, the L-valyl ester of aciclovir, is an oral pro-drug that is well absorbed when given by mouth to release aciclovir into

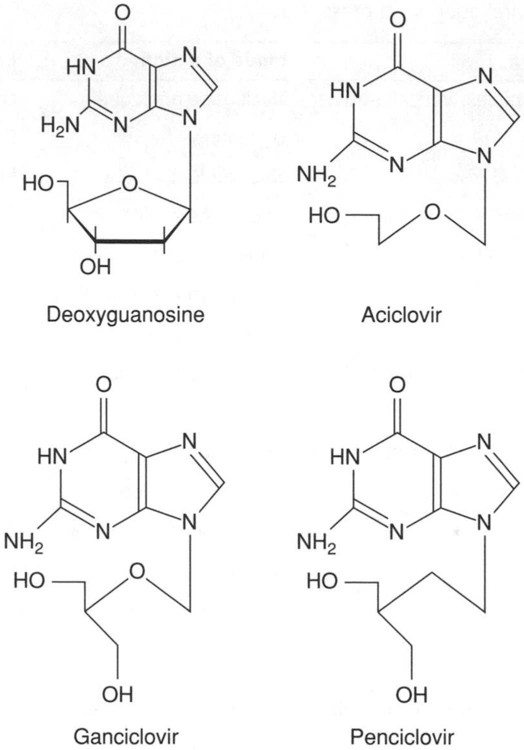

Fig. 4.2 Structures of deoxyguanosine and three antiviral agents that act as analogues of the nucleoside: aciclovir, ganciclovir, and penciclovir.

the bloodstream. A similar relationship exists between famciclovir and penciclovir; the former is metabolized into the latter after oral administration. Penciclovir (Fig. 4.2) exhibits antiviral activity very similar to that of aciclovir, but the half-life within cells is considerably longer, so fewer doses are necessary to achieve an antiviral effect.

Although aciclovir and its analogues are undoubtedly successful antiviral drugs, their clinical usefulness is limited by their narrow spectrum of activity. They are active only against a subgroup of herpesviruses—herpes simplex and varicella zoster viruses—that can perform the first phosphorylation step. It is particularly disappointing that these otherwise excellent drugs have no activity against cytomegalovirus, a herpesvirus that does not encode its own thymidine kinase enzyme.

Ganciclovir

Ganciclovir (dihydroxypropoxymethylguanine, DHPG, Fig. 4.2) is a derivative of aciclovir that shows useful activity against cytomegalovirus, an opportunist pathogen that causes severe and even life-threatening disease in immunosuppressed patients such as transplant recipients and HIV-infected individuals. Ganciclovir must be activated by phosphorylation, but cytomegalovirus uses a virally encoded phosphotransferase, encoded by gene UL97, that differs from thymidine kinase of herpes simplex or varicella zoster. Subsequent phosphorylation to the triphosphate generates a compound that acts as a viral DNA polymerase inhibitor. Unfortunately, cellular enzymes also phosphorylate ganciclovir, so that active drug is generated in uninfected cells. Thus the toxicity of ganciclovir is considerably greater than that of aciclovir. The most frequent unwanted effects, leucopenia and thrombocytopenia, arise from a toxic effect on the function of the bone marrow, particularly affecting the production of neutrophils. Ganciclovir treatment can also result in a rise in serum creatinine. It is poorly absorbed (<10%) when given orally, and has to be administered intravenously. The valyl ester of ganciclovir, valganciclovir, is much better absorbed orally (40%), and serum concentrations are close to those arising from intravenous ganciclovir therapy. Despite its drawbacks, ganciclovir can be sight or life saving in immunosuppressed patients with severe cytomegalovirus infections (see Chapter 32).

Resistance to ganciclovir through point mutations in the UL97 phosphotransferase gene arises fairly commonly in clinical practice. Fortunately, the viral mutants remain sensitive to foscarnet (see below). Although less common, mutations in the cytomegalovirus DNA polymerase (encoded by gene UL54) gene may also confer resistance, and such viruses may also be cross-resistant to foscarnet and cidofovir (see below).

Cidofovir

The difficulty in achieving the first phosphorylation step of aciclovir-like compounds is avoided by acyclic nucleoside phosphonates, a class of compounds of which cidofovir (Fig. 4.3) was the first to be developed and licensed for clinical use. The phosphonate group acts as a phosphate mimetic, and is attached to the acyclic nucleoside moiety through a stable P–C bond that cannot be split by cellular hydrolases. These agents need only two phosphorylation steps to reach the active triphosphate form, and cellular enzymes perform these steps. Thus, active drug may arise in both infected and uninfected cells, but a selective antiviral activity is maintained since the triphosphate exhibits a higher affinity for viral DNA polymerases than for the corresponding cellular enzymes. Like aciclovir triphosphate, the drugs act as chain terminators and competitive inhibitors.

Cidofovir is an acyclic cytosine analogue, with potent activity against cytomegalovirus. It is administered by intravenous infusion in the treatment of cytomegalovirus retinitis. It has a prolonged half-life such that dosing is required only once a week or less. It is, however, nephrotoxic in a dose-dependent manner, and must be administered with probenecid to prevent irreversible renal damage.

The mechanism of action of this class of drugs raises the possibility that they may have a much broader spectrum of activity than aciclovir and its derivatives, potentially against all viruses with a DNA polymerase function. Cidofovir is indeed active against all herpesviruses, as well as adeno-, polyoma-, papilloma-, and poxviruses, although clinical use in these infections is limited by drug toxicity. However, other class members such as adefovir and tenofovir have useful inhibitory activity against either or both the reverse transcriptase of HIV, and the DNA polymerase of hepatitis B virus

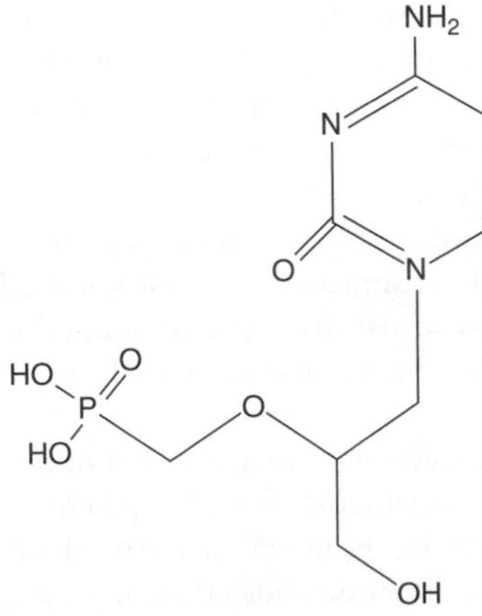

Fig. 4.3 Structure of cidofovir.

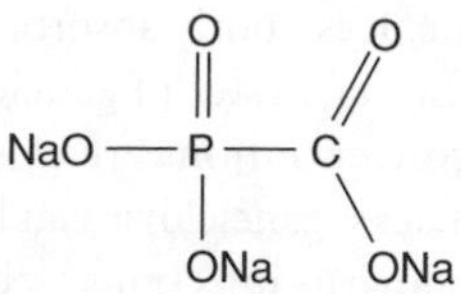

$$NaO-\overset{\displaystyle O}{\underset{\displaystyle ONa}{\|}}P-\overset{\displaystyle O}{\|}C\overset{\diagdown}{\underset{\diagdown ONa}{}}$$

Fig. 4.4 Structure of foscarnet.

(see Chapters 5 and 6). This class of drugs thus offers great promise for the treatment of a wide range of virus infections.

In theory, resistance to cidofovir and its congeners may arise through mutations in the viral DNA polymerases and time will tell how much of a problem this will become.

Foscarnet

Unlike the drugs discussed so far, foscarnet (Fig. 4.4) is not a nucleoside analogue; it is trisodium phosphonoformate, a derivative of phosphonoacetic acid, and is therefore a pyrophosphate analogue. It does not require phosphorylation. It forms complexes with DNA polymerases, and prevents cleavage of pyrophosphate from nucleoside triphosphates, resulting in inhibition of further DNA synthesis. It shows some selective toxicity for viral rather than host cell enzymes, and is active against all the herpesviruses, including cytomegalovirus. It is used as an alternative to ganciclovir in the treatment of serious cytomegalovirus infection, as well as in the treatment of aciclovir-resistant herpes simplex infection. Like ganciclovir, oral bioavailability is poor, and it has to be administered by intravenous injection. It is nephrotoxic, and can cause acute renal failure. Other side effects include symptomatic hypocalcaemia, and penile ulceration.

Fomivirsen

Fomivirsen is an oligonucleotide, 21 bases in length. It is not marketed in the European Union, but is available in some countries for the treatment of cytomegalovirus retinitis by intravitreous injection. It is an anti-sense molecule: the mirror image of a section of cytomegalovirus-derived mRNA encoding regulatory proteins. Binding of the drug to this region prevents translation of the RNA into protein.

Ribavirin

Ribavirin is a synthetic nucleoside in which ribose is linked to a triazole derivative (Fig. 4.5). Like other nucleoside analogues, it has to be activated intracellularly by phosphorylation. The precise mode of action has proved elusive, though there are several theories including the possibilities that it inhibits an essential step (5′ capping) in the processing of viral mRNA or that it causes lethal mutations in viral nucleotides.

Ribavirin has an unusually broad spectrum of activity, against both RNA and DNA viruses, at least in vitro. Its main use is in the treatment of severe lower respiratory tract infection in young children, caused by respiratory syncytial virus. The compound is administered by inhalation of an aerosolized solution. Oral ribavirin has also been used successfully in the treatment of Lassa fever.

Although ribavirin itself is ineffective in the treatment of chronic hepatitis C, combination therapy with interferon (especially peginterferon; see Chapter 6) produces a considerable improvement in response rates compared with the use of interferon alone.

The most commonly encountered serious side effect of prolonged ribavirin use is haemolytic anaemia.

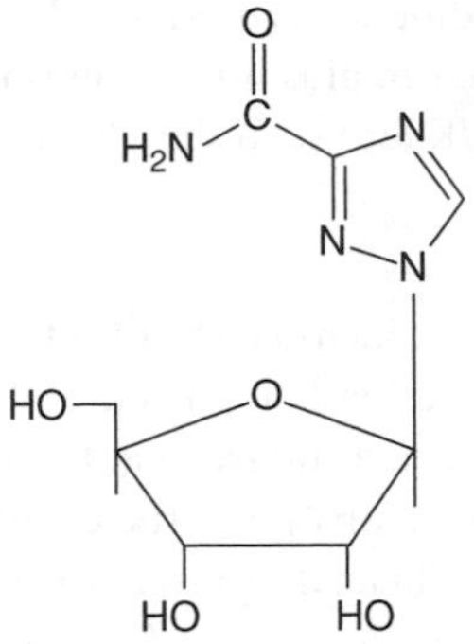

Fig. 4.5 Structure of ribavirin.

Older nucleoside analogues

Nucleoside analogues have been used for many years as antiviral agents, but the older ones are very toxic and have been eclipsed by later developments. Idoxuridine and trifluridine are still available in many countries for topical application in recurrent herpes simplex infections, but are no longer recommended. Cytarabine (cytosine arabinoside; ara-C) and vidarabine (adenine arabinoside; ara-A) are cytotoxic drugs of limited availability that are sometimes used as agents of last resort in life-threatening and otherwise untreatable viral infections.

Amantadine and rimantadine

Amantadine (Fig. 4.6) is a tricyclic amine derivative of adamantane, a compound that originally aroused interest because of its symmetrical three-dimensional structure, which is composed entirely of carbon atoms and is thus related to the crystalline array of natural diamonds. The antiviral activity of amantadine was first described in 1964. Rimantadine is a closely related substance that is available in some countries.

The activity of both amantadine and rimantadine is restricted to influenza A virus. Other influenza viruses are virtually unaffected at therapeutically achievable concentrations. These compounds block a viral matrix protein ion channel, thereby interfering with uncoating of the viral nucleic acid within the infected cell. Resistance readily arises by mutation in the matrix protein, which is then unable to bind the drugs.

Amantadine has dopaminergic effects and may cause restlessness, insomnia, agitation, and confusion, especially in the elderly, one of the groups who stand to benefit most from an effective anti-influenza drug. Rimantadine gives rise to fewer side effects and is generally favoured in countries where it is available.

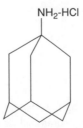

Fig. 4.6 Structure of amantadine.

Combination therapy of amantadine with interferon has been used in patients with chronic hepatitis C virus infection, but ribavirin plus interferon is more effective and is now preferred. Amantadine is also licensed in the UK for use in shingles, but this has few advocates.

Oseltamivir and zanamivir

These drugs belong to a class of anti-influenza compounds that selectively inhibit viral neuraminidase, one of the two proteins (the other being haemagglutinin) present on the surface of all types of influenza viruses. Viral neuraminidase enables budding influenza virus particles to break away from an infected cell by hydrolyzing the cellular sialic acid residues to which the haemagglutinin binds. It may also facilitate the passage of virus particles through mucus to reach epithelial cell surfaces, thereby aiding infection of new cells. Oseltamivir and zanamivir act extracellularly to inhibit the release and propagation of infectious influenza viruses from the epithelial cells of the respiratory tract. Unlike amantadine, they act against both influenza A and B viruses, and inhibit all the known neuraminidase subtypes of influenza A viruses. Oseltamivir is administered by mouth, while zanamivir is formulated for oral inhalation. They appear to be generally safe, but zanamivir occasionally causes bronchospasm in patients with underlying lung disease.

These drugs bind to the active site of neuraminidase, which is highly conserved among different strains of influenza virus. Oseltamivir has a more bulky side chain than zanamivir (see Fig. 4.7). High-level resistance to oseltamivir may arise through a single point mutation (H275Y) within its binding site, although such viruses remain sensitive to zanamivir. New neuraminidase inhibitors are in development, including peramivir.

Interferon

Interferon (IFN) was described in 1957 as an antiviral compound in chick embryo cells. It turns out that the activity is associated with a family of species-specific glycosylated proteins produced *in vivo* in response to viral or antigenic challenge. When IFNs were discovered, they were hailed

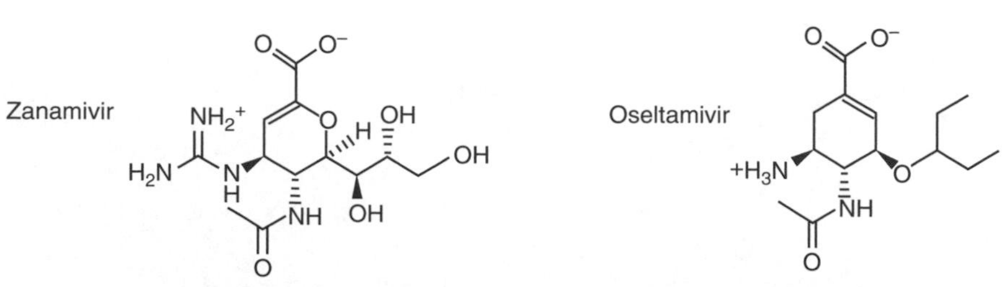

Fig. 4.7 Structure of sialic acid, zanamivir, and oseltamivir. Adapted from Ferraris, O and Lina B, 'Mutations of neuraminidase implicated in neuraminidase inhibitors resistance', *Clinical Virology*, 2008; **41**(1): 13–19, with permission from Elsevier.

as the antiviral equivalent of penicillin. As these substances were produced by cells as a natural defence in response to a wide range of virus infections, it seemed reasonable to imagine that when used as therapeutic agents, they would exhibit a broad antiviral spectrum, and that their toxic effects on host cells would be minimal. However, clinical trials of IFNs as a treatment for a range of viral infections have in general been disappointing, with the notable exception of their use in the management of patients with chronic hepatitis B or C infection. The interferons are therefore discussed in more detail in Chapter 6.

Prevention of virus infections

Prevention rather than cure plays such an important part in the control of viral diseases that an appreciation of the methods used is essential to understanding the complementary role of antiviral agents. The scourge of smallpox has been removed by appropriate use of vaccinia vaccine and certain other viral infections may be similarly eradicated. The World Health Organization campaign to eliminate polio is progressing towards a successful conclusion, and in many developed countries measles, mumps, and rubella are becoming rare.

Passive immunization

Immune globulin

The transfer of preformed antibodies from one individual to another can be achieved with human gammaglobulin derived from the blood of healthy individuals known to have high antibody titres. In the days before an effective vaccine against hepatitis A became available, normal human immunoglobulin obtained from pooled routine blood donations was widely used for the protection of individuals visiting countries where the virus is common. Other types of immunoglobulin are obtained specifically from known hyperimmune individuals. Those in current use include immuno-globulin preparations against hepatitis B, varicella zoster, and rabies viruses.

Monoclonal antibody

Techniques allowing the production of monoclonal antibodies with their exceptional intrinsic specificity have led to investigation of such compounds in the prevention of viral infection. The only one presently available, palivizumab, is a monoclonal antibody directed against respiratory syncytial virus. It is administered by intramuscular injection to vulnerable infants (those with underlying chronic lung disease, congenital heart disease, or immunodeficiency) at monthly intervals during the autumn and winter—seasons of greatest risk of infection with the virus.

Active immunization

The host can be stimulated to produce a protective immune response by vaccination with a form of the infectious agent that does not cause disease. Vaccines can be alive or dead. Live vaccines consist of attenuated forms of the infectious agent. Examples include measles, mumps, rubella, and live poliovirus (Sabin) vaccines.

Dead vaccines may consist of the whole agent, grown in the laboratory and subsequently killed by some means, or of a subunit of the agent, usually prepared by recombinant DNA technology. Dead vaccines have the advantage that there is no risk of reversion to virulence. However, they are less immunogenic than live vaccines, and therefore more doses need to be given to achieve a satisfactory response. Examples of such vaccines include the Salk polio vaccine (now generally preferred to the live Sabin vaccine), rabies virus, hepatitis A and hepatitis B virus vaccines; the latter is a subunit vaccine, consisting only of the surface protein (HBsAg), prepared by cloning and expressing the appropriate gene in yeast cells.

Key points

- Viruses are obligate intracellular parasites which rely to a greater or lesser extent on host cell functions for their replication.
- Nevertheless, a number of viral targets have been successfully exploited in the development of effective antiviral agents.
- Aciclovir and derivatives are nucleoside analogues that require initial phosphorylation by a virally encoded enzyme (thymidine kinase, TK), and subsequently act to inhibit viral DNA polymerase (DNA pol). Resistance may arise through mutations in TK or DNA pol.
- Cidofovir and derivatives are nucleotide analogues which are further phosphorylated by host enzymes and act to inhibit viral DNA pol.
- Foscarnet is a pyrophosphate analogue which inhibits viral DNA pol.
- Ribavirin is a nucleoside analogue with an unknown mechanism of action, but has a broad spectrum of activity *in vitro*.
- Zanamivir and oseltamivir are neuraminidase (NA) inhibitors and therefore prevent release of mature influenza virus particles from infected cells. Resistance, particularly to oseltamivir, may arise through point mutations in the NA gene.

Further reading

Yin, MT, Brust, JCM, Tieu HV, Hammer SM (2009), Antiherpesvirus, anti-hepatitus virus, and anti-respiratory virus agents, in *Clinical Virology* (3rd edn). Richman DD, Whitley RJ, Hayden FG (eds). Washington DC: ASM Press, 217–264.

Chapter 5

Antiretroviral agents

The first human immunodeficiency virus (HIV) was identified and characterized as a retrovirus in 1983. Long-term infection with HIV leads to inexorable destruction of the host immune system, and the development of the acquired immune deficiency syndrome (AIDS). Since that momentous discovery, considerable progress has been made in devising novel anti-retroviral agents, which, by inhibiting HIV replication, can prolong the time to the development of AIDS. Unfortunately, the concept of 'curing' a patient of HIV infection remains an elusive and as yet unattainable goal.

The fact that HIV belongs to the retroviral family identified the first and most obvious target in the search for anti-HIV drugs—the enzyme reverse transcriptase. This enzyme, which copies an RNA template into DNA, is not present within host cells, which have no need to perform this 'backwards' synthetic process. The enzyme is encoded within the HIV genome, and the protein itself is an essential component of infectious viral particles.

Initially, anti-HIV drugs were all nucleoside analogues. Subsequently, it became clear that compounds with other structures could also act as reverse transcriptase inhibitors. Further advances came with the development of drugs that target completely different steps within the viral life cycle (see Fig. 5.1), including processing of the viral polyprotein, binding of the virus particle to target cells, fusion of the viral envelope with host cell membranes leading to cell entry, and integration of the proviral DNA into the host chromosome. Thus, there are currently a number of classes of antiretroviral drugs licensed for clinical use: nucleoside and non-nucleoside reverse transcriptase inhibitors, protease inhibitors, binding-blockers, fusion inhibitors and integrase inhibitors (Table 5.1). Various other potential targets have been identified, and it is hoped that the number of anti-HIV drugs will continue to expand.

Antiretroviral drugs are commonly formulated as combination products in the hope of suppressing the development of resistance, to simplify the often complex dosage regimens that are required for effective therapy and, in some cases, to exploit possible synergistic interactions. However, the frequent occurrence of toxic interactions between various antiretroviral compounds demands careful selection of such drug permutations.

Reverse transcriptase inhibitors (RTIs)

(i) Nucleos(t)ide analogues (NRTIs)

Zidovudine

Zidovudine (azidothymidine; often simply called AZT; Fig. 5.2) was originally investigated for use as an anticancer agent. However, when the HIV epidemic arose in the 1980s, it was tested along with many other drugs for activity against the virus. It was found to inhibit the reverse transcriptase activity of retroviruses at concentrations considerably lower than those needed to interfere with synthesis of host cell DNA.

Molecules such as zidovudine are referred to as 2′-3′-dideoxy nucleoside analogues, since they lack hydroxyl groups at both the 2′ and 3′ positions of the deoxyribose ring. Like other nucleoside

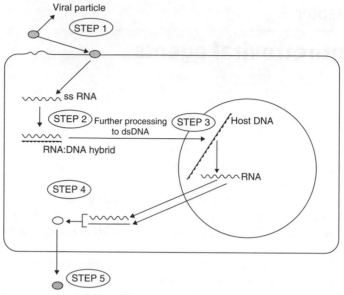

Fig. 5.1 HIV replication cycle and targets for antiretroviral drugs.

Step 1. Viral entry

Step 2. Reverse transcription of ssRNA into RNA:DNA hybrid

Step 3. Integration of dsDNA provirus into host DNA

Step 4. +ssRNA plus translated polyproteins form immature viral particles

Step 5. Protease processing of polyproteins results in maturation and release of virus particles

Table 5.1 Antiretroviral agents in clinical use in the UK and/or US (2011)

Nucleos(t)ide reverse transcriptase inhibitors	Non-nucleoside reverse transcriptase inhibitors	Protease inhibitors	Other antiretrovirals
Abacavir	Efavirenz	Atazanavir	Enfuvirtide (fusion inhibitor)
Didanosine (ddI)	Etravirine	Darunavir	Maraviroc (CCR5 binding inhibitor)
Emtricitabine	Nevirapine	Fosamprenavir[a]	Raltegravir (Integrase inhibitor)
Lamivudine (3TC)		Indinavir	
Stavudine (d4T)		Lopinavir[b]	
Tenofovir[c] (TDF)		Nelfinavir	
Zidovudine (AZT)		Ritonavir	
		Saquinavir	
		Tipranavir	

[a] A pro-drug formulation;

[b] Formulated as a combination tablet with low dose ritonavir;

[c] A nucleotide rather than a nucleoside analogue.

Abbreviations in brackets are often used to describe these compounds. They are derived from the chemical structures: didanosine is 2′,3′-dideoxyinosine; lamivudine is 2′-deoxy-3′-thiacytidine; stavudine is 2′,3′-didehydro-3′-deoxythymidine; zidovudine is 3′-azido-2′,3′-dideoxythymidine. TDF is tenofovir disoproxil fumarate, a pro-drug.

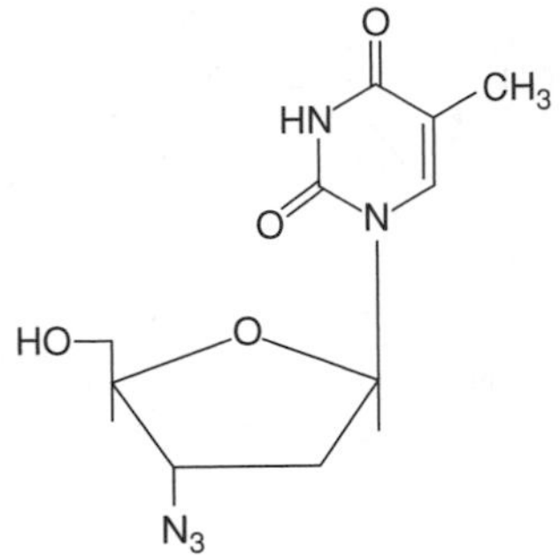

Fig. 5.2 Structure of azidothymidine (AZT).

analogues, these compounds are activated by phosphorylation to the triphosphate form, these steps being carried out by cellular enzymes. As with aciclovir (p. 52), incorporation of the triphosphate into a growing DNA chain will result in chain termination, as there is no 3' hydroxyl group available for formation of the next 5'-3' phosphodiester linkage.

Non-specific side effects such as headache, anorexia, and nausea are common with zidovudine therapy, but these effects often abate after two to three weeks. More serious toxicity to bone marrow cells is dose-related, and hence much effort has been directed at defining the minimum dose that exhibits effective antiviral action. Combination therapy with ganciclovir, although desirable, since many HIV-infected patients also suffer serious CMV infection, is complicated by an additive effect on the bone marrow.

Other nucleos(t)ide analogues

The success of zidovudine, albeit with limitations, at least showed that it was possible for anti-HIV drugs to be therapeutically useful. The pharmaceutical industry was therefore encouraged to design and test other potential nucleoside analogues. Currently there are, six further drugs of this type licensed for use in the USA and some other countries (Table 5.1). One of these compounds, tenofovir, is phosphorylated and is thus, like cidofovir (p. 55), a nucleotide, rather than a nucleoside analogue, but its mode of action is similar to that of true nucleoside analogues: it is converted to a triphosphate form that acts as a chain terminator and competitive inhibitor of HIV-derived reverse transcriptase.

The most frequent adverse reaction with all of these drugs is gastrointestinal disturbance, including nausea, vomiting, abdominal pain, and diarrhoea. More serious and potentially life-threatening effects include lactic acidosis and hepatomegaly. Abacavir is associated with life-threatening hypersensitivity reactions in patients with the HLA allele, HLA-B*5701. Thus, the presence of this allele must be excluded before initiating abacavir therapy. Among the many side effects more commonly associated with individual compounds are: peripheral neuropathy (didanosine, stavudine); pancreatitis (didanosine); elevation of liver transaminases (stavudine); increased serum phosphate levels and renal failure (tenofovir); and pruritus (emtricitabine).

(ii) Non-nucleoside analogue reverse transcriptase inhibitors (NNRTIs)

The recognition that compounds with a range of dissimilar structures could also act as inhibitors of reverse transcriptase led to the categorization of a new class of anti-HIV agents: the non-nucleoside analogue reverse transcriptase inhibitors. In contrast to the nucleoside analogues,

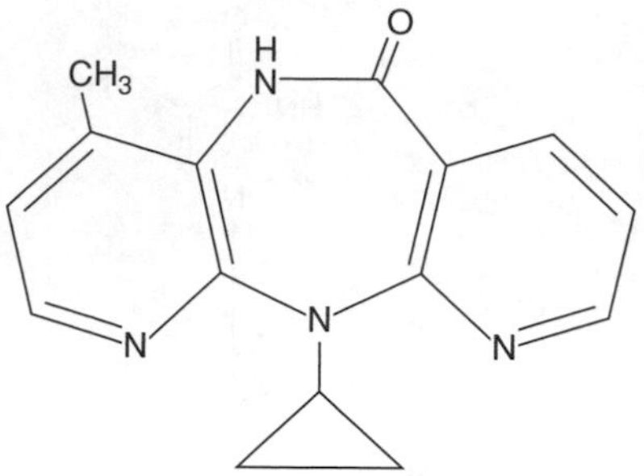

Fig. 5.3 Structure of nevirapine.

these agents bind specifically to a non-substrate binding site of reverse transcriptase located close to the substrate-binding site. These drugs inhibit the reverse transcriptase of HIV-1 but not that of HIV-2. Many chemical classes of non-nucleoside compounds that act as reverse transcriptase inhibitors have been described, but only three drugs are currently used extensively in the treatment of HIV infection: nevirapine (Fig. 5.3), efavirenz, and etravirine.

Rashes, which can be severe (e.g. Stevens–Johnson syndrome), hepatotoxicity, and numerous other side effects of varying frequency and severity are associated with the use of this class of compounds.

Protease inhibitors

The development of drugs acting on a viral target other than reverse transcriptase represented a major breakthrough in therapy for HIV-infected patients. When HIV replicates, it produces poly-cistronic mRNA, which is translated into a series of polyproteins that must be cleaved to yield the component proteins for infectious viral particles. This function is performed by a virally encoded aspartyl protease. Although mammalian cells also contain aspartyl proteases, these do not cleave HIV polyproteins efficiently.

Nine drugs that specifically inhibit HIV protease are currently licensed for use (Table 5.1). They are complex molecules and most are structurally related. All have important side effects. Besides gastrointestinal problems (particularly prominent with ritonavir), the most worrying adverse effect of protease inhibitors arises from their interference with fat and carbohydrate metabolism, leading to hyperlipidaemia, glucose intolerance (even frank diabetes mellitus), and peripheral lipodystrophy (abnormal body fat distribution) with increased abdominal fat, 'buffalo humps', and breast hypertrophy. The frequency and pathophysiology of these reactions are unclear, as is the long-term risk of other complications such as ischaemic heart disease. Indinavir may cause nephrolithiasis, by precipitation in the renal tubules.

Ritonavir has the useful property of boosting the activity of other protease inhibitors by pro-longing plasma concentrations, possibly by competing for liver enzymes that metabolize these drugs. The effect is obtained with low doses of ritonavir that lack intrinsic antiviral activity.

Fusion inhibitors

The process of fusion whereby viral particles gain entry into the CD4 T cell following the initial attachment process is an attractive target for selectively active antiretroviral drugs. Various synthetic peptides have been designed to mimic part of the viral envelope glycoprotein gp41, which is involved in the fusion of the virus to the membrane of the target cell, and several of them efficiently prevent viral infection of cells *in vitro*. Only one of these compounds, enfuvirtide (formerly pentafuside) has so far been approved for therapeutic use. As a peptide, enfuvirtide is digested when taken by mouth and it is therefore administered by subcutaneous injection twice daily. Enfuvirtide is licensed for use in patients who are intolerant of other antiretroviral drugs or are not responding to preferred regimens. Side effects of the drug are common, but are not normally serious.

CCR5 binding inhibitors

The primary cellular receptor for HIV is CD4. However, binding to CD4 alone is not sufficient to allow viral entry into a target cell. A number of essential co-receptors have been identified, the two most important ones being the chemokine receptors CCR5 and CXCR4. The observation that individuals homozygous for deletions in their CCR5 gene exhibit no significant clinical disease despite their lack of functional CCR5, but are highly resistant to infection with CCR5-tropic HIV, led to the development of small-molecule CCR5 antagonists aimed at blocking binding of HIV to target cells. Maraviroc is the leading agent in this class of compounds. Given this mode of action, it is necessary to confirm that a patient is infected with CCR5- (and not CXCR4-) tropic virus before prescribing this drug.

Integrase inhibitors

The latest target exploited for the development of antiretroviral drugs is the virally encoded integrase enzyme, which mediates integration of the DNA provirus into the host cell chromosome. Although an obvious target, it proved difficult to delineate the structure of this enzyme in order to design appropriate inhibitors, but raltegravir, the leading agent in this class of drugs, was licensed for clinical use in 2008.

Resistance to anti-HIV drugs

Unfortunately, optimism encouraged by the emergence of effective anti-HIV drugs has had to be tempered by the realization that the virus can rapidly acquire resistance to these agents. The enzyme reverse transcriptase is considerably more error-prone than other DNA polymerases. Thus, generation of large numbers of viral mutants is part of the natural replication cycle of HIV: it has been estimated that, within a single patient, every possible base substitution could occur at every possible nucleotide position in the viral genome every day! Clearly, the vast majority of these mutations will be deleterious and result in non-viable virus. However, the potential is there for mutations to occur that do confer benefit to the virus, especially if those mutations result in decreased efficacy of an antiviral drug. Experience with all anti-HIV drugs used thus far indicates that resistance is an inevitable consequence of drug usage, at least if the suppression of virus replication is not absolute.

Isolates of HIV derived from patients who have been taking zidovudine for at least six months are invariably less sensitive to the drug *in vitro* than isolates taken from the same patient at the initiation of therapy. This arises from mutations in the gene coding for reverse transcriptase, leading to reduced binding of zidovudine triphosphate. Resistance arises as a series of sequential point mutations within the reverse transcriptase gene, each additional mutation resulting in an increase in the dose of drug necessary to inhibit the virus. This relative resistance is of considerable clinical importance. Trials of zidovudine monotherapy conducted in the late 1980s showed early promise: increasing CD4 cell counts and prolonging survival in treated patients. However, as these patients were followed for longer periods, it became clear that the therapeutic efficacy of the drug was limited to a period of about six months, after which it was of no benefit. This loss of efficacy coincided with emergence of highly resistant viruses in treated patients.

Resistance to other nucleoside analogues similarly arises through mutations in the reverse transcriptase gene. In general, cross-resistance between zidovudine and the other nucleoside analogues is not a problem, as the positions of the mutations conferring resistance to zidovudine differ from those giving rise to resistance to, for instance, didanosine. In contrast, mutations causing resistance to didanosine overlap with those causing lamivudine resistance.

The news concerning resistance mutations may not be all bad, however. Mutation at position 184 in the reverse transcriptase gene results in increasing resistance to lamivudine, but paradoxically causes an increase in sensitivity to zidovudine in virus previously resistant. Thus, in theory at least, a combination regimen of zidovudine plus lamivudine should be of benefit, a hope reflected by the availability of a tablet that contains both agents.

Yet another set of mutations in the reverse transcriptase gene confers resistance to the non-nucleoside reverse transcriptase inhibitors, and several such changes have been reported. Some, but not all, lead to cross-resistance among the different drugs of this type, but they are distinct from those leading to resistance to the nucleos(t)ide analogues.

As with the reverse transcriptase inhibitors, resistance to the protease inhibitors may arise through point mutations in the gene coding for the target protein. Various mutations in the protease gene have been described. Many of these map at similar points in the genome of virus from patients receiving different protease inhibitors, indicating that cross-resistance between these drugs is common. Continued use of a given protease inhibitor leads to the accumulation of mutations, with a concomitant increase in resistance. Tipranavir and darunavir, so-called second-generation protease inhibitors, were introduced because they are active against strains resistant to other protease inhibitors.

Although the use of combination therapy substantially reduces the chance of treatment failure due to the emergence of drug resistance, there are disturbing reports of simultaneous resistance developing to two or more classes of antiretroviral drug. The spread of multiresistant strains of the virus clearly constitutes a major threat and it is important to minimize this possibility. Tests for drug resistance on isolates from patients receiving treatment are valuable in directing appropriate changes in therapy. These usually require sequencing of the appropriate viral gene to identify drug resistance mutations. Since resistant strains may revert to susceptibility when therapy is discontinued, a prompt switch to alternative agents is often helpful.

Anti-HIV drugs in development

Despite the clinical successes achieved by use of the above agents, there is a desperate need for new drugs with different sites of action, and different toxicity profiles in the fight against HIV infection. Much investigation continues into safer and more effective alternatives for existing classes of antiretroviral compounds.

Optimal therapy for patients with HIV infection may involve treatment with other drugs that do not necessarily exhibit antiviral activity. Immunomodulatory agents such as interleukin-2 have their advocates. Initially encouraging reports of the use of hydroxyurea, which blocks cellular activation necessary for viral replication in resting CD4-positive T cells have unfortunately not been confirmed.

Key points

- A detailed understanding of the replication cycle of HIV has led to the development of a number of classes of antitretroviral drugs acting at a number of different steps.

- Reverse transcriptase inhibitors include nucleos(t)ide analogues, referred to as NRTI, and non-nucleoside analogues (NNRTI). These act to prevent the synthesis of proviral DNA from the genomic RNA template.

- Protease inhibitors prevent the cleavage of the HIV polyproteins generated by the polycistronic mRNA transcribed from the proviral DNA, and hence prevent the maturation of nascent viral particles.

- Fusion inhibitors act to inhibit a very early step in the viral entry process. Another class of drugs acting at the viral entry stage is the CCR5 antagonists, which prevent binding of the viral gp120 to the CCR5 secondary co-receptor.

- Integrase inhibitors target the viral integrase enzyme responsible for integrating proviral DNA into the host cell chromosomes.

- The emergence of resistance to any of the above antiretroviral drugs may arise through spontaneous mutations within the target gene (reverse transcriptase, protease, gp120, integrase).

Further reading

Sobieszczyk ME, Taylor BS, Hammer SM (2009), 'Antiretroviral agents', in *Clinical Virology* (3rd edn). Richman DD, Whitley RJ, Hayden FG (eds). Washington DC: ASM Press, 167–216.

Chapter 6

Drugs used in the treatment of viral hepatitis

The World Health Organization estimates that there are over 350 million individuals chronically infected with hepatitis B virus, and over 200 million chronically infected with hepatitis C virus. Another way of looking at this is to say that one in 12 inhabitants of earth is infected with one of these two hepatotropic viruses. Between 15 and 40% of individuals with chronic viral hepatitis will develop complications of disease such as the development of cirrhosis, with all its attendant life-threatening complications, or hepatocellular carcinoma, the fourth commonest cause worldwide of death due to malignant disease. HBV infection is thought to account for around one million deaths per year, and the toll from chronic HCV infection is likely to be of similar magnitude.

In the face of such morbidity and mortality, and in the knowledge of the huge potential market for any successful drugs generated in this area, there have been extensive efforts to develop effective therapy for patients with chronic viral hepatitis. Initial efforts to treat chronic HBV infection were focused on interferon, a naturally produced cytokine with multiple modes of action. However, a better understanding of the molecular biology of HBV replication has led to a revolution in the management of chronic HBV infection in the past 10 years. Similarly, a detailed understanding of the molecular biology of HCV has resulted in the identification of several potential targets for antiviral drugs, with several new molecules now in late-stage clinical trials.

Drugs used in the treatment of chronic HBV infection

(i) Interferon-alpha

There are three classes of human IFN: class 1 includes IFN-α, produced by many cell types, and IFN-β, produced by fibroblasts; class 2 comprises IFN-γ (sometimes referred to as immune interferon) produced by T lymphocytes. Class 3 includes IFN-λ 1, 2, and 3. IFN-α and IFN-β share 30% structural homology, but they are quite distinct from IFN-γ, which shares only about 10% homology in its amino acid sequence. Moreover, there are over 15 different forms of IFN-α, each differing by a few amino acids, and, possibly, two forms of IFN-β.

Interferons have a wide range of biological effects. They activate several different biochemical pathways within a cell, with the result that the cell is rendered resistant to virus infection. The relative importance of each of these pathways differs between different IFNs, and indeed between different cells stimulated by the same IFN. One pathway results in the activation of a ribonuclease that digests viral RNA. Another results in phosphorylation of a protein known as an initiation factor; phosphorylation of this factor, the normal function of which is to assist in the initiation of transcription of mRNA into protein, effectively prevents production of viral proteins.

IFNs also have various effects on cells of the immune system. As with their antiviral properties, these immunomodulatory effects vary in detail between different IFNs, but they include stimulation of natural killer cells, induction or suppression of antibody production, stimulation of T-cell activity, and stimulation of expression of HLA class I and II molecules on the surface of cells.

Finally, IFNs affect cell proliferation, which has led to their successful use in the management of certain malignant tumours.

Early studies of the clinical efficacy of IFN therapy were hampered by difficulties in obtaining sufficient quantities of IFNs to conduct clinical trials. This problem has been solved by recombinant DNA technology, which has allowed cloning and expression of the relevant genes. Unexpectedly, clinical trials revealed that patients receiving IFN experienced flu-like side effects: fever, headache, and myalgia. This led to the realization that individuals suffering from influenza complain of flu-like symptoms precisely because of the induction of IFNs by the virus. Most patients become tolerant to these effects after the first few doses.

Chronic HBV infection was the first infection in which interferon-alpha was shown in appropriate clinical trials to be of clear therapeutic benefit. The standard regimen involved intramuscular administration three times a week for a minimum period of six months. Pegylated interferon (PEG-IFN) is a preparation in which IFN-α is covalently cross-linked to polyethylene glycol. This formulation has an extended half-life, leading to more prolonged therapeutic levels of the drug, and therefore requiring only once weekly injection (Fig. 6.1). PEG-IFN is better tolerated and, most importantly, produces a much superior virological response, and has therefore replaced the use of standard IFN. The evidence suggests that, in the context of chronic HBV infection, IFN exerts its therapeutic effect through immunomodulation rather than by acting directly as an antiviral agent. This is discussed further in Chapter 34.

(ii) Nucleoside and nucleotide analogues

There has been significant progress in the management of chronic HBV infection in the past 15 years, entirely due to the emergence of detailed information about the extraordinary and unique replicative cycle of the virus. Whilst the virus carries a partially double-stranded DNA genome, once within the cell a full-length RNA copy of the genome is transcribed (the RNA pre-genome), along with transcripts from the four open reading frames (surface, core, polymerase, and X ORFs). The RNA pre-genome is packaged within newly synthesized core protein, together with copies of the viral polymerase enzyme. The latter has reverse transcriptase activity, and copies the RNA pre-genome into single-stranded DNA, after which there is partial synthesis of the complementary DNA strand, resulting in the partially double-stranded DNA genome of the mature virus particle.

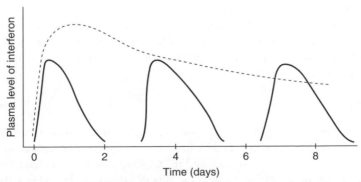

Fig. 6.1 Plasma levels of interferon and pegylated interferon. The solid lines show the IFN concentrations achieved after 3 individual injections of standard interferon. The dotted line shows the levels achieved after a single injection of pegylated interferon.

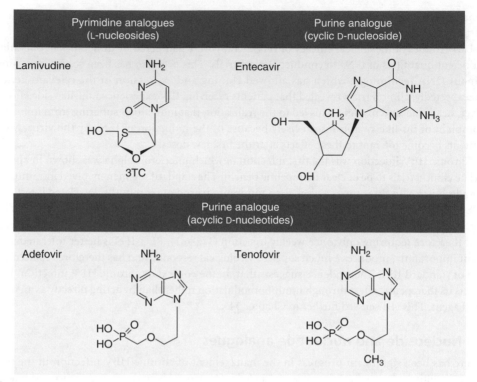

Fig. 6.2 Structure of nucelos(t)ide analogues used in the treatment of chronic hepatitis B virus infection.

Reverse transcriptase was formerly believed to exist only within the *Retroviridae*, so the elucidation of the convoluted replication strategy of HBV was a major surprise. The recognition of the key role of this enzymic activity within the HBV life cycle provided an obvious potential target for antiviral drugs, and, thanks to the epidemic of infection with the human immunodeficiency viruses which emerged in the 1980s, a variety of reverse transcriptase inhibitors were already available for appropriate clinical trials. Not all anti-HIV drugs have activity against the reverse transcriptase of HBV, and the same is true in reverse, i.e. there are some agents active against HBV but not HIV. The potency of some of these drugs in inhibiting HBV DNA production has revolutionized the management of these patients.

Historically lamivudine and adefovir were the first two agents to be licensed for the treatment of chronic HBV infection. However, due to relative lack of potency, and, more pertinently, much lower thresholds for the development of resistance, these two agents have now been replaced by entecavir and tenofovir.

Lamivudine

This agent (3-thiacytidine, Fig. 6.2), developed as a nucleoside analogue reverse transcriptase inhibitor (see Chapter 5) was the first RT inhibitor shown to inhibit HBV replication. It is triphosphorylated in the cell by cellular enzymes, and the triphosphate acts as a chain terminator and DNA polymerase inhibitor. Whilst treatment results in a dramatic decline in HBV viral loads, resistance has emerged as a major problem. After five years of therapy, over 80% of patients with hepatitis B harbour resistant virus, evidenced by rebound of HBV DNA to pre-treatment levels, and the presence of specific drug resistance mutations within the viral polymerase gene.

Adefovir

This acyclic adenine analogue (Fig. 6.2) is formulated as the dipivoxil ester for the oral treatment of chronic hepatitis B infection. As the first phosphate group is already present on the acyclic ring, this is a phosphonate nucleotide analogue. This agent has no anti-HIV activity, but does inhibit HBV replication. Although resistance does not emerge to quite the same extent as with lamivudine, nevertheless prolonged therapy does result in the induction of drug resistance mutations (DRMs) and loss of efficacy. The adefovir DRMs are distinct from those associated with lamivudine, so this drug is useful in patients with lamivudine resistance.

Entecavir

Entecavir is a nucleoside analogue based on guanosine (Fig. 6.2), but differs from aciclovir and ganciclovir in that carbon replaces oxygen in the modified ribose substituent, which retains a cyclic arrangement. It is a potent inhibitor of HBV replication, several hundredfold more so than lamivudine. In treatment-naïve patients receiving entecavir, emergence of resistance is very unusual, despite prolonged therapy. However, resistance may arise rapidly in patients who harbour virus containing lamivudine-resistance mutations, and therefore the dose recommended for lamivudine-experienced patients is twice the usual dose. It is administered orally.

Tenofovir

This more potent derivative of adefovir (Fig. 6.2) is formulated as tenofovir disoproxil fumarate. Not only does it demonstrate enhanced potency in viral suppression compared to adefovir, resistance mutations to this drug have not been identified to-date, indicating a very high barrier to resistance.

Drugs used in the treatment of chronic HCV infection

Interferon-alpha

Even before the identification of hepatitis C virus (HCV) as the causative agent of chronic non-A non-B hepatitis (NANBH), in the light of the moderate success achieved by interferon-alpha therapy of chronic HBV infection, such therapy was also applied to NANBH patients. This resulted in normalization of liver function tests and apparent cessation of disease progression in a minority of patients. HCV was characterized in 1989, so subsequent trials of IFN therapy were able to monitor the virological response, as opposed to the biochemical or histological responses to treatment. Standard IFN-alpha, given as thrice weekly injections for a minimum period of six months, led to clearance of virus in around 10% of infected patients (Fig. 6.3).

Ribavirin

Many other antiviral agents were tested empirically as possible therapy for chronic HCV infection. Ribavirin (RV, see Chapter 4) used as monotherapy had very little effect on the viral load detectable in peripheral blood, although it did normalize liver function in some patients. However, trials of combination therapy consisting of RV and standard IFN-alpha proved to be much more successful than the use of either drug alone, and this became the standard of care for patients with chronic HCV infection from the mid-1980s onwards. The overall response rate to IFN and RV combination therapy can reach as high as 40% (Fig. 6.3), although this is dependent on a number of host and viral factors (age, gender, degree of underlying liver damage, viral load, and, most especially, viral genotype) discussed in more detail in Chapter 34.

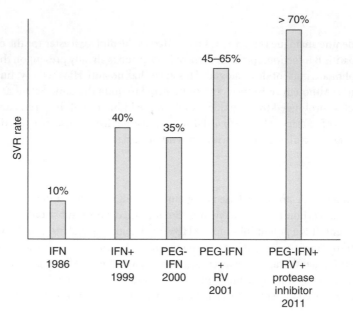

Fig. 6.3 Response rates to evolving therapies in chronic HCV infection.

Pegylated interferons

The next significant advance in the therapy of chronic HCV infection was the emergence of the pegylated interferons (see above). Indeed, PEG-IFNs were first trialled in the context of chronic HCV (as opposed to chronic HBV) infection. The dramatic effect that pegylation has on the maintenance of plasma levels of interferon, compared with standard IFN, is shown in Fig. 6.1.

PEG-IFN alone, given as once weekly injections for at least six months, achieved viral clearance rates similar to those from standard IFN plus RV combination therapy (Fig. 6.3).

Pegylated interferon and ribavirin combination therapy

Given the improvement in response rates seen with PEG-IFN, the natural next step was to set up clinical trials of PEG-IFN/RV combination therapy. Overall response rates increased yet again, to around 50% (Fig. 6.3), the exact figure again being dependent on the particular characteristics of the treated population, especially the infecting viral genotype. This regimen therefore replaced standard IFN/RV as the standard of care from 2001 onwards, and remains so at the time of writing.

Both drugs are associated with adverse effects. Interferon injections result in fever, myalgia, and headache. This can be controlled by paracetamol use, and after the first few doses, patients become tolerant to these effects. More serious effects include bone marrow suppression (neutropaenia, thrombocytopaenia), and depression which may result in suicidal ideation—patients may require psychiatric assessment before commencing therapy, and ongoing support with anti-depressives. Autoimmune manifestations may emerge on therapy, particularly autoimmune thyroid disease. Ribavirin causes a haemolytic anaemia. Combination therapy is therefore difficult, and patients may require extensive support and help in order to complete their course—especially in genotype 1 infection, where therapy should be continued for one year. Patient compliance is a problem— all clinical trials report at least a 10% patient drop-out rate.

It should be noted that although PEG/RV combination therapy can cure around half of all patients with chronic HCV infection, the mode of action(s) of either drug in this context remains unknown. The biochemical response to IFN therapy in chronic HCV infection is different from that in chronic HBV, and therefore it is unlikely that the action is entirely due to immunomodulation. There are a number of theories as to how RV might potentiate the response to IFN, but none have thus far been proven.

Genotype 1 virus is undoubtedly more resistant to therapy than any of the other genotypes (see Chapter 34), but in the absence of any understanding of how the drugs work, it has not been possible to discern at the molecular level why this should be, or what viral sequences in which genes confer resistance to either IFN or RV. An 'interferon sensitivity determining region' in the non-structural gene 5a has been reported in the literature, although this is controversial, and there is no practical benefit to be gained from sequencing the virus before therapy.

There has been much recent interest in identifying host genetic factors linked with response/non-response to PEG/RV therapy. Genome-wide association studies have identified a number of polymorphisms close to the gene encoding IL-28B (also known as interferon-lambda 3) on chromosome 19 which define responder and non-responder phenotypes, especially for genotype 1 infection. The distribution of these polymorphisms differs in populations of different ethnic origins, which explains the clinical observations that African-Americans have much lower overall response rates than do European-Americans—as the latter group has a much higher prevalence of the good-responder alleles (over 80%) than does the latter (around 50%). It is not possible yet to state whether pretreatment determination of the IL-28B polymorphisms will be clinically useful in assisting decision making about when and whom to treat.

Directly acting antivirals

In the 20 years or so since HCV was first characterized and sequenced, understanding of the molecular biology of the virus has increased dramatically. A number of potential viral (and host) targets within the viral replication cycle have been identified, and a wide range of drugs designed to act at those targets are undergoing clinical trials. This has led to the concept of treating patients with directly acting antivirals (DAA), also known as specifically targeted antiviral therapy for hepatitis C, or STAT-C drugs. A detailed map of the HCV genome is shown in Fig. 6.4, illustrating the known functions of the various components of the genome, and the potential targets for DAA.

Drugs

The most clinically advanced DAA are the NS3 protease and NS5b polymerase inhibitors. The protease inhibitors telaprevir and boceprevir have completed phase 3 clinical trials, and have achieved licenses for clinical use in late 2011. Whilst monotherapy with either of these agents induces a considerable decline in viral load within a few days of onset, viral rebound occurs associated with specific drug resistance mutations (DRMs) in the NS3 gene, so the clinical trials of these molecules have been conducted as triple therapy, with a PEG/RV backbone. In genotype 1 infection, where response rates to PEG and RV are around 45%, the addition of a protease inhibitor increases response to 65–70%. Similar response rates to triple therapy have been reported in patients who have previously failed PEG/RV therapy. Each of these drugs may cause severe adverse effects in a minority of patients—telaprevir is particularly associated with development of a rash, whilst boceprevir may cause anaemia. On the plus side, the added antiviral effect of these agents may mean that even for genotype 1 infection, the course of PEG and RV may only be necessary for six, as opposed to 12 months.

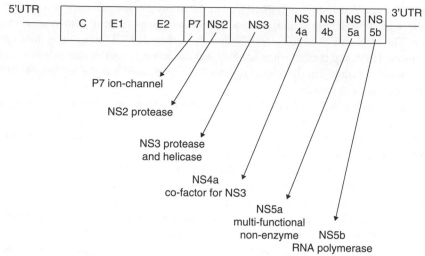

Fig. 6.4 HCV genome structure and potential targets for directly acting antivirals.

The polymerase inhibitors are perhaps a year or two behind in development. There are a number of different classes of NS5b inhibitors, binding to different regions (the so-called palm, thumb, and finger domains) of the target molecule. As would be expected, monotherapy with these molecules generates a range of DRMs within the NS5b gene. However, it is hoped that the availability of drugs acting at multiple sites within the viral life cycle may allow combinations of DAA to be used without the PEG/RV backbone. There are published data illustrating that combined use of protease and polymerase inhibitors can reduce the viral load below detectable levels within a few weeks. Data on the long-term sustainability of this response are eagerly awaited.

A number of other drugs acting at yet other sites are currently in development. A particularly promising target is NS5a. This is a multifunctional protein essential for successful execution of several steps within the viral life cycle. NS5a inhibitors are the most potent antiviral agents available—a single dose of the investigational compound known as BMS-790052 results in over a 3 log drop in viral load within 24 hours. The recognition that NS5a binds cyclophilin A, a host cell molecule, has led to a different class of anti-NS5a drugs, namely the cyclophilin antagonists (e.g. Debio-025, also known as alisporivir). As these agents are acting on a host molecule, it is hoped that it will be difficult for the virus to generate mutations resulting in resistance to this class of drugs. Other targets include the p7 protein, which is thought to act as an ion channel that is important in viral uncoating and/or production of mature virus particles, NS2 protease, the NS4b protein (which forms the membranous web within the cell that acts as a scaffold for viral replication), and the internal ribosomal entry site (IRES) within the 5' non-coding region (NCR). Again, a host factor, micro RNA 122 (miR-122) is known to be an essential co-factor for proper IRES binding, and anti-sense RNA molecules targeting miR-122 have shown some promise in reducing viral load in a chimpanzee model of infection.

The management of chronic HCV infection has already undergone several seismic shifts since the virus was first identified in 1989. We are now on the verge of another major paradigm change—the use of DAA, hopefully without the need for a PEG/RV backbone. The next five to 10 years will be a time of intense study and interest, with the likely outcome of a dramatic improvement in the prognosis for HCV-infected patients.

Key points

- The management of chronic HBV and HCV infections has changed dramatically in the last 10 years, concomitant with an increased understanding of the replication cycles of both viruses.

- There are two modes of therapy for chronic HBV infection—immunomodulation with interferon-alpha (now available in pegylated form), or inhibition of the viral reverse transcriptase activity by nucleos(t)ide analogues such as lamivudine, adefovir, entecavir, and tenofovir.

- The nucleos(t)ide analogues differ in both potency and their genetic barrier to the development of resistance. Tenofovir and entecavir have superceded lamivudine and adefovir, as they are more potent drugs and have high genetic barriers to resistance.

- Treatment of chronic HCV infection has evolved from standard interferon alone, to combination therapy with pegylated interferon (PEG) and ribavirin (RV). The latter combination achieves sustained viral clearance in around 50% of patients.

- Directly acting antiviral agents are in late stages of development for the treatment of chronic HCV infection. Telaprevir and boceprevir, both NS3 protease inhibitors (PI), have recently been licensed. Triple therapy (i.e. PEG/RV/PI) achieves around 70% viral clearance in patients infected with genotype 1 virus.

- Long term, it is hoped that combination of various DAAs will obviate the need for the PEG/RV backbone, and will require shorter duration of therapy.

Further reading

Balagopal A, Thomas DL, Thio CL (2010), 'IL28B and the control of hepatitis C virus infection', *Gastroenterology*, **139**: 1865–1876.

Webster DP, Klenerman P, Collier J, Jeffery KJ (2009), 'Development of novel treatments for hepatitis C', *Lancet Infectious Diseases*, **9**: 108–117.

Yuen LKW, Locarnini SA (2009), 'Genetic variability of hepatitis B virus and response to antiviral treatments: Searching for a bigger picture', *Journal of Hepatology*, **50**: 445–448.

Yin MT, Brust JCM, Tieu HV, Hammer SM (2009), 'Antiherpesvirus, anti-hepatitis virus, and anti-respiratory virus agents', in *Clinical Virology* (3rd edn), Washington DC: ASM Press, 217–264.

Antifungal agents

Fungi may cause benign but unsightly infection of the skin, nail, or hair (dermatophytosis), relatively trivial infection of mucous membranes (thrush), or systemic infection causing progressive, often fatal disease. The taxonomy of fungi is highly complex, but for medical purposes they are commonly considered in four morphological groups:

- yeasts that reproduce by budding (e.g. *Cryptococcus neoformans*);
- yeasts that produce a pseudomycelium (e.g. *Candida albicans*);
- filamentous fungi (moulds) that produce a true mycelium (e.g. *Aspergillus fumigatus*);
- dimorphic fungi that grow as yeasts or filamentous fungi, depending on the cultural conditions (e.g. *Histoplasma capsulatum*).

In addition, *Pneumocystis jiroveci*—formerly *P. carinii*, an important opportunist pathogen, especially of patients with AIDS—is now regarded as a fungus. Fungi are eukaryotic organisms, and antibacterial agents are generally ineffective against them. Specialized antifungal agents must therefore be used, and some are quite toxic. In order to minimize problems of toxicity, superficial lesions are usually treated by topical application, but deep mycoses, which are serious life-threatening infections, need vigorous systemic therapy. The polyene amphotericin was formerly the mainstay; choice also includes flucytosine, azole derivatives (mainly triazoles), and a group of semi-synthetic antibiotics, the echinocandins. *P. jiroveci* is insusceptible to conventional antifungal agents, and alternative treatment regimens are used.

The differential activity of the main antifungal agents in common use is summarized in Table 7.1. Precise assessment of the activity of antifungal agents *in vitro* is beset with methodological difficulties and susceptibility tests are not generally available, except in reference centres.

Polyenes

The polyenes are naturally occurring compounds exhibiting a complex macrocyclic structure. All act by binding to sterols in the fungal cell membrane, thereby interfering with membrane integrity and causing leakage of essential metabolites. The only one that can be administered parenterally is amphotericin (Fig. 7.1). Among related polyenes available for topical treatment in some countries are nystatin, natamycin (pimaricin), and trichomycin (hachimycin).

The activity of the polyenes embraces a variety of pathogenic fungi; yeasts are particularly susceptible. Nystatin has been extensively used for treating *Candida* infections of the mucous membranes, but has largely been replaced by imidazoles (see below). Most polyenes are restricted to topical use, but intravenous amphotericin remains an important agent for the treatment of systemic fungal infections, including disseminated candidiasis, cryptococcosis, aspergillosis, and deep mycoses caused by dimorphic fungi. Amphotericin can also be administered orally for the treatment of oral, oesophageal, and intestinal candidiasis, but azole derivatives are now preferred.

Toxicity is a major problem in systemic therapy with amphotericin and it needs to be used with care. The drug is highly insoluble and for parenteral use it is normally formulated in a surfactant vehicle. Various ways have been tried to minimize toxicity problems. Lipid-complexed colloidal formulations

Table 7.1 Summary of the differential activity of antifungal agents against the more common pathogenic fungi

Fungus	Principal diseases caused	Polyenes	Flucytosine	Griseofulvin	Azoles	Allylamines	Echinocandins
Yeasts							
Cryptococcus neoformans	Meningitis	+	+	–	+	–	–
Candida albicans	Thrush; systemic candidiasis	+	+	–	+	±	+
Filamentous fungi							
Trichophyton spp.	Infection of skin, nail or hair ('ringworm')	–	+	+	+	–	–
Microsporum spp.							–
Epidermophyton floccosum							–
Aspergillus fumigatus	Pulmonary aspergillosis	+	–	–	(+)[a]	+	+
Dimorphic fungi							
Histoplasma capsulatum	Histoplasmosis	+	–	–	+	(+)[b]	–
Coccidioides immitis	Coccidioidomycosis						–
Blastomyces dermatitidis	Blastomycosis						–

+, useful activity; –, no useful activity.

[a] Variable activity; itraconazole and voriconazole are most active.

[b] Clinical efficacy not established.

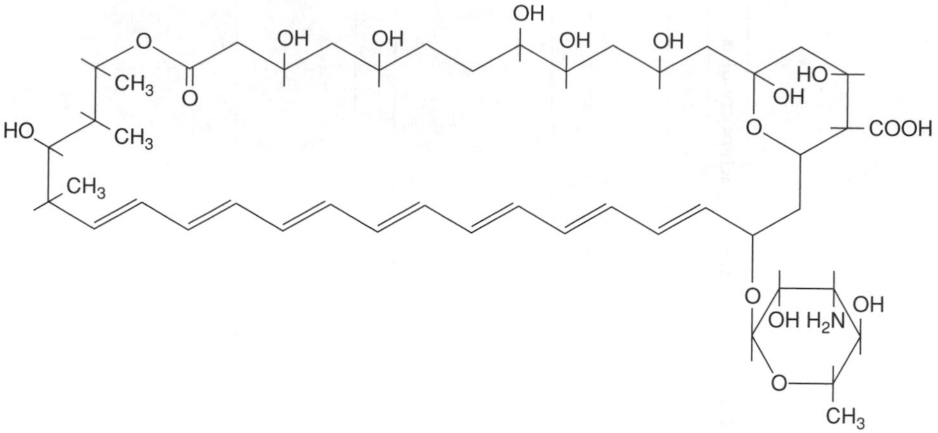

Fig. 7.1 Structure of amphotericin.

exhibit improved safety. Alternatively, phospholipid vesicles (liposomes) are used as carriers of the drug. Packaged in this way, the drug is delivered to the site of infection and this allows the use of higher doses without compromising safety. Another occasional approach, at least in systemic candidiasis, is to administer amphotericin in reduced dosage in combination with flucytosine (see below).

Azoles

Many imidazole and triazole derivatives display antifungal activity and, in fact, these compounds offer the nearest approximation to broad-spectrum antifungal agents. They act selectively against fungi (and some protozoa) by interfering with the demethylation of lanosterol during the synthesis of ergosterol, which is the principal sterol in the fungal cell membrane.

Imidazoles   Topical use only

Antifungal imidazoles are most widely used for topical application in superficial fungal infections and vaginal candidiasis. Indeed, these are virtually the only useful roles for bifonazole, butoconazole, clotrimazole, econazole, fenticonazole, isoconazole, miconazole, oxiconazole, sulconazole, and terconazole, all of which have very similar properties and indications. One antifungal imidazole, tioconazole, is also available in a formulation that is painted on infected nails, but is unlikely to be effective alone in severe nail infections, for which better treatment is available.

The only imidazole to be used in the oral therapy of systemic fungal infections is ketoconazole. This derivative achieves therapeutic concentrations for several hours after oral administration. However, early enthusiasm for ketoconazole waned when it was realized that it was occasionally implicated in fatal hepatotoxic reactions. It has been largely replaced by triazoles for the treatment of systemic mycoses. It should not be used for trivial dermatophyte infections.

Triazoles   For serious systemic mycoses

The triazoles, fluconazole (Fig. 7.2), itraconazole, and voriconazole are well absorbed after oral administration. They have many properties in common, but also display some distinctive features:

- fluconazole and voriconazole achieve higher plasma concentrations than itraconazole and penetrate into cerebrospinal fluid in therapeutically useful concentrations;

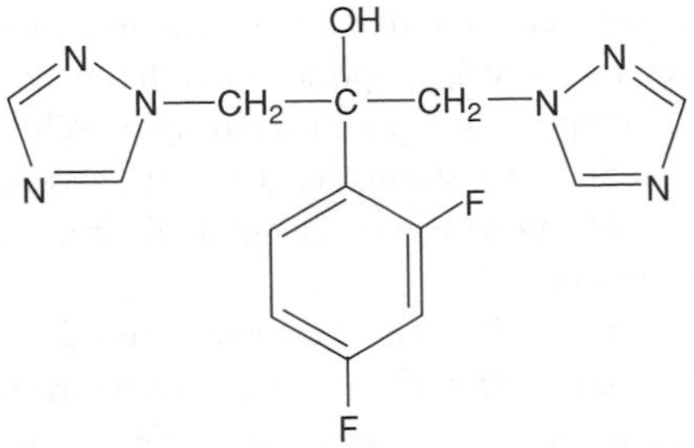

Fig. 7.2 Structure of fluconazole.

- itraconazole and voriconazole exhibit much better activity than fluconazole against *Aspergillus* spp., and against *C. krusei* and *C. (Torulopsis) glabrata*, yeasts that are seen with increasing frequency in immunocompromised patients and are often resistant to fluconazole;

- fluconazole and itraconazole have long plasma half-lives (20–30h), properties that make them suitable for once-daily administration;

- fluconazole is less extensively metabolized and protein bound than the other two triazoles and is less prone to side effects.

Triazoles are used in many forms of systemic mycosis. Fluconazole is widely used in the treatment of systemic *Candida* infections and, because of its ability to penetrate into cerebrospinal fluid, cryptococcal meningitis. It is also widely used in chemoprophylactic regimens in patients vulnerable to systemic mycoses. Itraconazole is now largely used as a topical antifungal. In contrast, voriconazole is the preferred agent to treat infections with *Aspergillus* spp. and a reserve drug for yeasts resistant to fluconazole.

Fluconazole and itraconazole can be used to treat superficial *Candida* infections if oral therapy is thought to be necessary or more acceptable than, for example, vaginal pessaries. Oral itraconazole is also effective in dermatophyte infections, including those involving nail.

Resistance to triazoles is increasing, and extensive use of these compounds could compromise their value in the long term.

Flucytosine (5-fluorocytosine) `Severe yeast infections only`

Flucytosine is a pyrimidine analogue originally developed as an anticancer drug, but found to have considerable activity against yeasts; it has no useful activity against filamentous fungi. The activity depends on its being converted intracellularly to 5-fluorouracil, which is incorporated into fungal RNA. The drug can be given orally or parenterally, but resistance develops readily and sometimes emerges during treatment. For this reason flucytosine is normally administered together with amphotericin, an arrangement that has the additional advantage of allowing a lower dose of amphotericin to be used. Amphotericin, by interfering with the permeability of the fungal membrane, may also facilitate entry of flucytosine into the fungal cell.

Flucytosine is usually well tolerated, but marrow toxicity can occur, particularly if the drug is allowed to accumulate in patients with impaired renal function. Adjustment of dosage according to the results of drug assays is therefore indicated.

Echinocandins `Severe systemic mycoses only`

Caspofungin was first of this relatively new class of antifungal drugs—the echinocandins. It was soon followed by related compounds, micafungin and anidulafungin. The echinocandins have recently become available for the treatment of systemic and invasive candidiasis resistant to the azoles and amphotericin. They are cyclic lipopeptides and interfere with fungal cell wall synthesis. They include anidulofungin, caspofungin, and micafungin. While resistance is uncommon among *Candida* spp., when it occurs, such strains are generally cross-resistant to all echinocandins. *Aspergillus* spp. are also inhibited by these agents. Caspofungin is used as alternative salvage treatment in severe invasive aspergillosis.

Clinical experience with echinocandins is now extensive and these agents have found a place in the treatment of systemic mycoses; caspofungin has become the preferred agent for invasive candidiasis and for the salvage treatment of invasive aspergillosis; micafungin is an alternative for serious systemic infection with *Candida*.

Griseofulvin   Dermatophyte infections only

Griseofulvin was the first antifungal antibiotic to be described. It is well absorbed when administered orally, particularly if a fine-particle formulation is used, and serious side effects are uncommon. The mode of action has not been definitively established, but activity appears to be directed against the process of mitosis, perhaps by interfering with the microtubules of the mitotic spindle. Use of griseofulvin is confined to the treatment of dermatophyte infections of the skin, nail, or hair. In the case of nail infections, treatment is prolonged. The failure rate is high so alternative drugs, especially terbinafine (see below) are usually preferred.

Allylamines   Dermatophyte infections only

Allylamines, like the antifungal azoles, interfere with ergosterol synthesis, but act at an earlier stage by inhibiting the formation of squalene epoxide, a precursor of lanosterol. The most important compound of this type, terbinafine, exhibits broad-spectrum antifungal activity and is almost completely absorbed when given orally. It accumulates in keratin, where it persists after treatment is stopped. This is particularly important in dermatophyte infections of the toenails, which are notoriously refractory to therapy.

The broad spectrum of activity of terbinafine includes *Aspergillus* spp. and dimorphic fungi, but it does not appear to offer a useful alternative to older antifungal agents in these conditions. *C. albicans* is more susceptible in the mycelial phase than in the yeast form and, whereas the drug is generally fungicidal, the action against *Candida* is fungistatic. Terbinafine is the drug of choice for fungal infections of the toenail, and offers an alternative to griseofulvin and azoles for the treatment of other dermatophyte infections if systemic therapy is indicated. An earlier allylamine, naftifine, is insufficiently active to be useful systemically, but is marketed in some countries for topical use.

Pneumocystis jiroveci (P.carinii)

Originally encountered as a rare cause of interstitial pneumonia in infants, *P. jiroveci* (formerly *P. carinii*) was later recognized as an infection of severely immunocompromised individuals, in whom it can cause a life-threatening pneumonia, most notably in individuals suffering from HIV/AIDS. The incidence of pneumocystis pneumonia has declined among these patients since the advent of highly active antiretroviral therapy (p. 331). Prophylaxis, usually with the antibacterial agent, co-trimoxazole (p. 41) has also been successful in reducing the incidence of this disease.

Co-trimoxazole is the drug of choice for treatment of established pneumocystis infection, but patients suffering from AIDS are often intolerant of the high doses used. Other combinations that have found favour in some units are trimethoprim with the antileprosy drug dapsone (p. 36) or clindamycin (p. 36) with the antimalarial agent primaquine (p. 85). The diamidine derivative, pentamidine isethionate (p. 332) is also active against *P. jiroveci*, but the intravenous infusion carries problems of toxicity, which may be severe, and the drug is sometimes (at least in prophylactic use) administered directly into the lungs by nebulizer in an effort to reduce systemic toxicity. Atovaquone (p. 332), appears to be a safe alternative to co-trimoxazole and pentamidine, and is sometimes used in patients intolerant of the older drugs.

Use of these agents in treatment and prophylaxis of pneumocystis infection is discussed in Chapter 31.

Topical antifungal agents

Apart from the azole, polyene, and allylamine derivatives that are available for topical use, a range of other agents is available in some countries for the treatment of ringworm and other superficial fungal infections. These include tolnaftate, haloprogin, and ciclopirox. None of these agents exhibits useful activity against *Candida* spp. A variety of ointments containing benzoic acid (e.g. Whitfield's ointment: benzoic acid, and salicylic acid in an emulsifying base) have been used traditionally for treating dermatophyte infections of the skin. Though old-fashioned and a little messy, they are cheap and effective. The monounsaturated fatty acid, undecylenic (undecenoic) acid is also widely used in proprietary preparations for conditions such as 'athlete's foot'.

A morpholine derivative, amorolfine, which is active against *Candida* and the dermatophytes, is marketed for the topical treatment of fungal infections of the skin and, in the form of a lacquer, for application to infected nails. Its action is said to persist so that it needs to be applied to infected nails only once or twice a week.

Key points

Antifungal agents: prescribing choices

- *Topical imidazoles ('any-onazole')*: good standby for mild fungal infections of skin and mucous membranes.

- *Oral terbinafine*: first choice for infections of finger and toenails.

- *Triazoles, amphotericin, echinocandins*: leave to the experts when treating serious systemic diseases in hospitals.

Further reading

Hay RJ (2010), 'Fungal infections', in *Oxford Textbook of Medicine* (5th edn). Oxford: Oxford University Press, 998–1018.

Warnock DW (2010), 'Antifungal agents', in *Antibiotic and Chemotherapy* (9th edn). London: Elsevier Saunders, 104–109.

Chapter 8

Antiprotozoal and anthelminthic agents

Pathogenic protozoa and helminths are among the most important causes of morbidity and mortality in the world. An estimated 700 million people suffer from malaria, filariasis, and schistosomiasis alone, and two-thirds of the world's population lives in conditions in which parasitic diseases are unavoidable.

Some parasitic diseases were among the first to be treated by specific remedies; indeed, cures for malaria, amoebic dysentery, and tapeworm infection have been known for centuries. Nevertheless, the therapeutic armamentarium for parasitic infection remains severely restricted. Many of the antiparasitic drugs that are available leave much to be desired in terms of efficacy and safety, and a few parasitic infections remain for which there is no effective remedy at all.

Protozoa

Protozoa are unicellular organisms. Those of medical importance are conveniently classified into four groups: amoebae, flagellates, sporozoa, and 'others' (Table 8.1). The agents used for treatment are very varied and often specific to the particular organism involved. Consequently, antiprotozoal agents defy formal classification and are best considered in the context of the organisms against which they are used. The mode of action is often poorly characterized.

Amoebae

Parasitic amoebae

Several species of parasitic amoebae are found in man. Only one, *Entamoeba histolytica*, the causative parasite of amoebic dysentery and amoebic liver abscess, is commonly incriminated in disease. Invasive infection is caused by the motile trophozoite form, but the disease is transmitted by non-motile cysts, which represent a more resistant resting phase. Occurrence of a morphologically identical, but non-pathogenic, species, *E. dispar*, makes laboratory identification of cyst excreters problematic.

An effective treatment for amoebiasis has been available for many years in the form of emetine, an alkaloid of ipecacuanha root. Emetine, and its less toxic derivative dehydroemetine, act by inhibiting protein synthesis in amoebae. Chloroquine provides a third alternative in the treatment of amoebic liver abscess where nitroimidazoles fail, or are inappropriate. These drugs have been superseded by metronidazole (or one of the other 5-nitroimidazoles) (p. 44), which is very effective in acute amoebiasis and amoebic liver abscess.

Other useful drugs include diloxanide furoate, which is particularly effective for the elimination of cysts from symptomless excreters. Two antibiotics, tetracycline and the aminoglycoside paromomycin, also have some activity against amoebae.

Free-living amoebae

Although *E. histolytica* is, to all intents and purposes, the only parasitic amoeba pathogenic to man, certain species of free-living amoebae, including *Naegleria fowleri* and *Balamuthia mandrillaris* are

Table 8.1 Principal pathogenic protozoa infecting man, and the drugs commonly used in treatment

Species	Diseases caused	Useful drugs
Amoebae		
Entamoeba histolytica	Amoebic dysentery; invasive amoebiasis	Metronidazole (diloxanide furoate)
Naegleria fowleri	Meningo-encephalitis	Amphotericin
Acanthamoeba spp.	Amoebic keratitis	Propamidine (topical)
Flagellates		
Trypanosoma brucei ssp.	Sleeping sickness	Melarsoprol; eflornithine;[a] (pentamidine; suramin)
Trypanosoma cruzi	Chagas' disease	Nifurtimox; benznidazole
Leishmania spp.	Kala azar, etc.	Sodium stibogluconate; miltefosine; liposomal amphotericin
Trichomonas vaginalis	Vaginitis	Metronidazole
Giardia lamblia	Diarrhoea; steatorrhoea	Metronidazole
Sporozoa		
Plasmodium spp.	Malaria	Quinine, chloroquine, etc. (see p. 357)
Toxoplasma gondii	Toxoplasmosis	Pyrimethamine + sulfadiazine; spiramycin
Cryptosporidium parvum	Diarrhoea	Nitazoxanide; (azithromycin; paromomycin)
Cyclospora cayetanensis	Diarrhoea	Co-trimoxazole
Others		
Balantidium coli	Balantidial dysentery	Tetracycline; metronidazole
Babesia spp.	Babesiosis	Clindamycin + quinine
Microsporidia	Microsporidiosis	Albendazole

[a] Eflornithine is not active against *T. brucei rhodesiense*. Drugs shown in brackets have limited usefulness (see text).

rare causes of primary amoebic meningoencephalitis. The condition is almost invariably fatal and only amphotericin, an antifungal agent (p. 76), has shown any useful *in vitro* activity. Free-living amoebae of the *Acanthamoeba* group are occasionally involved in serious eye infections (amoebic keratitis) following contamination of contact lenses. Suitable antimicrobial chemotherapy for this condition remains to be defined, but local application of propamidine and neomycin is often used.

Flagellates

Trypanosomes

Trypanosomes are transmitted by insects, and their distribution is restricted to areas where the vector is found. In tropical Africa, tsetse flies transmit *Trypanosoma brucei*, of which two subspecies (*T. brucei gambiense* and *T. brucei rhodesiense*) cause 'sleeping sickness', a disease that is inexorably fatal if untreated.

Organic arsenicals, though extremely toxic, have been used for many years to treat all forms of sleeping sickness. Melarsoprol (Mel B) is the derivative usually used. Melarsoprol affects glycolysis, and also forms a complex with trypanothione, which replaces glutathione in these organisms. Resistance may occur and is thought to be due to reduced uptake of the drug.

T. brucei gambiense infection responds to eflornithine (α-difluoromethyl-ornithine), which has shown to be effective in the late stages of the disease complicated by meningoencephalitis; but *T. brucei rhodesiense* is resistant. Eflornithine is an irreversible inhibitor of ornithine decarboxylase, an essential enzyme in polyamine synthesis. Differences in enzyme turnover have been proposed to account for the differential activity on the two *T. brucei* subspecies. If treatment can be started before the trypanosomes invade the central nervous system, suramin—which, like melarsoprol, interferes with glycolysis—may be curative. Because of toxicity, it is often used in a two to three dose regimen before melarsoprol in *T. brucei rhodesiense* meningoencephalitis. The diamidine pentamidine is also effective in the early stages of *T. brucei gambiense* infection but ineffective in *T. brucei rhodesiense*. Various targets have been proposed for this drug, but its primary site of action has proved elusive.

South American trypanosomiasis, Chagas' disease, is a chronic condition affecting heart muscle and other organs. It is caused by *T. cruzi* and is transmitted by reduviid bugs, nicknamed 'kissing bugs' because of their predilection for feeding round the mouths of sleeping persons. Currently nifurtimox, and the imidazole benznidazole are standard agents. However, they both have serious drug associated toxicities. Both drugs have some success in the acute phase of the disease. Benznidazole is the preferred agent. In the chronic phase of the disease, prolonged treatment with either benznidazole or nifurtimox is recommended.

Leishmania

Leishmania, which are related to the trypanosomes, also cause a variety of clinical conditions and are also transmitted by biting insects, in this case sandflies. Cutaneous leishmaniasis (oriental sore) caused by *Leishmania tropica* or *L. major* is usually self-limiting, but visceral leishmaniasis (kala azar) in which the reticulo-endothelial system is infected by *L. donovani* or *L. infantum*, is potentially fatal. Leishmaniasis occurs in the Middle East, India, parts of Africa, and countries on the south European coast of the Mediterranean. Various species of *Leishmania* have also been incriminated in disease in Central and South America, including *L. braziliensis* (mucocutaneous leishmaniasis, or espundia), *L. mexicana* (Chiclero's ulcer, a form of cutaneous leishmaniasis), and *L. chagasi* (visceral leishmaniasis).

Two related and effectually interchangeable antimonial compounds, sodium stibogluconate and meglumine antimonate, are traditionally used for the treatment of leishmaniasis. Resistance has, however, become a problem in many parts of the world. More recently most success has been achieved with the antifungal amphotericin (p. 76), especially when administered in a liposomal formulation that carries the drug into macrophages. The antifungal azoles (p. 78), the aminoglycoside, paromomycin, and pentamidine also exhibit some activity against leishmania and offer alternatives in recalcitrant cases. Much hope for leishmaniasis sufferers rests with an oral phosphocholine analogue, miltefosine, which has undergone successful trials in visceral leishmaniasis in India and also shows signs of benefit in cutaneous forms of the disease.

Other flagellates

Two other flagellates cause disease in man: *Giardia lamblia* (also known as *G. intestinalis*)—a common cause of diarrhoea, abdominal pain, and steatorrhoea—and *Trichomonas vaginalis*, a common cause of vaginitis or, more rarely, urethritis. *G. lamblia* is transmitted in the cyst form, often in infected water; *T. vaginalis* is transmitted sexually. Both of these parasites are susceptible to nitroimidazoles such as metronidazole (p. 44). Resistance is uncommon. Mepacrine (known in the USA as quinacrine), and the anthelminthic benzimidazole albendazole also exhibit effective antigiardial activity, but there are few alternatives for refractory trichomoniasis—except, perhaps, polyenes such as natamycin and trichomycin (p. 76), which are available in some countries.

Sporozoa

The sporozoa are all parasitic; they have a complex life cycle involving alternate sexual and asexual phases. Among important human parasites are the malaria parasites and the coccidia.

Malaria parasites

Malaria is the most important of all parasitic diseases. It remains the commonest cause of fever in the world and is a major cause of morbidity and mortality in areas of high endemicity throughout the tropical belt. Four species infect man. *Plasmodium falciparum* is the most dangerous, since primary infections are often rapidly fatal if left untreated. *P. vivax* and *P. ovale*, which cause benign tertian malaria, and *P. malariae*, which causes quartan malaria, rarely kill but give rise to debilitating infections. The most common species worldwide is *P. falciparum*, which accounts for over 90% of infections in tropical Africa; in some parts of the world, notably the Indian subcontinent, *P. vivax* is the dominant species.

The malaria parasite is transmitted by the bite of infected female *Anopheles* mosquitoes. The parasites first infect liver cells; then after one to two weeks the liver parasites mature and infect circulating red blood cells to commence the cycle of erythrocytic schizogony, which is responsible for the overt signs of disease. *P. vivax* and *P. ovale* can also set up a cryptic infection in the liver, which may cause the relapse of symptoms up to two years after the infection is acquired. A proportion of erythrocytic parasites differentiate into male and female gametocytes, which do not develop further in the mammalian host but complete the sexual phase of development in the anopheline vector when ingested during a blood meal.

The traditional mainstay of the treatment of malaria is quinine, but various other effective antimalarials have been developed. These include the 4-aminoquinolines chloroquine and amodiaquine, which act on erythrocytic parasites, and the 8-aminoquinolines primaquine, bulaquine (a primaquine analogue available in India) and tafenoquine (an investigational compound with an extended half-life), which are selectively active against the liver forms. Quinine and the 4-aminoquinolines are thought to achieve their effect by preventing the polymerization of haem (ferriprotoporphyrin IX), a reaction that is needed to detoxify this product of parasite metabolism within red blood cells. Primaquine appears to act in a different way, possibly by interfering with mitochondrial enzymes.

A group of compounds collectively known as 'antifolates' are also used, usually in combination, especially for antimalarial prophylaxis. These include pyrimethamine, proguanil, (and chlorproguanil) the long-acting sulphonamides, sulfadoxine and sulfalene (sulfametopyrazine), and dapsone (p. 47). Pyrimethamine, a dihydrofolate reductase inhibitor related to trimethoprim (p. 41), exhibits a selectively high affinity for the plasmodial form of the enzyme and interacts synergistically with sulphonamides. Proguanil and chlorproguanil are biguanides that are metabolized in the body to compounds closely related to pyrimethamine, and have an identical mode of action. Surprisingly, some pyrimethamine-resistant mutants retain susceptibility to these closely related compounds. Chlorproguanil (Lapudrine) combined with dapsone—'lapdap'—is being promoted in parts of Africa as a relatively cheap treatment for malaria with a reduced propensity to generate resistance. Proguanil itself is used solely for prophylaxis, usually together with chloroquine. A combination with atovaquone (a hydroxynaphthoquinone that acts on the respiratory chain of some protozoa) is available for treatment and prophylaxis.

Resistance to chloroquine and most other antimalarial agents is now common in *P. falciparum* in many parts of the world. Quinine remains reliably active against most strains, and this old compound is still widely used for the treatment of falciparum malaria, but derivatives of artemisinin, the active principle of an ancient Chinese herbal remedy, qinghaosu, are more rapidly effective and are widely used. Formulations include the water-soluble artesunate, and the oily solutions, artemether, and artemotil (β-arteether) and dihydroartemisinin, all of which are suitable for parenteral administration. Artesunate can also be given intravenously and by mouth. Some formulations, including artemisinin itself, can be administered rectally. Combination therapy is increasingly being used, especially for drug-resistant disease. For example, dihydroartemisinin with piperaquine and, for oral administration, artemether with lumefantrine (see below). Certain antibiotics, notably tetracyclines and clindamycin, have antimalarial activity and are used as adjuncts to artemisinin or quinine therapy in chloroquine-resistant falciparum malaria. Chloroquine-resistant strains usually remain susceptible to mefloquine and halofantrine, quinoline derivatives developed by the Walter Reed Army Institute of Research in Washington, but resistance to these agents is also beginning to appear. Lumefantrine (formerly known as benflumetol), appears to lack the cardiotoxicity of halofantrine.

Coccidia

Phylogenetically related to the malaria parasites are the coccidia, which share many features of the complex life cycle, but are not transmitted by insect vectors. Several species, including *Cryptosporidium parvum, Isospora belli*, and *Cyclospora cayetanensis* cause diarrhoea in man. Infection is usually self-limiting, but in immunocompromised patients, especially those suffering from AIDS, they may cause severe and protracted symptoms. Nitazoxanide, a nitrothiazole derivative, which is converted in the body to the active form, tizoxanide, seems to offer effective therapy against *C. parvum* if antimicrobial treatment is necessary. Infections with *I. belli* and *Cyclo. cayetanensis* respond to co-trimoxazole, though antimicrobial therapy is seldom required.

The most important human coccidian parasite is *Toxoplasma gondii*. Intrauterine infections with this organism are an important cause of congenital malformations and stillbirth throughout the world. AIDS sufferers may develop toxoplasma encephalitis, apparently by reactivation of latent infection. Cats often harbour the parasite and liberate the infectious oocysts in their faeces; this probably represents a major reservoir of infection, although undercooked meat is also a recognized source. Pyrimethamine, in combination with a sulphonamide (usually sulfadiazine) is the treatment of choice in symptomatic toxoplasmosis. Clindamycin and the macrolide antibiotic spiramycin have also been successfully used, especially in combination with pyrimethamine. Spiramycin has been recommended during pregnancy, when antifolates are best avoided.

Other protozoa

Babesia spp., like malaria parasites, infect red blood cells, but they are unrelated. They are predominantly animal parasites that are occasionally transmitted to man by the bite of ixodid ticks. Recorded European cases have mostly been in splenectomized patients and have usually been caused by *B. divergens*. Infection with *B. microti* occurs in previously healthy persons in parts of North America.

Balantidium coli is a ciliate, cosmopolitan in distribution, which is a rare cause of severe diarrhoea. *Encephalitozoon cuniculi* and some other microsporidia occasionally cause infection, usually in immunocompromised patients. Although these protozoa have ribosomes of the prokaryotic type, inhibitors of bacterial protein synthesis do not seem to work.

Treatment of babesiosis and infection with assorted intestinal protozoa is generally ill-defined. Options for therapy are considered in Chapter 35.

Helminths

Helminths are parasitic worms. They often have a complex life cycle involving a period of development outside the definitive host either in soil or in an intermediate host. Helminths of medical importance fall into three major groups: nematodes (roundworms), trematodes (flukes), and cestodes (tapeworms) (Table 8.2).

Little work is done on the development of anthelminthic agents for use in human beings, and most agents in present use have emerged through application of drugs originally intended for the treatment of animals. Despite this, a wide variety of compounds is available for use in worm infections of which three compounds—ivermectin, praziquantel, and albendazole—between them cover virtually the whole helminthic spectrum. Resistance to these agents is known to occur in animals, and there are reports of failures of treatment in man, but difficulties in testing limit knowledge of the prevalence of resistance or its mechanisms.

Information on the means by which anthelminthic agents achieve their effect is also relatively limited. The neuromuscular system of worms seems to be peculiarly susceptible to chemotherapeutic attack: many important anthelminthic agents, including piperazine, praziquantel, ivermectin, levamisole, and pyrantel appear to act by paralysing the worms. In contrast, the benzimidazoles interfere with the polymerization of tubulin in the formation of microtubules in the cytoskeleton of the worm.

Nematodes

The most important group of nematodes are the filarial worms, among which are *Wuchereria bancrofti*, which causes elephantiasis throughout the tropics, *Onchocerca volvulus*, the cause of river blindness in West Africa, and *Loa loa*, the African 'eye worm'. Infection is transmitted by biting insects.

Less important, but extremely common worldwide, are the intestinal nematodes, which include the hookworms *Ancylostoma duodenale* and *Necator americanus*, the common roundworm *Ascaris lumbricoides*, the threadworm *Enterobius vermicularis*, and the whipworm *Trichuris trichiura*.

Filarial worms

Diethylcarbamazine, a relative of piperazine, has been used for many years in filariasis, but its use has been steadily eroded by a remarkable compound, ivermectin, an antibiotic produced by *Streptomyces avermitilis*, which has activity against a number of helminths and some arthropods. Use of ivermectin does not seem to be accompanied by the severe side effects (Mazzotti reaction) associated with the administration of diethylcarbamazine and a further bonus is the concomitant expulsion of some intestinal worms. Ivermectin was originally developed for use in animals, and it is still used extensively in veterinary practice, together with related derivatives, including doramectin. It is active against many of the arthropod ectoparasites that cause problems in animal husbandry as well as helminths, and is effective in the treatment of human scabies.

Among other drugs that have been investigated for antifilarial activity, the most important is the benzimidazole albendazole, which turns out to have useful activity, particularly against *W. bancrofti* and other blood-borne filarial worms. Surprisingly, tetracyclines also appear to have an effect against filarial worms, apparently by killing endosymbiotic bacteria that are essential to the helminths.

Diethylcarbamazine and ivermectin act on the larval forms (microfilariae) but do not reliably kill the adult worms. This can be achieved with the antitrypanosomal drug suramin, but it is too toxic for routine use.

Roundworms other than filariae that invade tissues include *Trichinella spiralis*, now an uncommon cause of human infection, and the Guinea worm, *Dracunculus medinensis*. Anthelminthic therapy is of unproven benefit in these infections, but benzimidazoles have some activity against both parasites.

Table 8.2 Principal helminth parasites of man and the drugs commonly used in treatment

Species	Intermediate host	Geographical distribution	Useful drugs
Nematodes			
Wuchereria bancrofti	Mosquitoes	Tropical belt	
Loa loa	*Chrysops* spp.	Tropical Africa	Diethylcarbamazine; albendazole; ivermectin + doxycycline
Brugia malayi	Mosquitoes	South-east Asia	
Onchocerca volvulus	*Simulium* spp.	Tropical Africa; central America	Ivermectin
Dracunculus medinensis	*Cyclops* spp. (water flea)	Tropical Africa, Yemen	Benzimidazoles
Trichinella spiralis	Pig, etc.	World-wide	Benzimidazoles
Ancylostoma duodenale	None (soil)	Tropics and sub-tropics	
Necator americanus	None (soil)	Tropics and sub-tropics	
Ascaris lumbrlcoldes	None (soil)	World-wide	
Trichuris trichiura	None (soil)	World-wide	Albendazole, etc. (see Table 35.1, p. 358)
Strongyloldes stercoralis	None (soil)	Tropics and sub-tropics	
Enterobius vermicularis	None	World-wide	
Trematodes			
Schistosoma mansoni	Snail	Africa, West Indies, South America	
Schistosoma haematobium	Snail	Africa	Praziquantel
Schistosoma japonicum	Snail	Far East	
Fasciola hepatica	Snail/vegetation	World-wide	Triclabendazole
Clonorchis sinensis	Snail/freshwaterfish	Far East	
Paragonimus westermani	Snail/crabs, crayfish	Far East, West Africa, South America	Praziquantel
Fasciolopsis buski	Snail/water chestnut	Far East	
Cestodes			
Echinococcus granulosus	Sheep, man	World-wide	Albendazole
Taenia saginata	Cattle	World-wide	
Taenia solium	Pig	World-wide	Niclosamide, praziquantel
Hymenolepis nana	None	Mainly tropics and sub-tropics	
Diphyllobothrium latum	*Cyclops* spp./fish	Mainly northern Russia, Finland	

Guinea worm infection, lymphatic filariasis, and onchocerciasis are the target of elimination programmes by the World Health Organization. Guinea worm, which is transmitted via the water flea *Cyclops*, has been much reduced in prevalence by health education and the provision of clean water in infected areas. Drug donation schemes from the pharmaceutical industry are facilitating the other two campaigns: albendazole (in combination with ivermectin or diethylcarbamazine) for lymphatic filariasis; and ivermectin in onchocerciasis.

Intestinal nematodes

With the exception of *E. vermicularis*, intestinal worms are associated with poor standards of hygiene and sanitation. Treatment has traditionally relied on a variety of compounds of variable efficacy, including piperazine, levamisole, and pyrantel pamoate (see Table 35.1, p. 358). Benzimidazoles are more reliable and are active against most intestinal roundworms. Albendazole exhibits the broadest spectrum of activity and is the drug of choice for the elimination of intestinal roundworms. Mebendazole is also sometimes used, but the first of the benzimidazoles to be introduced into human medicine, tiabendazole (thiabendazole), has now been largely abandoned because of its side effects.

Larvae of the dog ascarid, *Toxocara canis*, sometimes infect children who come into contact with dogs. Albendazole is the agent of choice. Mebendazole is a less effective alternative. Piperazine or, preferably, fenbendazole are used to de-worm infected dogs.

Trematodes

Trematodes (flukes) generally have a complex life cycle involving a stage of development in a snail and, usually, a secondary intermediate host, as well as in the definitive host in which the mature adult forms develop.

Most important are the schistosomes, which cause human infection in many parts of Africa as well as the Far East, the West Indies, and South America. Infection is acquired when cercaria (the infective form) penetrate the skin following exposure to water inhabited by infected snails. Mature adults develop in the portal vessels from where they migrate to the small veins of the rectum (*Schistosoma mansoni*, *S. japonicum*, *S. mekongi*, and *S. intercalatum*) or the bladder (*S. haematobium*). Eggs are then passed through the rectal or bladder mucosa into the faeces or urine.

For many years, treatment relied on highly toxic antimony derivatives of which sodium (or potassium) antimony tartrate (tartar emetic) was the mainstay. Other compounds were later introduced. They include metrifonate (known as trichlorfon in America), which was originally developed as an organophosphate insecticide and is active against *S. haematobium*, and oxamniquine, a quinolinemethanol used to treat *S. mansoni* infection. These drugs have been superseded by praziquantel, which is highly active against all forms of human schistosomiasis. Praziquantel appears to cause schistosomes to release their hold within the venules, and to expose surface antigens that are normally protected from host attack.

Praziquantel is also the drug of choice for most other trematode infections. These include *Clonorchis sinensis* (Chinese liver fluke) infection, which is acquired from eating uncooked freshwater fish and is extremely common in parts of the Far East where raw fish is widely eaten, and *Paragonimus westermani* (lung fluke) infection, which is acquired from raw or under-cooked crabs and crayfish.

Praziquantel is not, however, effective against the liver fluke *Fasciola hepatica*, a parasite of sheep encountered in sheep-rearing areas of the UK and elsewhere. Bithionol was formerly used in treatment, but the veterinary anthelminthic, triclabendazole is now the preferred drug of choice. Nitazoxanide provides an alternative less-effective choice.

Cestodes

By far the most important tapeworms are *Echinococcus granulosus* and the closely related *E. multilocularis* (the hydatid worms). These parasites are unusual in that man is an intermediate host, harbouring the larval form in hydatid cysts that arise, usually in the liver, following ingestion of eggs from an infected dog. The internal wall of the hydatid cyst consists of a germinal layer from which 'brood capsules' containing protoscolices develop. Hydatid disease occurs in many countries, including limited rural parts of the UK, where sheep and sheepdogs maintain the cycle of infection.

There is no reliable chemotherapy for hydatid disease, although some success has been obtained with albendazole or praziquantel. However, chemotherapy remains an adjunct to surgical removal, which is not without risk from the spillage of viable protoscolices into the peritoneal cavity.

Other tapeworms infecting man include *Taenia saginata* (the beef tapeworm), *T. solium* (the pork tapeworm), *Hymenolepis nana* (the dwarf tapeworm), and *Diphyllobothrium latum* (the fish tapeworm). Despite their reputation, none of these well-adapted parasites causes much mischief under normal circumstances, although autoinfection with the larval form of *T. solium* can cause an epileptiform condition known as cerebral cysticercosis.

The ancient, and effective treatment for tapeworm infection is extract of male fern (*Dryopteris filix-mas*); the acridine dye mepacrine (quinacrine) was also successfully used. These old drugs have now been replaced by niclosamide or praziquantel, both of which are very effective. Niclosamide treatment causes disruption of the worm and in *T. solium* infection there is a theoretical risk of cysticercosis caused by autoinfection with liberated eggs. Cerebral cysticercosis may respond to treatment with praziquantel given together with steroids. Albendazole is also effective and, since it penetrates better into the cerebrospinal fluid, it may be preferable.

Key points

Antiprotozoal drugs: notes for prescribers

- *Quinine*: emergency treatment for suspected falciparum malaria.
- *Chloroquine*: treatment of vivax, ovale and quartan malaria.
- *Primaquine*: prevention of relapse; vivax and ovale malaria.
- *Metronidazole*: first choice for trichomoniasis, giardiasis, amoebiasis.
- *All other protozoal infections*: leave to the experts.

Anthelminthic drugs: notes for prescribers

- *Albendazole*: most intestinal worms.
- *Piperazine*: alternative for threadworm or ascaris.
- *Praziquantel*: fluke infections and tapeworms.
- *All other worm infections*: leave to the experts.

Further reading

Lalloo DG, Shingadia D, Pasvol G, Chiodini PL, Whitty CJ, Beeching NJ, Hill DR, Warrell DA, Bannister BA, for the HPA Advisory Committee on Malaria Prevention in UK Travellers (2007), 'UK malaria treatment guidelines', *Journal of Infection*, 54: 111–121.

Cook GC, Zumla A (2002), *Manson's Tropical Diseases* (21st edn). London: Saunders.

Cook GC (2008), *Manson's Tropical Diseases: Expert Consult*. London: Saunders.

Resistance to antimicrobial agents

Chapter 9

The problem of resistance

What is resistance?

Bacterial isolates have been categorized as being susceptible or resistant to antibiotics ever since they became available. Some of the criteria on which this categorization has been based are discussed in Chapter 12, where the concepts of the minimum inhibitory concentrations (MIC) and minimum bactericidal concentrations of an antibiotic are described. Unfortunately, making an accurate judgement about microbial susceptibility or resistance is somewhat less straightforward than this traditional working definition, since there is usually no simple relationship between the MIC (or minimum bactericidal concentrations) of an antibiotic and clinical response. Therapeutic success depends not only on the concentration of the antibiotic achieved at the site of infection (i.e. its pharmacokinetic behaviour) and its activity against the infecting organisms encountered there (i.e. its pharmacodynamic behaviour), but also on the contribution that the host's own defences are able to make towards clearance of the offending microbes. Furthermore, it is clear that, particularly in life-threatening infections, outcome is worse if antibiotic therapy is not commenced within one to four hours of the onset of symptoms.

The decision as to whether a given bacterial isolate should be termed susceptible or resistant depends ultimately on the likelihood that an infection with that organism can be expected to respond to treatment with a given drug, but microbiologists and clinicians have become accustomed to the idea that an organism is 'resistant' when it is inhibited *in vitro* by an antibiotic concentration that is greater than that achievable *in vivo*. Importantly, the concentration of antibiotic that is achievable will vary according to the site of infection, dosage, and route of administration. For example, some antibiotics, such as trimethoprim, are excreted primarily via the kidneys and therefore achieve, in the context of urinary tract infections, advantageously high concentrations in urine. Furthermore, the intrinsic activity of an antibiotic against some bacteria (e.g. staphylococci) may be greater than for others (e.g. *Escherichia coli*) because of the effect of cell envelope structure on achievable intracellular antibiotic concentrations. These issues mean that several different thresholds (breakpoint concentrations) are often used to define susceptibility to an antibiotic. For example, an *Esch. coli* strain for which the MIC of ampicillin is 32 mg/l might be classed as susceptible if isolated from the urine of a patient with presumed urinary tract infection, while the same bacterium causing a bloodstream infection would be classified as ampicillin-resistant. These differences in definition of susceptibility relate to the variations in achievable concentrations at the site of infection: thus, an ampicillin concentration of 32 mg/l can reliably be achieved in urine, but not in blood.

Intrinsic resistance

If whole bacterial species are considered, rather than individual isolates, it is apparent immediately that they are not all intrinsically susceptible to all antibiotics (Table 9.1); for example, a coliform infection would not be treated with erythromycin, or a streptococcal infection with an aminoglycoside, since the organisms are intrinsically resistant to these antibiotics. Similarly, *Pseudomonas aeruginosa* and *Mycobacterium tuberculosis* are intrinsically resistant to most of the

Table 9.1 Effective antimicrobial spectrum of some of the most commonly used antibacterial agents

Organism	Penicillins	Cephalo-sporins	Amino-glycosides	Tetra-cyclines	Macrolides	Chloram-phenicol	Fluoro-quinolones	Sulpho-namides	Trimethoprim	Metronidazole	Glyco-peptides
Gram-positive bacteria											
Staph. aureus	V	(S)	(S)	(S)	(S)	(S)	V	(S)	(S)	R	S
Str. pyogenes	S	S	R	(S)	S	S	V	(S)	S	R	S
Other streptococci	S	S	R	(S)	S	S	V	(S)	S	R	S
Enterococci	V	R	R	(S)	S	S	V	(S)	(S)	R	(S)
Clostridium spp.	S	S	R	S	S	S	V	(S)	R	S	S
Gram-negative bacteria											
Esch. coli	V	V	(S)	(S)	R	(S)	(S)	(S)	(S)	R	R
Other enterobacteria	V	V	(S)	(S)	R	(S)	(S)	(S)	(S)	R	R
Ps. aeruginosa	V	V	V	R	R	R	(S)	R	R	R	R
H. influenzae	V	V	R	(S)	S	S	S	(S)	(S)	R	R
Neisseria spp.	V	S	R	(S)	S	S	(S)	(S)	R	R	R
Bacteroides spp.	Ft	V	R	(S)	S	S	V	(S)	R	S	R
Other organisms											
Mycobacteria	R	R	V	R	R	R	(S)	R	R	R	R
Chlamydiae	R	R	R	S	S	S	S	S	R	R	R
Mycoplasmas	R	R	R	S	S	S	S	R	R	R	R
Fungi	R	R	R	R	R	R	R	R	R	R	R

S, usually considered susceptible; R, usually considered resistant; (S), strain variation in susceptibility; V, variation among related drugs and/or strains.

agents used to treat more tractable infections. Such intrinsically resistant organisms are sometimes termed non-susceptible, with the term resistant reserved for variants of normally susceptible species that acquire mechanism(s) of resistance.

A microbe will be intrinsically resistant to an antibiotic if it either does not possess a target for the drug's action, or it is impermeable to the drug. Thus, bacteria are intrinsically resistant to polyene antibiotics, such as amphotericin, as sterols that are present in the fungal but not bacterial cell membrane, are the target for these drugs. The lipopolysaccharide outer envelope of Gram-negative bacteria is important in determining susceptibility patterns, since many antibiotics cannot penetrate this barrier to reach their intracellular target. Fortunately, intrinsic resistance is therefore often predictable, and should not pose problems provided that informed and judicious choices of antibiotics are made for the treatment of infection. Of greater concern is the primarily unpredictable acquisition or emergence of resistance in previously susceptible microbes, sometimes during the course of therapy itself.

Acquired resistance

Introduction of clinically effective antibiotics has been followed invariably by the emergence of resistant strains of bacteria among species that would normally be considered to be susceptible. Acquisition of resistance has seriously reduced the therapeutic value of many important antibiotics, but is also a major stimulus to the constant search for new and more effective antimicrobial drugs. However, while the emergence of resistance to new antibiotics is inevitable, the rate of development and spread of resistance is not predictable.

The first systematic observations of acquired drug resistance were made by Paul Ehrlich between 1902 and 1909 while using dyes and organic arsenicals to treat mice infected experimentally with trypanosomes. Within a very few years of the introduction of sulphonamides and penicillin (in 1935 and 1941 respectively), micro-organisms originally susceptible to these drugs were found to have acquired resistance. When penicillin came into use, less than 1% of all *Staphylococcus aureus* strains were resistant to its action. By 1946, however, under the selective pressure of this antibiotic, the proportion of penicillin-resistant strains found in hospitals had risen to 14%. A year later, 38% were resistant, and today, resistance is found in more than 90% of all *Staph. aureus* strains. In contrast, over the same period, an equally important pathogen, *Streptococcus pyogenes*, has remained uniformly susceptible to penicillin, although there is no guarantee that resistance will not spread to *Str. pyogenes* in future years.

There is no clear explanation for the marked differences in rate or extent of acquisition of resistance between different species. Possession of the genetic capacity for resistance does not always explain its prevalence in a particular species. Even when selection pressures are similar, the end result may not be the same. Thus, although about 90% of all strains of *Staph. aureus* are now resistant to penicillin, the same has not happened to ampicillin resistance in *Esch. coli* under similar selection pressure. At present, apart from localized outbreaks involving epidemic strains, about 50% of *Esch. coli* strains are resistant to ampicillin, and this level has remained more or less steady for a number of years. However, since an increasing incidence of resistance is at least partly a consequence of selective pressure, it is not surprising that the withdrawal of an antibiotic from clinical use may often result in a slow reduction in the number of resistant strains encountered in a particular environment. For example, fluoroquinolone-resistant strains of *Ps. aeruginosa* that emerged in some hospitals as ciprofloxacin or levofloxacin were used more frequently were replaced by more susceptible strains following restriction of removal of these drugs. Conversely, sulphonamide-resistant *Esch. coli* strains that became commonplace when the sulphonamide-containing combination drug co-trimoxazole was widely used are still prevalent. This is probably because the selection pressure still exists for other antibiotics, such as ampicillin, and the genes coding for sulphonamide and ampicillin resistance are often closely linked on plasmids; hence, use of one antibiotic can select or maintain resistance to another.

The introduction of new antibiotics has also resulted in changes to the predominant spectrum of organisms responsible for infections. In the 1960s semi-synthetic 'β-lactamase-stable' penicillins and cephalosporins were introduced which, temporarily, solved the problem of staphylococcal infections. Unfortunately, Gram-negative bacteria then became the major pathogens found in hospitals and rapidly acquired resistance to multiple antibiotics in the succeeding years. In the 1970s the pendulum swung the other way with the first outbreaks of hospital infection with multiresistant staphylococci that were resistant to nearly all antistaphylococcal agents. Outbreaks of infection caused by such organisms have occurred subsequently all over the world.

Gram-negative bacteria are once again assuming greater importance, particularly in hospitals. Resistance to newer cephalosporins—mediated by extended-spectrum β-lactamases—and fluoroquinolones in *Esch. coli* and other enterobacteria has increased or is continuing to increase, depending on geographical locale, rendering these commonly used antibiotics less effective. Multiresistant Gram-negative bacteria (such as *Acinetobacter* species) have emerged that are resistant to most and, occasionally, all approved antibiotics. The recent emergence of carbapenemase producing enterobacteria is a most worrying development given the 'last line of defence' status of the carbapenem class of antibiotics.

Types of acquired resistance

Two main types of acquired resistance may be encountered in bacterial species that would normally be considered susceptible to a particular antibacterial agent.

Mutational resistance

In any large population of bacterial cells a very few individual cells may spontaneously become resistant (see Chapter 10). Such resistant cells have no particular survival advantage in the absence of antibiotic, but after the introduction of antibiotic treatment susceptible bacterial cells will be killed, so that the (initially) very few resistant cells can proliferate until they eventually form a wholly resistant population. Many antimicrobial agents select for this type of acquired resistance in many different bacterial species, both *in vitro* and *in vivo*. The problem has been recognized as being of particular importance in the long-term treatment of tuberculosis with antituberculosis drugs.

Transmissible resistance

A more spectacular type of acquired resistance occurs when genes conferring antibiotic resistance transfer from a resistant bacterial cell to a sensitive one. The simultaneous transfer of resistance to several unrelated antimicrobial agents can be demonstrated readily, both in the laboratory and the patient. Exponential transfer and spread of existing resistance genes through a previously susceptible bacterial population is a much more efficient mechanism of acquiring resistance than the development of resistance by mutation of individual susceptible cells.

Mechanisms by which transfer of resistance genes takes place are discussed in Chapter 10. Here it is sufficient to stress that however resistance appears in a hitherto susceptible bacterial cell or population, resistance will only become widespread under the selective pressures produced by the presence of appropriate antibiotics. Also, the development of resistant cells does not have to happen often or on a large scale. A single mutation or transfer event can, if the appropriate selective pressures are operating, lead to the replacement of a susceptible population by a resistant one. Without selective pressure, antibiotic resistance may be a handicap rather than an asset to a bacterium.

Cross-resistance and multiple resistance

These terms are often confused. Cross-resistance involves resistance to a number of different members of a group of (usually) chemically related agents that are affected alike by the same resistance mechanism. For example, there is almost complete cross-resistance between the different tetracyclines (although not necessarily the closely related tigecycline; see p. 32), because tetracycline resistance results largely from an efflux mechanism that affects all members of the group. The situation is more complex among other antibiotic families. Thus, resistance to aminoglycosides may be mediated by any one of a number of different drug-inactivating enzymes (see Table 10.4, p. 112) with different substrate specificities, and the range of aminoglycosides to which the organism is resistant will depend on which enzyme it produces. Cross-resistance can also be observed occasionally between unrelated antibiotics. For example, a change in the outer membrane structure of Gram-negative bacilli may concomitantly deny access of unrelated compounds to their target sites.

In contrast, multiple drug (multidrug) resistance involves a bacterium becoming resistant to several unrelated antibiotics by different resistance mechanisms. For example, if a staphylococcus is resistant to penicillin, gentamicin, and tetracycline, the resistances must have originated independently, since the strain destroys the penicillin with a β-lactamase, inactivates gentamicin with an aminoglycoside-modifying enzyme, and excludes tetracycline from the cell by an active efflux mechanism.

It is, however, not always clear whether cross-resistance or multiple resistance is being observed. Genes conferring resistance to several unrelated agents can be transferred en bloc from one bacterial cell to another on plasmids (see Chapter 10), thereby giving the appearance of cross-resistance. In such cases, detailed biochemical and genetic analysis may be required to prove that the resistance mechanisms are distinct (multiple resistance), although the genes conferring resistance are linked and transferred together on one plasmid. The end result may be the same (i.e. resistance to multiple agents), but the risk of the spread is greater for plasmid mediated resistance.

The clinical problem of drug resistance

Concerns about resistance have been raised at regular intervals since the first introduction of antimicrobial chemotherapy, but awareness of the antibiotic resistance problem has probably never been greater than it is today. It has been suggested that antibiotic resistance is becoming so commonplace that there is a danger of returning to the pre-antibiotic era. It is important not to understate or overstate the problem; the situation is presently becoming serious, but is not yet desperate since most infections are still treatable with several currently available agents. This may, however, mean that the only antibiotics that are still active are more toxic or less effective (or both) than those to which bacteria have acquired resistance. For example, it is generally accepted that glycopeptide antibiotics are less effective in the treatment of *Staph. aureus* infection than are antistaphylococcal penicillins (e.g. flucloxacillin); since the latter cannot be used against meticillin-resistant *Staph. aureus* (MRSA), this may partly explain the poorer outcome, including increased risk of death, that is seen in such cases in comparison with infection caused by meticillin-susceptible strains.

There is good evidence that if the antibiotic regimen chosen is subsequently shown to be inactive against the pathogens causing infection, then patient outcome is worse (Fig. 9.1). This means that clinicians are likely to opt for unnecessarily broad-spectrum therapy particularly in critically ill patients. Unfortunately, repeated use of such regimens against bacteria that harbour resistance genes intensifies the selective pressure for further resistance development, notably in hospital, where the most vulnerable patients are managed.

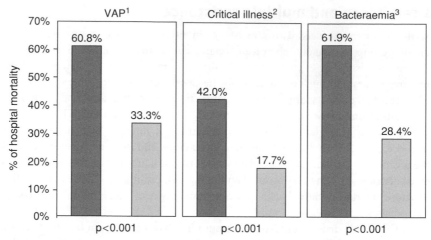

Fig. 9.1 Mortality recorded in three separate studies for patients who received antibiotic treatment that was subsequently shown to be inactive (dark grey) or active (light grey) against pathogens isolated. VAP, ventilator associated pneumonia. Data from: [1]Kollef MH, Ward S (1998) 'The influence of mini-BAL cultures on patient outcomes: implications for the antibiotic management of ventilator-associated pneumonia', *Chest* 1998; 113: 412–420; [2]Kollef MH Sherman G, Ward S, Fraser VJ (1999) 'Inadequate antimicrobial treatment of infections: a risk factor for hospital mortality among critically ill patients', *Chest* 115: 462–474; [3]Ibrahim EH, Sherman G, Ward S, Fraser VJ, Kollef MH. 'The influence of inadequate antimicrobial treatment of bloodstream infections on patient outcomes in the ICU setting'. *Chest* 2000; 118: 146–155.

In many less-developed countries of the world, the therapeutic options may be severely restricted for economic reasons. There is no doubt that the problem of antibiotic resistance is a global issue, and in future years there is a real possibility that physicians will be faced increasingly with infections for which effective treatment is not available. There are many examples of the inter-continental spread of resistant pathogens, and so the judicious use of antibiotics has global as well as local relevance. Some of the organisms in which resistance is a particular problem are summarized below.

Enteric Gram-negative bacteria

The prevalence of resistance in hospital strains of enteric Gram-negative bacteria has been rising steadily for the past 40 years, particularly in large units. Although cephalosporins, quinolones, and aminoglycosides have been developed to cope with the problem, resistance to these newer compounds has increased in most countries. Outbreaks of infection caused by multi-resistant *Klebsiella* strains and extended-spectrum β-lactamase-producing enterobacteria in general are reported increasingly often, both in high dependency areas of hospitals and in urinary tract isolates from patients in the community. The latter phenomenon is consistent with more widespread dissemination of these strains and their carriage in faecal flora. Whilst absolute numbers of carbapenemase (e.g. NDM-1 and KPC) producing Gram-negative enteric bacteria are still low, there has been an exponential increase in reported isolates in the UK in the last three years, with *Klebsiella* strains notably prominent.

Widespread resistance in enteric bacteria is a particular problem in less-developed areas of the world where heavy and indiscriminate use of antibiotics may combine with a high prevalence of drug-resistant bacteria in the faecal flora, poor standards of sanitation, and a high incidence of diarrhoeal disease to encourage the rapid emergence and spread of multiresistant strains of enteric bacteria. Epidemics of diarrhoeal disease caused by multiresistant strains of intestinal pathogens, including *Vibrio cholerae*, shigellae, salmonellae, and toxin-producing strains of *Esch. coli*, have occurred around the world.

Acinetobacter

These organisms cause hospital-acquired infections especially in patients in intensive care units, e.g. ventilator-associated pneumonia. Such infections are usually extremely difficult to treat because of the multiple classes of antibiotic resistance found in these bacteria. Very few antibiotics are now reliably effective for treatment of acinetobacter infections. Even with carbapenems such as imipenem or meropenem, resistance has emerged. Colistin, a relatively toxic old antibiotic that has largely been abandoned for systemic administration, is used to treat some strains that are resistant to all other licensed antibiotics. Many multiresistant *Acinetobacter* spp. strains are currently susceptible to the new antibiotic tigecycline, although again resistance to this agent has already become more common.

Staphylococci and enterococci

MRSA is endemic in many hospitals and nursing homes. The proportion of *Staph. aureus* isolates causing serious sepsis, such as bloodstream infection, that are resistant to meticillin reached 40 to 50% in the UK and some countries in southern Europe, although recent improvement in infection control practice have reduced their prevalence. The prevalence is even higher in countries in the Far East and USA. Clones of MRSA associated with community infections, typically skin sepsis, have spread rapidly in the USA. MRSA infections have often been treated with glycopeptides, and isolates with low-level resistance to these antibiotics can be found. Very occasional MRSA strains with high-level resistance to glycopeptides have also been reported. Several newer antibiotics, including linezolid, daptomycin, and tigecycline, are active against these strains, but occasional reports of resistance have already occurred.

Coagulase-negative staphylococci and enterococci are often multiresistant and cause infections typically in patients with indwelling prosthetic material, such as catheters, vascular grafts, joints and heart valves. A combination of antibiotics may be required to treat serious enterococcal infections, but the emergence of high-level aminoglycoside resistance may seriously limit this option. Enterococci carrying genes conferring high-level resistance to glycopeptides have emerged (Chapter 10). Linezolid has been used successfully to treat infection caused by such strains, but resistance has some occurred in patients receiving long courses of therapy, particularly if the focus of infection has not been removed.

Streptococcus pneumoniae

Another major problem concerns the emergence of resistance in *Streptococcus pneumoniae*, the most common cause of community-acquired pneumonia and other respiratory infections. This organism used to be combated easily by treatment with penicillin and its derivatives. Unfortunately, isolates with resistance to most antibiotics can now be found in most countries of the world. Such infections are often treated with broad-spectrum cephalosporins, which can attain sufficient tissue concentrations to exceed the raised MIC for these strains. The prevalence of macrolide-resistant pneumococci tends to correlate with how often these antibiotics are used, especially in the community where most respiratory tract infections are treated. Newer fluoroquinolones such as moxifloxacin have increased activity against pneumococci. Some resistance emergence has developed in units where these agents have been used commonly.

Neisseria meningitidis

Decreased levels of susceptibility to penicillin have been seen in many countries, but high-level resistance is exceptionally rare. The emergence of resistance to penicillin in *N. meningitidis* has important strategic implications because of the need for immediate treatment of the life-threatening infections caused by these organisms. Currently penicillin is still used empirically in some cases of suspected meningococcal infection. The cephalosporins cefotaxime or ceftriaxone are often favoured for the empirical treatment of meningitis because the antibiotic concentration achieved in the cerebrospinal fluid more reliably exceeds the MIC for the pathogen in both meningococcal and pneumococcal infection.

Tuberculosis (TB)

Strains of *M. tuberculosis* that are resistant to two or more of the first-line drugs—isoniazid, ethambutol, rifampicin, and streptomycin—are increasingly common, particularly in HIV-infected patients. Multidrug-resistant TB (MDR-TB) is caused by bacteria that are resistant to the most effective anti-TB drugs (isoniazid and rifampicin). MDR-TB results from either primary infection or may develop in the course of a patient's treatment. Extensively drug-resistant TB (XDR-TB) is a form of TB caused by bacteria that are resistant to isoniazid and rifampicin (i.e. MDR-TB) as well as any fluoroquinolone and any of the second-line anti-TB intravenous antibiotics (amikacin, kanamycin, or capreomycin). These forms of TB do not respond to the standard six month treatment with first-line anti-TB drugs and can take two years or more to treat with drugs that are less potent, more toxic, and much more expensive. The resistant bacteria can be transmitted, for example in hospitals, prisons, and in the community, and represent a major public health issue. The emergence of resistance is associated with poor compliance with antituberculosis medication. Directly observed therapy is advocated therefore for patients in whom compliance may be unreliable (see Chapter 30).

The World Health Organization estimates that there were 440 000 MDR-TB cases and 150 0 deaths in 2008, with nearly half of all the world's cases occurring in China and India. The prevalence of MDR-TB is extremely variable: in parts of north-west Russia one in four new TB patients diagnosed has MDR-TB, compared with one in 50 in London. As of March 2010, 58 countries have reported at least one case of XDR-TB. About 5% of MDR-TB cases have XDR-TB, and about 25 000 of the latter are estimated to develop each year. Only an estimated 7% of all MDR-TB patients are diagnosed and notified as such. Nevertheless, approximately 60% of people with MDR-TB who are enrolled on treatment programmes are successfully treated.

Key points

+ The extent of antibiotic resistance does not reverse in some cases when antibiotics stop being used.

+ There is no clear explanation for the marked differences in rate or extent of acquisition of resistance between different bacterial species.

+ The recent emergence of carbapenemase-producing enterobacteria is a serious threat given the 'last line of defence' status of the carbapenems.

+ MDR-TB is caused by bacteria that are resistant to the most effective anti-TB drugs (isoniazid and rifampicin) and may occur because of poor compliance; directly observed therapy of TB is preferred when compliance is uncertain.

+ XDR-TB is defined as MDR-TB plus resistance to any fluoroquinolone and any of the second-line anti-TB intravenous antibiotics (amikacin, kanamycin, or capreomycin) and is increasing rapidly.

Further reading

British Society for Antimicrobial Chemotherapy. Available at: http://www.bsac.org.uk/.

Health Protection Agency. Available at: http://www.hpa.org.uk/Topics/InfectiousDiseases/InfectionsAZ/
AntimicrobialResistance/.

World Health Organization. Antimicrobial resistance. Fact sheet 194. February 2011. Available at:
http://www.who.int/mediacentre/factsheets/fs194/en/.

World Health Organization. *Multidrug and extensively drug-resistant TB (M/XDR-TB): 2010 global report on
surveillance and response.* Available at: http://www.who.int/tb/features_archive/m_xdrtb_facts/en/
index.html.

Centers for Disease Control and Prevention. Available at: http://www.cdc.gov/drugresistance/index.html.

Chapter 10

The genetics and mechanisms of acquired resistance

The mechanisms discussed in the second part of this chapter illustrate the diversity of ways that microbes can become resistant to the drugs deployed against them. However, attempts to limit the spread of drug resistance require not only knowledge of the mechanisms themselves, but also an understanding of the genetic factors that control their emergence and continued evolution.

Genetics of resistance

All the properties of a microbial cell, including its antibiotic resistance and virulence determinants, are determined ultimately by the microbial genome. The genome comprises the three possible sources of genetic information: the chromosome, plasmids, and bacteriophages. Resistance of bacteria to antibiotics may be either intrinsic or acquired (see Chapter 9). Intrinsic resistance is the 'natural' resistance possessed by a bacterial species and is usually specified by chromosomal genes. An example of a bacterial species with a high degree of intrinsic resistance is *Pseudomonas aeruginosa*. By contrast, acquired resistance occurs in formerly susceptible cells, either following alterations to the existing genome or by transfer of genetic information between cells. Thus, a basic knowledge of microbial genetics is essential to understand the development and spread of resistance to antimicrobial drugs.

The heritable information that specifies a bacterial cell, and passes to daughter cells at cell division, is carried in bacteria, as in all living cells, as an ordered sequence of nucleotide pairs along molecules of DNA. The process of transcription of this information into messenger RNA, and its subsequent translation into functioning proteins by ribosomes, is also similar in bacteria and in other cells.

The bacterial chromosome

Each bacterial cell has a single chromosome, which is the main source of genetic information, and usually comprises a closed circular DNA molecule. In *Escherichia coli*, the organism studied most intensively, this single DNA molecule comprises about 4×10^3 kb (kilobases) and is about 1.4 mm in length. Considering the average cell is about 1–3 mm in length, only by 'super-coiling' of DNA can the chromosome fit inside the bacterium. Enzymes known as DNA gyrases control the process of super-coiling DNA. Conversely, DNA uncoiling, which is necessary for messenger RNA production or chromosome replication, is controlled by DNA topoisomerases. The chromosome is found in the cytoplasm of the cell, not separated from it by a nuclear membrane. Transcription of DNA and translation of the resulting messenger RNA can therefore proceed simultaneously. Most bacterial chromosomes contain sufficient DNA to encode for 1000–3000 different genes. Not all of these genes need to be expressed at any one time, and indeed it would be wasteful for the cell to do so. Gene regulation is therefore necessary, and this can occur at either the transcriptional or translational level.

Chromosomal mutations to antibiotic resistance

Mutations result from rare mistakes in the DNA replication process and occur at the rate of between 10^{-4} and 10^{-10} per cell division. They usually involve deletion, substitution, or addition of one or only a few base pairs, which cause an alteration in the amino acid composition of a specific protein. Such mistakes are random and spontaneous. They occur continuously in cell genes and are independent of the presence or absence of antibiotics. The vast majority of mutations are repaired by the cell without any noticeable effect. In the presence of an antibiotic some of these occasional spontaneous antibiotic-resistant mutants that are present among a predominantly susceptible population of bacteria may be selected. In such a situation, the susceptible cells will be killed or inhibited by the antibiotic, whereas the resistant mutants will survive and proliferate to become the new predominant type. Most chromosomal resistance mutations result in alterations to permeability or specific antibiotic target sites, but some result in enhanced production of an inactivating enzyme or bypass mechanism. The latter types are mutations at the transcriptional or translational level in gene regulatory mechanisms.

Chromosomal mutations causing antibiotic resistance can be divided into single-step and multistep types.

Single large-step mutations

With these mutations, a single mutational change results in a large increase in the minimum inhibitory concentration of a particular antibiotic, and may lead to treatment failure if this drug is used alone. In some Gram-negative bacilli, mutations in the genetic regulatory system for the normally low-level chromosomal β-lactamase may result in a vast overproduction (sometimes referred to as 'derepression') of this enzyme with resulting slow hydrolysis of compounds such as cefotaxime and ceftazidime that are normally considered to be β-lactamase stable.

Multistep (stepwise) mutations

These are sequential mutations that result in cumulative gradual stepwise increases in the minimum inhibitory concentration of a particular antibiotic. They are clinically quite common, especially in situations where only low concentrations of antibiotic can be delivered to the site of an infection.

Plasmids

Many, perhaps all, bacteria in addition to the chromosome carry additional DNA molecules (usually 2–200 kb in size) known as plasmids. These normally replicate independently of the bacterial chromosome. Plasmids can carry genes that confer a wide range of properties on the host cell, which are usually not essential for survival but offer a survival advantage in unusual or adverse conditions. Examples of such properties are:

♦ fertility: the ability to conjugate with and transfer genetic information into other bacteria (see later);

♦ resistance to antibiotics: antibiotic resistance encountered clinically is often associated with plasmids;

♦ ability to produce bacteriocins: proteins inhibitory to other bacteria that may be ecological competitors;

♦ exotoxin production;

♦ immunity to some bacteriophages;

♦ ability to use unusual sugars and other substrates as foods.

'Compatible' plasmids can coexist in the same host cell, while 'incompatible' plasmids cannot, and so tend to be unstable and displace one another. There are at least 20 incompatibility (Inc) groups within the plasmids found in enteric Gram-negative bacilli, and similar incompatibility schemes are used to subdivide staphylococcal plasmids and those found in *Pseudomonas* spp.

Bacteriophages

The third possible source of genetic information in a bacterial cell is a bacteriophage. Bacteriophages (phages) are viruses that infect bacteria. Most phages will attack only a relatively limited range of bacteria, and can be divided into two main types:

- ◆ Virulent phages inevitably destroy by lysis any bacteria that they infect, with the release of numerous new phage particles from each lysed cell;

- ◆ Temperate (lysogenic) phages may either lyse or lysogenize infected bacterial cells. In the state of lysogeny, the phage nucleic acid is replicated in a stable and dormant fashion within the infected cell, often following insertion into the host cell chromosome. Such a dormant phage is known as a prophage. However, while in the prophage state, some prophage genes may be expressed and may confer additional properties on the cell. Once in every few thousand cell divisions, a prophage becomes released from the dormant state and enters the lytic cycle, with subsequent destruction of its host cell and release of new phage particles into the surrounding medium.

Naturally occurring phages have been used in limited settings (for example, the countries formerly part of the Soviet Union) for the treatment of some infections (phage therapy). Some companies are exploring such treatment modalities in response to the threat posed by antibiotic resistance pathogens.

Transfer of genetic information

There are three ways in which genetic information can be transferred from one bacterial cell into another: transformation, transduction, and conjugation.

- ◆ Transformation involves lysis of a bacterial cell and the release of naked DNA into the surrounding medium. Under certain circumstances, intact bacterial cells in the vicinity can acquire some of this DNA. This process has been much studied in the laboratory, but there are few convincing demonstrations of its occurrence *in vivo*. The process depends crucially on whether the recipient cells are competent for uptake of free DNA;

- ◆ Transduction involves the accidental incorporation of bacterial DNA, either from the chromosome or a plasmid, into a bacteriophage particle during the phage lytic cycle. The phage particle then acts as a vector and transfers the bacterial DNA to the next cell that it infects;

- ◆ Conjugation involves physical contact between two bacterial cells. The cells adhere to one another and DNA passes from one cell, termed the donor, into the other, the recipient. Ability to conjugate depends on carriage of an appropriate plasmid or transposon (see later) by the host cell.

These transfer mechanisms mean that bacteria do not have to rely solely on a process of mutation and selection for their evolution. They can, therefore, acquire and express blocks of genetic information that have evolved elsewhere. A bacterial cell can, for example, acquire by conjugation a plasmid that carries genes conferring resistance to several different antibiotics. As a result, within a very short time following the receipt of such a plasmid by a susceptible cell, the bacteria in a given niche may change from being predominantly susceptible to being resistant to multiple drugs.

Of course, the ability to transfer genes in this way does not eliminate the need for these to evolve; however, once they have evolved, it ensures their eventual widespread dissemination under appropriate selection pressures.

Evolution of new resistance gene combinations

The distinction between chromosomal and plasmid genes is not absolute. Where appropriate regions of DNA homology exist, classic ('normal' or 'homologous') recombination can occur, both between different plasmids and between plasmids and the chromosome. Although this process can lead to the formation of new antibiotic resistance gene combinations, it is relatively uncommon in bacteria because there are few regions of sequence homology between the bacterial chromosome and plasmids that can be exploited for this purpose. Homologous recombination is used by researchers to create 'knockout' cells in which the function of a specific gene is disrupted. A more important mechanism by which antibiotic resistance genes can pass naturally from one bacterial replicon to another is the 'illegitimate' recombination process known as transposition.

Transposons

Transposition depends on the existence of specific genetic elements termed transposons. These elements are discrete sequences of DNA capable of translocation (transposition) from one replicon (plasmid or chromosome) to another. Unlike classic ('normal') recombination, transposons do not share extensive regions of homology with the replicon into which they insert. In many cases, transposons consist of individual resistance genes, or groups of genes, bounded by DNA sequences called either direct or inverted repeats; that is, a sequence of bases at one end of the transposon that also appears, either in direct or reverse order, at the other end. These repeats may be relatively short, often of the order of 40 base pairs, but longer examples have been identified. It is likely that these DNA sequences provide highly specific recognition sites for certain enzymes (transposases) that catalyse the movement of transposons from one replicon to another, without the need for extensive regions of sequence homology. Depending upon the transposon involved, insertion may occur at only a few or at many different sites on the host replicon. Transposons may carry genes conferring resistance to many different antibiotics, as well as other metabolic properties, and most likely explain how a single antibiotic resistance gene can become disseminated over a wide range of unrelated replicons.

Isolated DNA sequences analogous to the terminal sequences of transposons can also move from one replicon to another, or be inserted in any region of any DNA molecule. Such insertion sequences appear to contain only genes that are related to insertion functions; however, in principle at least, two similar insertion sequences could bracket any assemblage of genes and convert it into a transposon. Thus, theoretically, all replicons are accessible to transposition and all genes are potentially transposable. This theory is of crucial evolutionary importance since it explains how genes of appropriate function can accumulate on a single replicon under the impact of selection pressure. Transposons and insertion sequences therefore play a vital part in plasmid evolution.

Integrons

Transposons may contain combinations of genes conferring resistance to various different antibiotics. An important question concerns the mechanism by which new combinations of antibiotic resistance genes are formed. It is now apparent that special molecular structures, termed integrons, may enable the formation of new combinations of resistance genes within a bacterial cell, either on a plasmid or within a transposon, in response to selection pressures.

Integrons appear to consist of two conserved segments of DNA located either side of inserted antibiotic resistance genes. Individual resistance genes seem to be capable of insertion or removal as 'cassettes' between these conserved structures. The cassettes can be found inserted in different orders and combinations. Integrons also act as an expression vector for 'foreign' antibiotic resistance genes by supplying a promoter for transcription of cassettes derived originally from completely unrelated organisms. Integrons lack many of the features associated with transposons, including direct or inverted repeats and functions required for transposition. They do, however, possess site-specific integration functions, notably a special enzyme termed an integrase.

Integrons can spread via site-specific insertion, following insertion into a transposon or via plasmids. The precise role of integrons in the evolution and spread of antibiotic resistance genes remains to be determined, but they have been found, together with their associated antibiotic resistance gene cassettes, in many different Gram-negative bacteria. More recently, chromosomal integron structures have been found in the genomes of hundreds of bacterial species. Notably, unrelated clinical isolates from different worldwide locations have been shown to carry the same integron structures, and it appears that these structures play a key role in the formation and dissemination of new combinations of antibiotic resistance genes.

Genotypic resistance and spread

The process of evolution and spread of antibiotic resistance genes continues. The origin of resistance genes carried by integrons, transposons, or plasmids, or even the origin of these elements themselves, is generally not known, but it has been possible to observe a steady increase in the numbers of resistant bacterial strains following the introduction of successive chemotherapeutic agents into clinical use. For example, the *qnrA* genes that encode plasmid-mediated quinolone resistance are embedded in complex integrons. Similar genes have been identified in the water-borne species *Shewanella algae*, emphasizing the potential for spread of resistance mechanisms from environmental bacteria. Furthermore, the discovery of a variant gene encoding an aminoglycoside modifying (acetyltransferase) enzyme that can mediate quinolone resistance highlighted the plasticity of resistance mechanisms. In this case, the new mechanism is all the more startling given that antimicrobial-modifying enzymes have traditionally been antibiotic class specific.

Chromosomal and plasmid-mediated types of resistance may be equally important in the antibiotic management of an individual patient. However, the plasmid-encoded variety has achieved greater notoriety because of the spectacular fashion in which bacteria may acquire resistance to a number of unrelated agents by a single genetic event. Furthermore, the potential for spread of plasmid-borne resistance to other species or genera highlights the importance of control of pathogens that are antibiotic resistant by virtue of such plasmid genes. Nevertheless, mutational resistance involving the bacterial chromosome is also a common cause of treatment failure with some compounds. Antibacterial agents for which resistance is not known to be encoded on plasmids (e.g. rifampicin and fusidic acid) generally suffer from mutational resistance problems instead.

Phenotypic resistance

Phenotypic resistance is due to changes in the bacterial physiological state. Bacteria in stationary phase (e.g. in biofilms) and spore forms are good examples of cells that are not actively dividing and thus relatively non-susceptible to antibiotics. By contrast, daughter cells released from a biofilm may be readily inactivated by antibiotics, and yet the biolfim 'source' remains viable. Once antibiotics are removed the biofilm bacteria may then continue to release daughter cells and thus cause infection recrudescence. The extent of phenotypic resistance to antibacterial agents is unclear, particularly as it is not always possible to be sure that phenotypic changes brought about in the micro-environment of a lesion do not contribute to insusceptibility of bacteria. In the laboratory, phenotypic resistance can sometimes be induced; for example, varying the conditions of growth of *Ps. aeruginosa* can alter the outer envelope, which affects susceptibility to polymyxins.

Another example is the failure of penicillins and cephalosporins to kill 'persisters' (those cells in a bacterial population that survive exposure to concentrations of β-lactam agents lethal to the rest of the culture). This does not result from a genetic event since the resistance is not heritable, and it is probable that the 'resistant' bacteria are caught in a particular metabolic state at the time of first encounter with the drug.

A peculiar form of phenotypic resistance is observed with mecillinam, a β-lactam antibiotic which, unusually, does not affect bacterial cell division. Mecillinam induces surface changes in susceptible Gram-negative bacilli which generally lead to cell death by osmotic rupture (p. 14–22). However, those cells in the population that happen to have low internal osmolality survive, and, as mecillinam lacks the ability to prevent growth and division, such bacteria continue to grow in a morphologically altered form. On withdrawal of the drug, the bacteria resume their normal shape and, in due course, revert to the same mixed susceptibility as the original parent culture.

The influence of antibiotic selection pressure

Antibiotic resistance genes, and the genetic elements that carry them, existed before the introduction of antibiotics into human medicine. However, it is clear that the emergence and survival of predominantly resistant bacterial populations is due to the selective pressure associated with the widespread use of antibiotics. Resistant cells survive in a given niche at the expense of susceptible cells of the same or other species. In some cases, however, there is a fitness cost to resistant bacterial cells that may mean that they are less able to compete once the selective pressure imparted by the antibiotic is removed. In such cases, any antibiotic susceptible progeny cells that remain may be counterselected in preference to these unfit mutants. Individual cells may lose their plasmids and chromosomal mutations may revert to being antibiotic susceptible. The implications of this process for efforts to control and limit the spread of bacterial drug resistance are discussed in Chapter 11.

Mechanisms of acquired resistance

Three conditions must be met in order that a particular antimicrobial agent can inhibit susceptible bacteria:

- the antibiotic must be able to reach the target in sufficient concentration and be metabolically active (e.g. optimal pH, redox potential);
- the antibiotic must not be inactivated before binding to the target;
- a vital target susceptible to the action of the antibiotic must exist in the bacterial cell.

The targets of individual antibiotics are often enzymes or other essential proteins. Most antimicrobial agents have to pass through the cell wall and outer membrane to reach their target, and many are carried into the cell by active transport mechanisms that usually transport sugars and other beneficial substances. Some of the differences in susceptibility of bacterial species are therefore related to differences in cell wall structure. For example, the cell envelope of Gram-negative bacteria is a more complex structure than the Gram-positive cell wall (see Chapter 1) and offers a relatively greater barrier to many antibiotics, including penicillins, glycopeptides, and macrolides. Polymyxins exert their effects at the cell surface by disrupting the Gram-negative cell membranes from the outside in a way that resembles the action of some detergents.

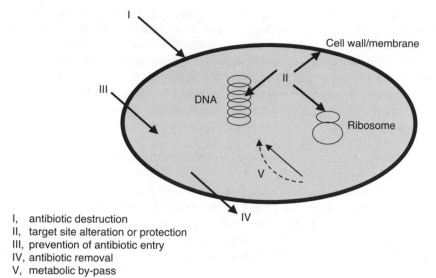

I, antibiotic destruction
II, target site alteration or protection
III, prevention of antibiotic entry
IV, antibiotic removal
V, metabolic by-pass

Fig. 10.1 Mechanisms of antimicrobial drug resistance.

The mechanisms by which resistance may occur can be divided into the following major groups:

◆ destruction or inactivation of the antibiotic (Fig. 10.1, I);

◆ alteration or protection of the target site to reduce or eliminate binding of the antibiotic to the target (Fig. 10.1, II);

◆ reduction in cell surface permeability or blockage of the mechanism by which the antibiotic enters the cell (Fig. 10.1, III), or removal from the cell (efflux) (Fig. 10.1, IV);

◆ acquisition of a replacement for the metabolic step inhibited by the antibiotic (Fig. 10.1, V).

It is worth emphasizing that certain resistance mechanisms overlap within these groups. Furthermore, bacteria can become resistant to an antibiotic by several different mechanisms; e.g. drug efflux, target protection, target alteration, and enzymatic inactivation may each afford resistance to tetracyclines.

Some of the known mechanisms of antibiotic resistance are summarized in Table 10.1.

Inactivation or modification mechanisms

These are probably the most important resistance mechanisms in clinical practice since they include the common modes of resistance to penicillins and cephalosporins, the therapeutic agents of widest use.

β-lactam antibiotics

There are many different agents in this group (see Chapter 1) and a correspondingly large number of β-lactamases that catalyse hydrolysis of the β-lactam ring to form an inactive product (Fig. 10.2). In addition, varying levels of β-lactamase production, variable properties of the enzymes, notably the breadth of activity, and differences in the permeability of the Gram-negative cell envelope, determine the differential susceptibilities of bacteria to these antibiotics.

Table 10.1 Important known resistance mechanisms for the major groups of antibiotics

Inactivation or modification	Altered or protected target site	Reduced permeability or access	Metabolic by-pass
β-Lactam antibiotics	β-Lactam antibiotics	Tetracyclines[d]	Trimethoprim
Chloramphenicol	Streptomycin	β-Lactam antibiotics	Sulphonamides
Aminoglycosides[a]	Chloramphenicol	Chloramphenicol	
	Erythromycin[b]	Quinolones[d]	
	Fusidic acid	Aminoglycosides	
	Quinolones		
	Rifampicin		
	Glycopeptides[b]		
	Tetracyclines[c]		

[a] Resulting in reduced drug uptake.
[b] Resulting from enzymic modification.
[c] Resulting from ribosomal protection.
[d] Resulting from an increased efflux.

All bacteria appear to contain enzymes capable of hydrolysing β-lactam antibiotics. Indeed, it has been suggested that the normal function and evolutionary origin of β-lactamases is to break a β-lactam structure that is a transitory intermediate in cell wall synthesis. These constitutive enzymes are encoded by the bacterial chromosome, and are normally bound closely to the cell membrane. In general, they are produced only in small amounts, they attack cephalosporins more readily than penicillins, and they act relatively slowly. In certain organisms, notably *Enterobacter* spp., *Acinetobacter* spp., *Citrobacter* spp., and *Pseudomonas aeruginosa*, gross over-production of these chromosomal enzymes has been associated with treatment failure, even with so-called 'β-lactamase-stable' cephalosporins and carbapenems. Resistance seems to result from a combination of the slow enzyme-mediated hydrolysis, and cell wall mutations that partially impede antibiotic entry into the bacterial cell.

The classification of β-lactamases has become extremely complex as more and more examples of these enzymes (now numbering more than 200), some differing from one another by only one or a few amino acids, have been described. Various characteristics are used to distinguish the

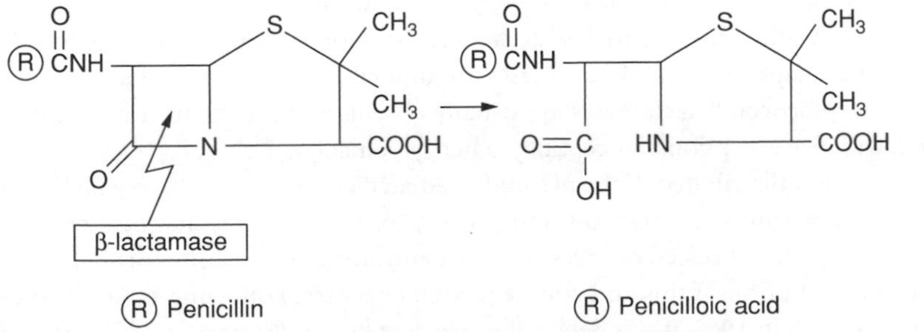

Fig. 10.2 β-Lactamase hydrolysis of penicillins to form the corresponding penicilloic acid, which is antibacterially inactive. Cephalosporins may be attacked in a similar fashion, but the resultant cephalosporoic acid is usually unstable and disintegrates into smaller fragments.

Table 10.2 Simplified categorization of the most common bacterial β-lactamases

Group	Molecular class	Preferred substrates	Inhibited by: Clavulanic acid	EDT^	Representative enzymes
1	C	Cephalosporins	No	No	Gram-negative chromosomal enzymes
2a	A	Penicillins	Yes	No	Staphylococcal β-lactamases
2b	A	Penicillins; cephalosporins	Yes	No	TEM series; SHV series; CTX-M
2c	A	Penicillins; carbenicillin	Yes	No	PSE series
2d	D	Penicillins; cloxacillin	Variable	No	OXA series
2e	A	Cephalosporins	Yes	No	Proteus cephalosporinase
2f	A	Carbapenems	Yes	Yes	IMI-1, KPC-2, SME-1
3	B	Most β-lactam antibiotics	No	Yes	Metallo-enzymes (carbapenemases) e.g. IMP-1, VIM-1

EDTA, ethylenediaminetetraacetic acid. Adapted and updated from the scheme of Bush K, Jacoby GA, Medeiros AA *Antimicrobial Agents and Chemotherapy* 1995; **39**: 1211–1233, and Bush K, Jacoby GA *Antimicrobial Agents and Chemotherapy* 2010; **54**: 969–976.

different enzymes, including substrate profile, and the action of enzyme inhibitors such as clavulanic acid and the ion-chelator, ethylenediaminetetraacetic acid (EDTA). Substrate profile refers to the hydrolytic activity of a β-lactamase preparation against a number of β-lactam substrates, often expressed as the ratio to a value for a reference substrate such as benzylpenicillin. Methods based on DNA–DNA hybridization or the polymerase chain reaction (PCR) to identify specific genes, have been used to distinguish newly recognized enzymes. A simplified classification of the common bacterial β-lactamases is shown in Table 10.2.

Gram-negative bacteria produce a greater variety of β-lactamases than Gram-positive bacteria. From a clinical point of view, most interest centres on the large number of plasmid-encoded enzymes, particularly given their potential for widespread dissemination. Plasmid-encoded enzymes are the major cause of bacterial resistance to penicillins and cephalosporins in clinical isolates. Some are located on transposons (see above), so allowing movement of genes between plasmids and the chromosome. This means that the distinction between plasmid-encoded and chromosome-encoded enzymes sometimes is blurred.

Among Gram-positive cocci, plasmid-encoded β-lactamases of clinical significance are found almost exclusively in staphylococci. These enzymes rapidly hydrolyse benzylpenicillin, ampicillin, and most other penicillins, but are less active against antistaphylococcal penicillins (p. 14) and cephalosporins. Staphylococcal β-lactamases are inducible exo-enzymes that are usually related closely. In streptococci, β-lactamases are usually absent, and these bacteria have consequently remained, with few exceptions, susceptible to benzylpenicillin.

The most widely distributed of the plasmid-mediated enzymes is TEM-1, which is encoded by many different plasmids (p. 103) and transposons (p. 105). The resultant genetic promiscuity, coupled with sustained selective pressure from antibiotic prescribing, probably explains the widespread distribution of this and closely related enzymes. Following the first recognition of TEM-1 in *Esch. coli* in 1965, it was detected in *Haemophilus influenzae* and *Neisseria gonorrhoeae* in the mid-1970s, and in *Neisseria meningitidis* in 1989.

There are more than 100 genetic TEM variants, some of which have an altered substrate spectrum. Some produce β-lactamases that can hydrolyse a wide variety of penicillins and cephalosporins (extended-spectrum β-lactamases). Extended-spectrum enzymes unrelated to TEM, have also been described, notably the plasmid-encoded cefotaxime-hydrolysing (CTX-M) class of β-lactamases that are found in some *Klebsiella* spp., *Esch. coli*, and salmonellae. They have become much more prevalent in the UK and other European countries, in particular causing urinary tract infections or septicaemia. The laboratory detection of these enzymes is not straightforward, and relies on a combination of clues obtained from the results of routine susceptibility testing and additional tests based on cephalosporin-induced β-lactamase production *in vitro*.

Other types of β-lactamases that are encountered in Gram-negative bacilli include: SHV-1 and its many variants—of which there are now more than 50—that are common in *Klebsiella* spp.; the OXA group of enzymes, which can hydrolyse meticillin and isoxazolylpenicillins; and the PSE group that hydrolyse carbenicillin at least as fast as benzylpenicillin, and which were thought originally to be confined to *Ps. aeruginosa*.

Control of resistance caused by TEM-1 and some other β-lactamases produced by Gram-negative organisms is afforded by 'β-lactamase-stable' cephalosporins, and the use of β-lactamase inhibitors, such as clavulanic acid. However, some plasmid-encoded β-lactamases inactivate even the newer 'β-lactamase-stable' β-lactam agents. Many of these novel enzymes seem to be derived by mutation from the widely distributed TEM-1 and SHV-1 β-lactamases.

Most β-lactamases have serine at the active site and are often referred to as serine β-lactamases. However, some β-lactamases require zinc, and thus are known as metallo-β-lactamases; these enzymes are inhibited by the chelating agent EDTA. Metallo-β-lactamases are found in diverse organisms including *Acinetobacter* spp., *Ps. aeruginosa*, and the *Bacteroides* group. They hydrolyse virtually all β-lactam compounds, including the carbapenems (p. 19) and enzyme inhibitors such as clavulanic acid do not offer protection (Table 10.3). Serine β-lactamases that inactivate carbapenems have also been described. Fortunately, strains that elaborate such enzymes are still relatively uncommon, although they are now being reported with increasing frequency from many different countries. Increasing numbers of outbreaks are reported involving multiresistant *Klebsiella* strains that have also acquired a carbapenemase, leaving very few therapeutic options.

Aminoglycosides

Resistance to aminoglycosides results largely from interference with the drug transport mechanism following modification of the antibiotic by one or more of a series of enzymes produced by the resistant bacteria. Such aminoglycoside-modifying enzymes are often plasmid-encoded, but have been associated increasingly with the presence of transposons (p. 105) and integrons (p. 105). They

Table 10.3 Examples of carbapenemases and their most common host bacteria

	Pseudomonas	Acinetobacter	Enterobacteria
KPC	–	–	+++
OXA	–	+++	+
GES	+	–	+
VIM*	++	+/–	+
IMP*	++	+/–	+
SPM*	+++	–	–
NDM*	–	–	++

*metallo-β-lactamases; others are serine β-lactamases.

Table 10.4 Examples of some of the most common aminoglycoside-modifying enzymes and their characteristic substrates

Enzyme	Typical substrates	Bacterial distribution	
		Gram-positive	Gram-negative
Acetyltransferases			
AAC (3)-I	Gen	−	+
AAC (3)-II	Gen, Tob, Net	−	+
AAC (3)-IV	Gen, Tob, Net	−	+
AAC (2′)	Gen, Tob	−	+
AAC (6′)-I	Tob, Amk, Net, Kan	+	+
AAC (6′)-II	Gen, Tob, Net	−	+
Nucleotidyltransferases			
ANT (4′)	Tob, Amk, Kan, Neo	+	(−)
ANT (2″)	Gen, Tob, Kan	−	+
Phosphotransferases			
APH (3′)-III	Kan, Neo	+	−
APH (3′)-VI	Neo, Kan, Amk	+	+
APH (2″)	Gen, Tob, Kan	+	−

(−) indicates that this activity is uncommon. Amk, amikacin; Gen, gentamicin; Kan, kanamycin; Neo, neomycin; Net, netilmicin; Tob, tobramycin. The figure in brackets indicates the site of modification according to the internationally accepted numbering system for the various parts of the complex aminoglycoside molecule (see Fig. 10.2).

are classified according to the precise type of modification performed, and by the site of modification on the aminoglycoside molecule. Over 30 such modifying enzymes and their variants have been identified by biochemical or nucleic acid-based methods, and these can be divided into three main groups: aminoglycoside acetylating enzymes; nucleotidyltransferase enzymes; and phosphorylating enzymes. Examples of the most widely distributed enzymes are listed in Table 10.4.

Figure 10.3 shows the structure of kanamycin A, a typical aminoglycoside, and indicates the various sites at which modification can take place. The presence or absence of available amino or hydroxyl groupings affects the susceptibility to various enzymes; this is the basis of variability within the aminoglycoside group. The steric configuration of the groupings is also important; thus, the semi-synthetic aminoglycoside amikacin is, structurally, related closely to kanamycin A, but is much less susceptible to enzymic modification because of a hydroxyaminobutyric acid side chain that alters the steric configuration of the molecule. The acetylating enzymes, of which there are at least 16 types, catalyse the transfer of acetate from acetyl coenzyme A to an amino group on the aminoglycoside molecule. These enzymes modify only deoxystreptamine-containing aminoglycosides (p. 26) and are, therefore, without effect on streptomycin or spectinomycin. By contrast, aminoglycoside nucleotidyltransferases use adenosine triphosphate or other nucleotides as substrates and attach the nucleotide to exposed hydroxyl groups, while phosphotransferases also modify hydroxyl groups, but by attachment of a phosphate molecule.

Various patterns of cross-resistance can be shown by bacteria that produce different enzymes (Table 10.4), but these are complicated further because many clinical isolates produce more than one enzyme at any one time. Susceptibility or resistance to any one agent cannot be predicted reliably from results obtained for another; thus, susceptibility tests must be performed with the agent that is to be used therapeutically.

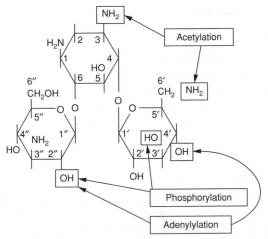

Fig. 10.3 Structure of kanamycin A, showing the sites at which enzymic modification can occur.

Although aminoglycosides exhibit poor activity against enterococci, they interact synergistically with β-lactam antibiotics to achieve a more rapid and complete bactericidal action. Unfortunately plasmid-mediated high-level aminoglycoside resistance, which abolishes synergy, has become much more prevalent in enterococci, so removing the possibility of synergistic β-lactam–aminoglycoside therapy in serious enterococcal infection caused by such strains.

When the aminoglycoside-modifying enzymes were first described, they were considered to be examples of drug-inactivating enzymes analogous to those responsible for resistance to β-lactam antibiotics and chloramphenicol. However, aminoglycoside-modifying enzymes mediate resistance by modifying only small amounts of antibiotic. They are strategically placed near the inner cytoplasmic membrane where they are accessible to acetyl coenzyme A and adenosine triphosphate. As soon as a few molecules of drug are modified, all further transport of drug into the cell becomes blocked.

Chloramphenicol

Resistance to chloramphenicol in both Gram-positive and Gram-negative bacteria is normally associated with production of an enzyme, chloramphenicol acetyltransferase, which converts the drug to either the monoacetate or diacetate. The acetylated drug will not bind to the bacterial ribosome, and so cannot block protein synthesis. Several different acetyltransferases have been described. Some appear to be genus- and species-specific; others, usually plasmid or transposon-associated, are more widespread. This variety is a little surprising since chloramphenicol has been used less widely than many other antibiotics because of its rare, but serious, toxic side effects.

Alteration or protection of the target site

Resistance arising from the selection of rare, pre-existent mutants from within an otherwise susceptible bacterial population has been described for many antibiotics. The mutations usually affect the drug target and often confer high-level resistance in a single step. The emergence of this type of resistance during therapy is an important cause of treatment failure with certain drugs, including rifampicin, the older quinolones, fusidic acid, and various antituberculosis drugs. Use of combinations of antibiotics can prevent the emergence of such resistance during therapy, since the likelihood of independent mutations conferring resistance to two or more unrelated antibiotics appearing simultaneously in the same cell is very small. This strategy has been crucial in antituberculosis therapy. Similarly, monotherapy of staphylococcal infection with rifampicin or fusidic acid should not normally be used.

Variants exhibiting low levels of resistance to almost any antibiotic can be isolated readily from most bacteria. In contrast to single-step mutants they usually develop in a stepwise fashion, and may be accompanied by other phenotypic changes (e.g. slower growth rate, colonial variation on solid media, reduced virulence). These so-called 'fitness costs' become more marked as the degree of resistance increases. It is likely that the shifts in penicillin susceptibility of gonococci and pneumococci that have occurred over the years result from such cumulative changes.

β-Lactam antibiotics

The major mechanism of resistance to β-lactam antibiotics is enzymic inactivation (see above), but mechanisms involving target site modification also occur. *Streptococcus pneumoniae* strains with reduced susceptibility to penicillin exhibit alterations in the target penicillin-binding proteins (PBPs; p. 19) that result in reduced ability to bind penicillin. Similarly, meticillin resistance in staphylococci is associated with the synthesis of a modified PBP (PBP 2′), which exhibits decreased affinity for meticillin and other β-lactam antibiotics. Low-level resistance to penicillin in *N. gonorrhoeae* has also been associated with alterations to PBPs. Such resistance appears to have developed by rare mutational events and to have become disseminated as a result of considerable antibiotic selection pressure.

Glycopeptides

Resistance to vancomycin and teicoplanin first emerged in enterococci only after the antibiotic had been available for 30 years. Expression of resistance depends on the presence or absence of several genes and two enzymes (a ligase and a dehydrogenase), which probably originated in non-human pathogens and were transferred to enterococci. The net effect of these is target site alteration. Glycopeptides bind to the D-alanyl-D-alanine terminus of the muramyl pentapeptide of peptidoglycan (p. 11). Enterococci that exhibit high-level resistance to glycopeptides produce a new dipeptide terminus, either D-alanyl-D-lactate or D-alanyl-D-serine. Such substitutions allow cell wall synthesis to continue in the presence of one or both of the currently available glycopeptides, vancomycin and teicoplanin. Several different glycopeptide resistance phenotypes have been described (Table 10.5). Glycopeptide resistance is usually inducible in those strains that posses the necessary genes and enzymes, but some essentially non-pathogenic enterococci (e.g. *Enterococcus gallinarum*, *E. casseliflavus*, and *E. flavescens*) are constitutively resistant to low to moderate levels of vancomycin.

The mechanism of the low-level resistance to glycopeptide antibiotics that has emerged in some *Staph. aureus* and coagulase-negative staphylococci has not been completely elucidated, but appears to be associated with overproduction of peptidoglycan precursors that require increased amounts of drug to saturate them. Very rare strains of *Staph. aureus* that are highly resistant (MIC >128 mg/l) to vancomycin and teicoplanin have been described. So far these have all possessed the *Van A* gene that confers the vanA glycopeptide resistance phenotype in enterococci. Some years before these clinical isolates were first seen, the *Van A* gene was successfully transferred from an enterococcal strain into *Staph. aureus in vitro*. It now appears that enterococci can also transfer the genes coding for high-level glycopeptide resistance to *Staph. aureus in vivo*. The hope is that such occurrences remain rare, and that highly glycopeptide resistant strains do not spread widely.

Table 10.5 Types of glycopeptide resistance in enterococci

Phenotype		vanA	vanB	vanC	vanD	vanE	vanG
Susceptibility to	vancomycin	R (high)	R (low or high)	R (low)	R (high)	R (low)	R (low)
	teicoplanin	R	S	S	S or R	S	S
Expression		Inducible	Inducible	Constitutive or inducible	Constitutive	inducible	Unknown
Gene location		Plasmid or chromosome	Plasmid or chromosome	Chromosome	Chromosome	Chromosome	Chromosome
Species commonly affected		E. faecalis, E. faecium	E. faecalis, E. faecium	E. gallinarum, E. casseliflavus, E. flavescens	E. faecium	E. faecalis	E. faecalis

R, resistant; S, susceptible.

Streptomycin

Streptomycin binds to a protein (S12) in the smaller (30 S) ribosomal subunit in bacteria. A single amino acid change in the structure of this protein can prevent the binding of streptomycin entirely, so rendering bacteria resistant to very high concentrations of the drug. The alteration is so specific that other aminoglycosides, such as gentamicin, are unaffected by the change.

Erythromycin and chloramphenicol

Changes in the proteins of the larger (50 S) ribosomal subunit have been implicated in resistance to chloramphenicol and macrolides such as erythromycin. However, erythromycin resistance in staphylococci and streptococci results more usually from methylation of the 23 S ribosomal RNA subunit by an inducible plasmid-encoded enzyme. Methylation of the ribosomal RNA also renders the bacteria resistant to other macrolides, lincosamides (p. 36), and streptogramins (p. 37) by reducing ribosomal binding of these drugs. Since erythromycin is a specific inducer of the methylating enzyme, bacteria carrying a plasmid encoding this property are resistant to the other drugs only in the presence of erythromycin. This phenomenon is known as dissociated resistance. Because of a similarity in the sites of action of macrolides and lincosamides, lincosamide resistance is more likely to emerge during treatment of infection caused by strains that are initially erythromycin resistant.

Fusidic acid

Fusidic acid inhibits translocation of the growing polypeptide chain. Resistance is occurs due to point mutations in the *fus A* gene, leading to altered structure of the protein that regulates this process (elongation factor G), or by expression of a protein that protects the drug target (Fus B and Fus C classes).

Quinolones

Intermediate levels of resistance to quinolones in Gram-negative rods are usually caused by chromosomal-encoded structural alterations to a subunit of the DNA gyrase target (p. 102). High levels of resistance are associated with additional mutations in the secondary target, topoisomerase IV. In Gram-positive cocci the situation is reversed, since topoisomerase IV is the primary target. In general, mutations that confer reduced susceptibility to older quinolones ('first stage mutations') may not reduce the effectiveness of newer more active versions, unless additional ('second' or 'third stage') mutations occur; an example of stepwise resistance. There is some evidence that quinolones differ in their propensity to select for resistance mutations. This observation has led to the concept of a 'mutant protection concentration'; that is, the concentration that prevents the growth of the least susceptible single-step mutant present in a bacterial population. It has been suggested that these differences between quinolones, related to their achievable tissue concentrations, may influence the likelihood of resistant mutant selection during therapy.

Quinolone resistance can be transferred by plasmids that may additionally code for resistance to other antibiotic classes. Two types of plasmid resistance occur with variable prevalence. One is mediated by the *qnr* gene, which encodes a protein that protects DNA gyrase and DNA topoisomerase from the action of quinolones. The other is a more recently discovered bifunctional aminoglycoside acetyltransferase (AAC(6')-Ib variant), which catalyzes the acetylation of fluoroquinolones and aminoglycosides.

Rifampicin

Resistance to rifampicin is invariably the result of a structural alteration in the *rpo* gene that encodes the β-subunit of RNA polymerase, which is involved in the transcription of DNA to messenger RNA; this reduces its binding affinity for rifampicin. The location of the *rpo* gene mutations is usually within a well-defined small area; molecular tests (Chapter 12) are now available for the direct detection of this gene (for example, in *Mycobacterium tuberculosis* strains).

Linezolid

This oxazolidinone antibiotic inhibits protein synthesis at the stage of ribosomal assembly (p. 25). A ribosomal mutation leads to linezolid resistance in both staphylococci and enterococci. More recently some strains have acquired a plasmid-mediated *cfr* gene, named because it caused resistance to chloramphenicol and florfenicol. This encodes a RNA methyltransferase, and affects the binding of at least five chemically unrelated antimicrobial classes: phenicols, lincosamides, oxazolidinones, pleuromutilins, and streptogramin A antibiotics. Linezolid resistance is currently very uncommon in *Staph. aureus* and is only occasionally seen in enterococci, usually associated with prolonged therapy and failure to remove or drain a focus of infection.

Interference with drug transport and accumulation

In addition to reduced drug accumulation resulting from enzymic modification of aminoglycosides (see above), interference with transport of drugs into the bacterial cell is of proven clinical importance as a cause of resistance to tetracyclines, β-lactam antibiotics, and quinolones.

Tetracyclines

Uptake of tetracyclines into cells normally involves an active transport mechanism that uses energy and results in accumulation of drug inside the cell. Plasmid or transposon-mediated resistance to tetracyclines is common in both Gram-positive and Gram-negative bacteria. Generally, there is complete cross-resistance, so a strain that is resistant to one tetracycline is resistant to all the others; exceptions to this rule may be found with minocycline. Tigecycline, which is related to minocycline, retains activity against bacteria that are resistant to other tetracyclines, possibly relating to higher affinity binding to the ribosome.

Tetracycline resistance is often associated with the synthesis of a membrane protein that mediates rapid efflux of antibiotic by an active mechanism; thus, drug entering the cell is removed almost simultaneously and so fails to reach an inhibitory level. Such resistance is normally inducible, and full expression of resistance is obtained only after cells have been exposed to subinhibitory concentrations of the drug.

Some bacteria produce a cytoplasmic protein that appears to have the function of protecting ribosomes from tetracycline attack. Also, tetracycline resistance in *Helicobacter pylori* is mediated by a modification to the ribosomal target.

β-Lactam antibiotics

The outer membranes of Gram-negative bacilli vary greatly in permeability to various penicillins and cephalosporins. Most β-lactam agents reach their targets in Gram-negative bacilli by passing through the water-filled pores (porins) that extend across the outer membrane bilayer. The rate of permeation is governed largely by the physical size of a particular β-lactam molecule in comparison with the size of the porin, but ionic charge also plays a part. In some bacteria, resistance can result from changes to the size or function of the porins, so that passage of the antibiotic is prevented. In a few instances, genes carried on plasmids encode non-specific changes in cell permeability to β-lactam antibiotics; these changes seem to affect the overall outer membrane structure of the cell. Resistance to carbapenems can be caused by loss of porins, sometimes exacerbated by β-lactamase production; e.g. imipenem resistance in *Ps. aeruginosa*.

Chloramphenicol

A few strains of chloramphenicol-resistant Gram-negative bacilli possess a plasmid that appears to confer the property of impermeability to chloramphenicol upon the host cell.

Quinolones

Gram-negative bacteria have been described in which resistance to quinolones is caused by impermeability associated with a decrease in the amount of the OmpF outer membrane porin protein. Such strains may simultaneously acquire resistance to β-lactam antibiotics and some other agents that gain access through the OmpF porin. Resistance caused by active efflux also occurs in some Gram-negative bacilli and staphylococci. This can be mediated by efflux pumps that are specific for quinolones or by non-specific transporter pumps.

Aminoglycosides

A mechanism of resistance to aminoglycosides, unrelated to enzymic modification, is associated with alterations in membrane proteins that affect active transport of the antibiotic into the cell.

Metabolic bypass

Most common resistance mechanisms can be accommodated in one or other of the three major groups described already. However, there are two known examples in which a plasmid or transposon provides the cell with an entirely new and drug-resistant enzyme that can bypass the susceptible chromosomal enzyme that is also present unaltered in the cell.

Sulphonamides

Sulphonamides exert their bacteristatic effect by competitive inhibition of dihydropteroate synthetase. Sulphonamide-resistant strains of Gram-negative bacilli synthesize an additional dihydropteroate synthetase that is unaffected by sulphonamides. The additional enzyme allows continued functioning of the threatened metabolic pathway in the presence of the drug. At least two such enzymes are widespread in Gram-negative bacilli throughout the world.

Trimethoprim

Trimethoprim blocks a later step in the same metabolic pathway by inhibiting the dihydrofolate reductase enzymes in susceptible bacteria. Resistant strains synthesize a new, trimethoprim-insensitive, dihydrofolate reductase as well as the normal drug-susceptible chromosomal enzyme. At least 14 groups of trimethoprim-insusceptible dihydrofolate reductases have been described in Gram-negative bacilli, and a further example is found in multiresistant isolates of *Staph. aureus*.

Key points

- Resistance genes located on plasmids have the greatest potential for spread within and between bacterial species.
- Co-location of resistance genes, especially on plasmids, means that bacteria can become resistant to multiple antibiotic classes.
- The widespread use of β-lactam antibiotics has led to the development of hundreds of different types of enzymes capable of rendering these drugs inactive.
- Carbapenemases (enzymes that destroy carbapenems) were once rare, but in some places are now becoming a common cause of resistance particularly in Gram-negative bacilli.
- Efflux systems can either be specific for an antibiotic or may eject multiple different classes of antimicrobial agents from the bacterial cell.

Further reading

Nature Reviews Microbiology. Available at: www.nature.com/nrg/index.html.

Nature Reviews Genetics. Available at: www.nature.com/nrmicro/index.html.

Chapter 11

Control of the spread of resistance and *Clostridium difficile* infection

The 60 year period during which antibiotics have been available has seen dramatic changes in the disease burden caused by infections. Outcomes from infections such as pneumococcal pneumonia, tuberculosis, and streptococcal puerperal sepsis, that used to cause considerable morbidity and mortality, are now frequently benign, at least in developed countries. We can also prevent much infection by using antibiotics during high-risk procedures, notably in the peri-operative period. The immense social, economic, and health benefits that are due to antibiotic use are, however, increasingly overshadowed by the issue of resistance. Indeed, the emergence and spread of multiresistant strains—sometimes referred to emotively as 'superbugs'—have raised the spectre of untreatable infection. The reality is that such instances remain extremely rare. However, resistance does limit antibiotic choice available to prescribers, sometimes meaning that less effective, more toxic, or more expensive drugs have to be used. For example, the antibiotics needed to treat multiresistant forms of tuberculosis are over 100 times more expensive than the first-line drugs used to treat disease caused by fully susceptible strains. Such excess costs mean that some infections can no longer be treated in poor communities where resistance to first-line drugs is widespread. Furthermore, significant slowing in the development of genuinely new antibiotics—that is,those with novel modes of action to which cross-resistance to older agents does not occur—has increased the potential for this threat to become a reality that once again compromises patient outcome.

Like resistance, *C. difficile* infection is a manifestation of collateral damage to the normal flora caused by use of antibiotics, which promotes colonization and subsequent infection. The solution to both problems lies in a combination of strategies to minimize collateral damage from use of antibiotics and promote use of infection control to minimize risk of colonization. Moreover *C. difficile* infection is a powerful stimulus to change because it is a very immediate threat to the patient who is receiving antibiotics, whereas selection of resistant bacteria may have no immediate impact on patients or their carers. Consequently control of *C. difficile* infection is now an integral component of most national antibiotic prescribing programs.

In 1945 during his Nobel Prize acceptance speech Sir Alexander Fleming said, 'It is not difficult to make microbes resistant to penicillin in the laboratory by exposing them to concentrations not sufficient to kill them, and the same thing has occasionally happened in the body.' This warning was evident less than a decade after the introduction of penicillin, when a particular penicillin-resistant *Staphylococcus aureus* strain started to cause outbreaks of post-operative and perinatal infection in hospitals across the world. Poor hospital cleaning, increasing dependence on antibiotics, and changing healthcare practices were blamed. Unfortunately, these issues are again topical, with frequent media headlines about 'superbugs' and their spread.

Compared with most other drugs of similar potency, antibiotics are remarkably safe, and they are also remarkably effective. This has inevitably led to liberal use so that within 10 years of the discovery, penicillin antibiotics were routinely being used to treat acute bronchitis despite the fact that treatment makes very little difference to the speed of recovery (Chapter 21). Evidence linking antibiotic use to increasing resistance in bacteria in the community and in hospitals led to calls for action from the European Union and the World Health Organization in the 1990s and to the establishment of systems for surveillance of antibiotic use and resistance. There is welcome evidence that efforts to control resistance are having an impact with reduction in MRSA (Fig. 11.1) and in penicillin resistance in *Strep. pneumoniae* in the past five years. However, at the same time resistance has been increasing in *Esch. coli* so there are no grounds for complacency.

Availability of antibiotics

Most developed countries have tightly regulated systems for the control of the manufacture, importation, distribution, sale, supply, and description of medicinal products, including antibiotics, for human and veterinary use (see Chapter 36). In the global market for medicines, licensing authorities will increasingly be required to ensure that there is a consistency of approach to medicines availability. Currently there are many examples of inconsistencies in the availability and recommendations for use of antibiotics throughout both the developed and developing world. The availability of antibiotics, notably newer, more expensive agents, is an issue in poorer countries. Pharmaceutical companies have a part to play in helping to ensure that antimicrobial agents, including critical antimalarial, antituberculosis, and antiretroviral drugs are priced and advertised appropriately in these markets.

While the sale and distribution of antibiotics are fairly tightly controlled in rich, developed countries, the marketing of these agents is much less restricted in the poorer, and numerically much larger, developing world. Paradoxically, the use of antibiotics in the developing countries

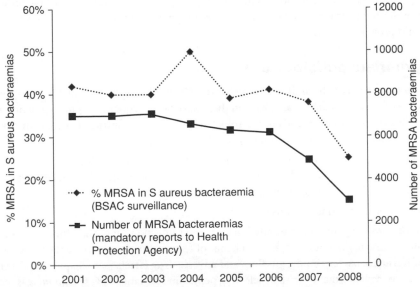

Fig. 11.1 Changes in MRSA over time in the UK measured by two different surveillance systems. The BSAC (British Society for Antimicrobial Chemotherapy) surveillance scheme collects bacterial isolates from blood and sputum samples from selected laboratories and tests them with a standardized method. The Health Protection Agency coordinates a mandatory reporting system for all cases of MRSA bacteraemias. Both systems show a downward trend from 2004 onwards Data from Alasdair MacGowan, Chair of the BSAC Working Party on Resistance Surveillance http://www.bsacsurv.org/.

needs to be extended, not restricted, if standards of health are to be brought up to those of the developed world. A key issue here is unregulated 'over-the-counter' availability of antibiotics. Controversy persists about striking a balance between making effective medicines available in a timely fashion to those who need them, against the potential detrimental effects of uncontrolled or indiscriminate use. This argument is most pertinent in the case of antimicrobial drugs, as there is no other example in therapeutics in which local misuse of an efficacious agent can lead to a general diminution in its effectiveness. It was no great surprise that chloramphenicol-resistant typhoid bacilli first emerged in South America and penicillin-resistant gonococci in south-east Asia, where unrestricted availability of antibiotics is commonplace. In some countries antibiotics can still be purchased easily as single tablets resulting in inappropriate use, suboptimal dosing, and the consequent encouragement of resistance.

In the UK, fluconazole and aciclovir have been available for over-the-counter purchase without the need for a prescription for more than a decade. There is no convincing evidence that this availability additional to prescribed courses has increased the emergence of resistance to these agents in the target pathogens—*Candida albicans* and herpes simplex virus—for which they are commonly used. This may, however, reflect inherent properties of these drugs uncommonly to select for resistant variants. There has been pressure to extend the availability of over-the-counter antibiotics to include drugs such as trimethoprim for use in urinary tract infections in order to reduce delay in access to treatment. However, the Council of the European Union in 2001 recommended restricting systemic antibacterial agents to prescription-only use. In the UK there has been extension of capacity to prescribe antibiotics (and other drugs) to other healthcare professionals, including pharmacists and nurses, which is intended to improve access to antibiotics for people with bacterial infections (Chapter 20). Consequently systemic antibacterial drugs remain prescription, only medicines in the UK, although the range of professionals who can issue prescriptions has increased.

Inappropriate antibiotic use

Attention has repeatedly been drawn to the worldwide public health problem of the spread and persistence of drug-resistant organisms, and there have been frequent calls for regulation to curb the unnecessary use and misuse of antimicrobial drugs in some countries. The following practices have been clearly identified as contributing to the present situation:

- **Inappropriate prescribing of antibiotics**—e.g. for ailments for which they are ineffective, such as for sore throats and bronchitis where they make very little difference to the speed of recovery or risk of complications (see Chapter 21).

- **Incorrect dose or duration of use**

  - *In therapy*—e.g. in uncomplicated urinary tract infection more than three days of antibiotic treatment does not increase the chance of success, but does increase the risk of selection of resistance bacteria in the gut flora and adverse drug effects (see Chapter 23). In children there is evidence that the risk of selecting penicillin resistant *Strep. pneumoniae* is increased by prescribing prolonged courses of treatment, particularly at low dose. *In prophylaxis*— e.g. for most types of surgery there is no value in giving more than one dose of antibiotic(s) and prophylaxis should never continue for >24 h after surgery (see Chapter 18). Excess antibiotic doses may encourage resistance emergence or side effects including antibiotic-associated diarrhoea and *C. difficile* infection.

- **Antibiotic use without prescription**—e.g. the uncontrolled availability of antibiotics 'over-the-counter', which can result in unnecessary use or intermittent, suboptimal dosing.

The increasing availability of antibiotics through the internet may exacerbate this risk. In some countries, poorly formulated or manufactured, counterfeited or expired antibiotics are sold and used for self-medication or prophylaxis.

◆ **Animal/agricultural use of antibiotics**—e.g using clinically useful antibiotics as growth promoters in animal feeds and on agricultural crops (see below).

Antibiotics use in animals

More than half of all antibiotics produced worldwide are used in animals, primarily as part of the food production chain. Two aspects of this use are particularly worrying. First, there is a large overlap between the types of antibiotics given to animals and those used to treat infection in man. Secondly, large quantities of antibiotics are used not to treat overt infection but instead as animal growth promoters to increase weight gain and therefore market value of animals or in prophylaxis of large numbers of animals to prevent infection. Combining these two issues, it is not surprising therefore that there is mounting evidence of resistant bacteria developing in animals and either infecting human beings or acting as a source of resistance genes for human pathogens. For example, avoparcin use in animals is linked to the development of resistance to glycopeptides in animal strains of enterococci and possibly also in human strains. Avoparcin was banned as a growth promoter in Denmark in 1995, at which point about 80% of Danish broiler chickens were colonized with vancomycin-resistant enterococci; the current prevalence is less than 5%. Similarly, fluoroquinolone use in animals has been clearly associated with the increase in prevalence of fluoroquinolone resistance in salmonella and campylobacter strains that infect man. Notably, a multiresistant *Salmonella enterica* serotype Typhimurium strain (DT104) has spread in animals, foods and, subsequently, in human beings. Recently use of a broad-spectrum cephalosporin (ceftiofur) in poultry farming has been associated with spread of ESBL resistance from *Esch. coli* in the gut flora to *Salmonella* Heidelberg with infections in humans (Fig. 11.2). In Canada, the antibiotic was being injected into all broiler eggs but there was a dramatic reduction in animal colonization and human infection with resistant *Salmonella* when this practice was discontinued (Fig. 11.2).

All use of antimicrobial agents for growth promotion is now banned in the European Union. There is some concern that the therapeutic use of antibiotics in animals may increase as use of antibiotic growth promoters is curtailed, but this is unlikely to have the same negative consequences as seen with unrestricted use of antibiotics in animals. Nonetheless, the experience from Canada shows that targeted interventions on mass prophylaxis can have important benefits for human health (Fig. 11.2).

Antibiotic prescribing in the community and hospital

The European Union, the US Food and Drug Administration, and the World Health Organization have initiated national and regional campaigns aimed at professionals and the public to reduce the unnecessary prescribing of antibiotics. Efforts have concentrated on prescribing in the community, not least because this accounts for 80% of all human use of antimicrobial drugs. Principles such as not prescribing antibiotics for viral sore throats, or simple coughs and colds, and avoiding the use of new and more expensive antibiotics—for example, quinolones and cephalosporins (see Fig. 19.4)—when standard and less expensive antibiotics remain effective have been emphasized. Prescribing of antibiotics started to fall in England in 1995–1996. The decrease subsequently stabilized, with a slight rise in 2003–2004 (Fig. 11.3). However, much greater reduction in antibiotic use was achieved in Belgium (Fig. 11.3) and in France where annual, national campaigns

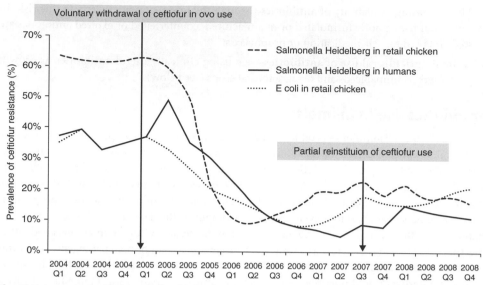

Fig. 11.2 Impact of withdrawal of ceftiofur for *in ovo* use in chickens in Quebec, Canada on the prevalence of resistant strains. Ceftiofur is a third generation cephalosporin licensed for veterinary use. Prior to the withdrawal it was injected *in ovo* to control *Escherichia coli* omphalitis in broiler chickens. Withdrawal coincided with reduction in the prevalence of resistant strains of *Salmonella* in humans as well as *Salmonella* and *E coli* in chickens. These strains exhibited multi-resistance mediated by ESBLs (extended spectrum β-lactamases). Redrawn from data in Figure 2 of Dutil, L, Irwin, R, Finley, R, Ng, LK, Avery, B, Boerlin, P, Bourgault, AM, Cole, L, Daignault, D, Desruisseau, A, Demczuk, W, Hoang, L, Horsman, GB, Ismail, J, Jamieson, F, Maki, A, Pacagnella, A, Pillai, DR (2010) Ceftiofur resistance in Salmonella enterica serovar Heidelberg from chicken meat and humans, Canada. *Emerging Infectious Diseases* **16**(1): 48–54.

targeted at public and professionals achieved 50% reduction over five years. The ESAC (European Surveillance of Antibiotic Consumption) project provides publicly accessible national comparisons of community antibiotic use in all European countries and has acted as an important stimulus to change in Belgium and France, which were amongst the highest users of antibiotics when ESAC began in 2001. In Sweden, use of antibiotics in 2010 was about half as much as in England and Belgium in 2005 (Fig. 11.3). Nonetheless in 2010 the Swedish Government announced a new initiative to reduce total use in the community by 36% by 2014 (Fig. 11.3).

Note that measurement of antibiotic use in Fig. 11.3 is in prescriptions per 1000 inhabitants per day. The World Health Organization's standard measure for drug use is defined daily doses (DDD) per 1000 inhabitants per day, but this is because some national data comes from drug wholesalers, who cannot provide information about the number of prescriptions. Measurement by number of prescriptions is a better guide to the number of people treated than DDD because the WHO DDD does not always equate to the actual prescribed dose, which can vary between countries. For example, when the data used in Fig. 11.3 were expressed in DDD/1000 inhabitants per day use in Belgium appeared to be 66% higher than in England in 2005 whereas the number of prescriptions was only 25% higher (Fig. 11.3). The explanation is that daily doses of penicillins in England are routinely lower than in Belgium.

It is estimated that up to 50% of antibiotic usage in hospitals is inappropriate and the problems of antimicrobial resistance and *C. difficile* infection are most likely to occur in hospital or in people who have recently been in hospital. Nonetheless, in comparison with community use information

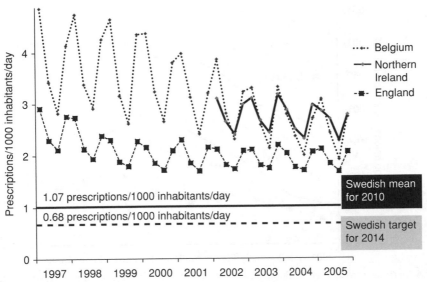

Fig. 11.3 Use of antibiotics in ambulatory care measured in prescriptions per 1000 inhabitants in Belgium, Northern Ireland, and England. The data show a marked downward trend in Belgium over the whole time period with an initial downward trend in England from 1997 to 2001. Data were only available for Northern Ireland from 2002 and showed very similar levels of use to Belgium from then on. Use in England in 2005 was nearly twice as high as in Sweden in 2010. Nonetheless the Swedish Government has set a target to reduce use to no more than 250 prescriptions per 1000 inhabitants per year by 2014, a reduction of 36% (http://en.strama.se/dyn/,84,.html) Redrawn from data originally published in Davey, P, Ferech, M, Ansari, F, Muller, A, Goossens, H, on behalf of the ESAC Project Group (2008) Outpatient antibiotic use in the four administrations of the UK: cross-sectional and longitudinal analysis. *Journal Antimicrobial Chemotherapy* **62**(6): 1441–1447.

about use of antibiotics in hospitals has been limited. For example the ESAC project can obtain data about community use from 30 countries but only 19 can provide national data about hospital use. The ESAC project has therefore focused on disseminating new methods for hospitals to measure their use through point prevalence surveys of treatment of individual patients and through longitudinal analysis of data from hospital pharmacies. The European Centre for Disease Control will co-ordinate the first Europe-wide point prevalence survey of antibiotic use and hospital-acquired infection in 2012. Interventions to improve antibiotic prescribing for hospital inpatients can be successful, and importantly may reduce antimicrobial resistance or hospital-acquired infections, such as *C. difficile* infection (Fig. 11.5). A key issue is choosing the most appropriate control methods for a given setting and ensuring that they are sustainable. The scope of measures that can be used to reduce inappropriate antibiotic prescribing is too large to consider in detail here, but can generally be grouped into restrictive versus non-restrictive approaches (see Chapters 19 and 20).

Appropriate antibiotic use

The World Health Organization advocates the following 12 key interventions to promote more rational use of medicines in general. All are applicable to antibiotic use:

♦ Establishment of a multidisciplinary national body to coordinate policies on medicine use;

♦ Use of clinical guidelines;

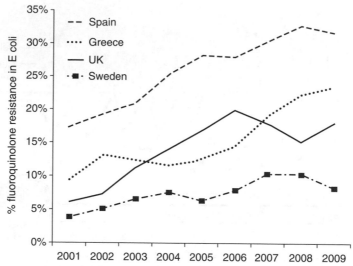

Fig. 11.4 Increase in resistance to fluoroquionlones in *Esch. coli* in Greece, Spain, Sweden and the UK. Data are for invasive isolates (blood or CSF). Drawn from data obtained from the EARS-NET on line Table Reports page http://ecdc.europa.eu/en/activities/surveillance/EARS-net/database/Pages/table_reports.aspx.

- Development and use of national essential medicines list;
- Establishment of drug and therapeutics committees in districts and hospitals;
- Inclusion of problem-based pharmacotherapy training in undergraduate curricula;
- Continuing in-service medical education as a licensure requirement;
- Supervision, audit, and feedback;
- Use of independent information on medicines;
- Public education about medicines;
- Avoidance of perverse financial incentives;
- Use of appropriate and enforced regulation;
- Sufficient government expenditure to ensure availability of medicines and staff.

In addition to these measures, good antimicrobial prescribing needs to be informed by timely and accurate information on the likely infecting pathogens. Delays in diagnosis occur through poor or non-existing sampling techniques, delay in transport, slow and laborious laboratory techniques, and unsatisfactory reporting methods (see Chapter 12). A major problem in dealing with patients in whom an infection is suspected is distinguishing between infection and colonization. Patients with an undiagnosed fever may well be colonized with potentially pathogenic micro-organisms, but may not be infected. The distinction is not always obvious, and under these circumstances it is understandable for a clinician to prescribe antibiotics. It is not rational, however, to treat patients merely because they have a raised temperature. Good practice dictates that all relevant samples for culture should ideally be collected before treatment, unless this requirement could compromise outcome (for example, in patients with suspected meningitis where prompt antibiotic therapy may be life saving). The initial choice of antimicrobial therapy will depend on the most likely infecting organism, the severity of the illness, and the type of patient (see Chapter 13). If the identity of the organism is known, then treatment can be specific and a single, narrow-spectrum antibiotic used. If the infecting organism can be targeted, then broad-spectrum antibiotics do not need to be used, thus leaving much of the body's normal flora undisturbed.

Initial (often empirical) antibiotic therapy is based on good surveillance and prompt guidance informed by accessible policies (see Chapter 19) or from infection specialists. Crucially, antibiotic prescriptions should be reviewed regularly to determine whether the drug or route of administration is still appropriate. Oral antibiotics tend to be considerably cheaper than intravenous alternatives and of course do not require an access device that itself may be a source of infection. For these reasons, intravenous antibiotics should be reviewed after 48–72 h and switched to a suitable oral formulation, which does not have to the same drug that was used intravenously. Some antibiotics are not available in oral formulation (e.g. gentamicin). Moreover, when the decision to switch to oral therapy is made, new microbiological or other information (e.g. fever defervescence for at least 24 h, marked clinical improvement; low C-reactive protein) should prompt a review of therapy and consideration of whether a switch to a narrow-spectrum alternative to intravenous therapy, or cessation of antibiotics (no infection present) is appropriate. Laboratory reports should contain information on a restricted number of antibiotic susceptibilities (see Chapter 12).

Antibiotic policies and resistance surveillance

The principles that should be followed in deciding which antibiotic, if any, to use in a given situation are discussed in Chapter 13. However, even in relatively straightforward clinical situations, there are often several equally effective agents that might be used. Choice may then be determined by a locally agreed set of guidelines for the rational use of antibiotics. The antibiotic formulary is a locally agreed list of available antibiotics, usually including some degree of restriction on particular agents. Guidance on the most appropriate use of antibiotics should not be too restrictive, should reflect local needs, and should be formulated with the agreement of the local users. Advice should of course facilitate the most effective treatment for the individual patient, but should take into account the potential consequences for the wider population. These issues are considered more fully in Chapters 19 and 20.

The best antibiotic policies are grounded in good microbiology laboratory surveillance, which is required to detect important change in bacterial resistance. Clinicians need to be aware of the local and changing patterns of infection and antibiotic resistance in their locality. Information about new agents, together with an assessment of their likely place in therapy, should be available. There are a number of caveats to pathogen and antibiotic surveillance data in general. Bias inherent in the way samples or pathogens are collected is a common problem. For example, uncomplicated urinary tract and respiratory tract infections are usually treated empirically and indeed without samples being submitted. General practitioners tend to reserve the submission of urine or sputum samples for those cases that have complicated courses or where recurrence of symptoms occurs. Thus, antibiotic treatment policies based entirely on the results of such samples and pathogens will tend to be skewed towards more antibiotic-resistant pathogens, and in turn may recommend unnecessarily broad spectrum or newer antibiotics. Such issues can be overcome by using sentinel (sometimes also called spotter) practices that submit samples from all patients with acute infections, usually for set periods of the year.

Local surveillance of resistance is limited by the reliability of susceptibility in routine laboratory practice and by limited numbers of organisms from samples other than urine. Collection of data from several laboratories overcomes these problems and allows further investigation of mechanisms of resistance. In the UK, surveillance of antibiotic resistance is conducted by the Health Protection Agency and Health Protection Scotland, with additional surveillance of blood and respiratory isolates co-ordinated by the British Society for Antimcirobial Chemotherapy. In Europe, data about resistance in invasive bacterial isolates (from blood and CSF) are made publicly available on the EARS-NET website. This is a network of national surveillance systems in the European countries. The national networks systematically collect data from clinical laboratories in their own countries. At present these include 900 public health laboratories serving over 1400 hospitals in Europe and providing services to an estimated population of 100 million European citizens. The national networks upload the data to a central database maintained at ECDC (The European Surveillance System——TESSy). After uploading, each country approves its own data and the results are made available from the ECDC website. The data are externally quality assured. The data allow analysis of trends in the occurrence of antimicrobial resistance over time and between different countries (Fig. 11.4). Data are available for seven bacterial pathogens commonly causing infections in humans:

- *Streptococcus pneumonia;*
- *Staphylococcus aureus;*
- *Enterococcus faecalis;*
- *Enterococcus faecium;*
- *Escherichia coli;*
- *Klebsiella pneumonia;*
- *Pseudomonas auruginosa.*

Antibiotic rotation

The selective pressure that results from relying on one or a few antibiotics has led some to explore whether antibiotic rotation (also called antibiotic cycling), particularly in the intensive care unit, can reduce or delay the emergence of resistance. However, this theory has several important unanswered issues: how often should antibiotics be rotated? Is the optimum period of usage the same for all antimicrobial drugs? Which antibiotics and classes should be rotated and in what order? What are the practicalities of ensuring compliance with a rotational policy? Current consensus is that routine antibiotic rotation should not be implemented. Indeed, several studies have been unable to demonstrate a reduction in the prevalence of resistance while antibiotic rotation was being used, and some have found that resistance actually increased during some parts of the cycle. Ironically, diverse antimicrobial prescribing may be associated with reduced emergence of resistance. This should not be interpreted as an argument for entirely unrestricted prescribing, as this is likely to be associated with suboptimal therapy for some patients.

Control of resistance and *C. difficile* infection: integration of antibiotic policies with infection control

It is essential that an active infection control programme is also in place, so that patients harbouring multiresistant bacteria are appropriately nursed, managed, and treated. While a full account of the optimal infection control procedure to minimize the risk of pathogen transmission

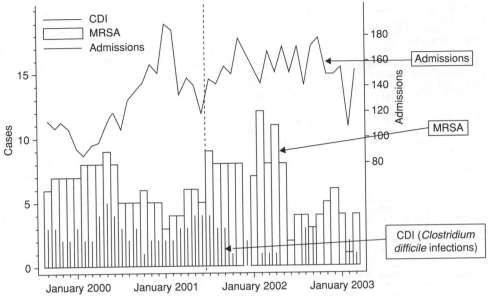

Fig. 11.5 Reduction in *C. difficile* infection associated with the introduction of a conservative antibiotic policy. Infection control practices remained unchanged after the intervention and there was no associated change in new cases of MRSA infection, which implies that the reduction in *C. difficile* infection was due to the antibiotic policy change.

is not appropriate here, some important principles are worth emphasizing. Hand hygiene is critical and should be monitored to ensure that both frequency and technique are maintained. Alcohol-based hand rubs need to be supplemented with hand washing when there is risk of *C. difficile* infection because the spores of this organism are resistant to alchohol and need to be washed off the hands. Wearing protective equipment (masks and aprons), isolation of patients at risk, and environmental decontamination are also critical. Although the need to isolate a patient may conflict with other pressures on healthcare delivery, this should not prevent infection control teams implementing this fundamental way of minimizing pathogen dissemination risk where appropriate. Patients may be isolated in single rooms or cohort-isolated in groups of beds or on dedicated units. Controversy still exists about the true control benefit of screening for specific potential pathogens such as MRSA. The role and benefit of new rapid screening methods, usually based on DNA detection, remain to be determined. Alternative approaches include targeted prophylaxis against such pathogens in patients undergoing high-risk procedures such as surgery.

The evidence base for antibiotic stewardship and infection control interventions is steadily growing but will be greatly strengthened by standardized reporting of interventions to manage outbreaks and to reduce endemic levels of resistance and *C. difficile* infection (Figs. 11.5 and 11.6). In addition to showing the impact of a conservative antibiotic policy on reducing *C. difficile* (Fig. 11.5) this work provides a demonstration of documentation of infection-control practices and patient demographics before and after the intervention (Fig. 11.6).

Setting: three acute-care words for the elderly (78 beds) in 1200 bed tertiary hospital with 0.3 WTE ICD and 4.5 WTE ICNs	Dates: 1 September 1999 to 31 March 2003	Population characteristics: 6129 unselected acute consecutive unselected elderly medical emergency admissions (80 years plus). Monthly length of stay 11.93–13.53 days. Endemic CDI and E-MRSA 15 and 16. No inter-hospital transfers.

Major infection control changes during the study: change from 'cephalosporin restrictive' antibiotic policy with audit and feedback every 2–3 months (Phase 1) to 'narrows-spectrum' antibiotic policy with audit and feedback as before and provision of laminated pocket-sized card with policy written on it (Phase 2)

	Antibiotic policy	Audit and feedback	Isolation policy CDI	Isolation policy MRSA
Phase 1: 21 months (1 September 1999 to 30 June 2001)	Cephalosporin restrictive (see below for details)	Two or three monthly feedback of antibiotic use in notional 7 day courses per 100 admissions per month and of monthly numbers of CDI and new MRSA cases	All proven cases isolated in side rooms. Aprons and gloves worn for contact	All cases of colonization or infection isolated in side rooms or four-bedded cohort in one ward. Aprons and gloves worn for contact
Phase 2: 21 months (1 July 2001 to 31 March 2003)	Narrow-spectrum antibiotic policy (Figure 2) Policy written on portable pocket-sized laminated card	As Phase 1	As Phase 1	As Phase 1

Cephalosporin restrictive antibiotic policy details (phase 1): community-acquried pneumonia (CAP), amoxicillin; urinary tract infection (UTI), trimethoprim: cellulitis, flucloxacillin and benzyl penicillin; community-acquired aspiration pneumonia, benzyl penicillin and metronidazole.

Ceftriaxone reserved for: (i) severe CAP; (ii) hospital-acquired aspiration pneumonia and (iii) UTI with renal failure, Gentamicin: UTI with shock, septicaemia with no apparent focus infection and intra-abdominal sepsis (with ampicillin and metronidazole); erythromycin; penicillin allergy

Isolation details (both phases): Ten side rooms available in the three wards. One four-bedded MRSA cohort in one ward. All other beds configured in four-bedded bays. Wall-mounted liquid soap and alcohol handrub dispenser and sink in each side room. One sink for each four-bedded bay with liquid soap and, from January 2002, one wall-mounted alcohol handrub dispenser per four-bedded bay

MRSA screening policy (both phases): admission screening (nose, perineum, wounds and devices) of admissions from nursing homes and of those with a past history of MRSA (both groups admitted to side room). Patients screened during admission if they had been in the same bay with a new case of MRSA

MRSA eradication policy (both phases): intranasal mupirocin and chlorhexidine body washes and shampoo for patient with no wounds. Clearance defined as three consecutive negative weekly swabs

Definition CDI (both phases): an episode of diarrhoea a sample of which was positive for toxin (I). No culture or typing performed

Definition of new MRSA acquisition (both phases): cases found on screening or clinical specimens taken > 48 h after admission. No routine typing performed but E-MRSA 15 and 16 endemic

Fig. 11.6 Description of population, clinical setting, nature, and timing of antibiotic prescribing and infection control interventions before (Phase 1) and after (Phase 2) introduction of: ICD, infection control doctor; ICN, infection control nurse; WTE, whole-time equivalent.

Key points

- Emergence and spread of antimicrobial resistance is an inevitable consequence of widespread use of antibiotics in medical and veterinary practice.

- The problem of *C. difficile* infection is another manifestation of collateral damage from antibiotic use that is a more immediate threat to patients than resistance.

- Surveillance of antibiotics and microbes are critical to the control of resistance and *C. difficile* infection.

- In the last 10 years there has been increasing evidence that both national campaigns and targeted interventions have been successful in reducing both resistance and *C. difficile* infection.

- Standardized methods for reporting are critical to building the evidence base and should always include details of changes in antibiotic use and infection control practices.

Further reading

BSAC Surveillance of blood and respiratory isolates. Available at: http://www.bsacsurv.org.

European Antimicrobial Resistance Surveillance Network (EARS-Net). Available at: http://www.ecdc.europa.eu/en/activities/surveillance/EARS-Net/.

European Surveillance of Antimicrobial Consumption(ESAC). Available at: http://app.esac.ua.ac.be/public/.

The **ORION** statement: Guidelines for transparent reporting of **O**utbreak **R**eports and **I**ntervention studies **O**f **N**osocomial infections. Available at: http://www.idrn.org/orion.php.

Part 3

General principles of usage of antimicrobial agents

Chapter 12

Laboratory investigations and the treatment of infection

This chapter covers the basic principles and limitations of using a microbiology laboratory to obtain information on the selection and control of antimicrobial therapy. It is not a comprehensive account of the clinical laboratory microbiology. The examples used refer primarily to bacteriological practice, but the principles apply to the investigation of any infection.

In the diagnostic microbiology laboratory the aim is to identify the presence of pathogens as rapidly as possible and to provide, where applicable, antimicrobial susceptibility data to the clinician. A wide range of techniques, including microscopy, culture, antigen or antibody detection, and nucleic acid detection methods are used in the diagnostic laboratory. There is an increasing trend to standardize the protocols used to detect micro-organisms and their antimicrobial susceptibility. Also, the use of automation is increasing markedly in microbiology laboratories, which offers the opportunity of more rapid diagnosis of infection. A key issue will be demonstrating that speedier diagnosis translates to more effective treatment and of course outcome.

The importance of clinical details

When using laboratory services, it is important to provide appropriate clinical details (e.g. travel history, antibiotic therapy) on the request form; without these the optimal use of diagnostic methods cannot be guaranteed. Clinical details may dictate the tests used and influence the interpretation of the result; e.g. in a patient treated for endocarditis with a penicillin and gentamicin the optimal serum aminoglycoside concentration is lower than that required in other infections.

Crucially, many diagnostic methods, in particular those involving microbial culture, are prone to biological variability, which may hinder the interpretation of results. Clinical details can play a key part in the correct interpretation of the micro-organisms recovered from samples; for example, knowing that a patient has symptoms of a urinary tract infection (as opposed to being asymptomatic) and whether the sample was collected as a clean catch specimen (rather than via a catheter), shifts the interpretation towards the result being a clinically significant pathogen. Bacteria commonly colonize foreign bodies, such as catheters, drains, and breathing tubes, and other sites including surgical wounds and ulcers. In the absence of specific symptoms of infection, recovered micro-organisms may simply reflect 'normal' flora at that site.

Interpretation of the results of specimens taken from areas of the body that have a resident microbial flora, and which may sometimes assume a pathogenic role, is particularly difficult. Culture results from respiratory sources are often the most difficult to interpret, given that sputum has to traverse sites with their own flora (e.g. the mouth) before reaching the specimen pot. *Candida albicans* is often a harmless commensal, although it can cause serious disease in immunocompromised patients. The ability of some organisms to strike while the host defences are down has given them the title opportunist pathogens. However, merely by looking at cultures of these opportunists, it is impossible to say in a particular case whether or not they are adopting a pathogenic role. The interpretation of their detection can be influenced by ancillary findings (e.g. presence or absence of pus; numbers of organisms isolated) and most importantly by clinical information provided on the request card. If the latter is absent, non-contributory, or misleading the report issued may be valueless. Conversely, demonstration of M. tuberculosis is always significant, and even in the absence of clinical disease the patient must be further examined and treated.

Although many diseases have a well-defined microbial aetiology, the clinical information and the results of specimen examination are often insufficient to form a definitive opinion as to the microbial cause in an individual case. Most patients with infection survive and many improve so rapidly that the significance of microbes isolated is never known. Thus, although we know from historical and epidemiological evidence that Str. pyogenes causes tonsillitis and is involved in the aetiology of rheumatic fever, when an individual patient presents with joint pains following a sore throat we cannot be absolutely sure that the Str. pyogenes in the throat is the cause of the illness, as opposed to representing the chance finding of asymptomatic colonization in someone with disease due to another cause. In such situations, additional investigations (such as raised antistreptolysin O antibodies in the serum in this case) may be needed in order to establish a causal relationship.

In the absence of sufficient supportive information, the laboratory can adopt one of two approaches: report any microbe isolated regardless of any possible significance, or report only common pathogens and dismiss all the others as 'normal flora'. The importance of this to antimicrobial therapy is that if the isolate is not considered 'significant', no further work (including antimicrobial susceptibility tests) will be carried out. The corollary is that many susceptibility tests may be carried out, some unnecessarily. This occurs more commonly than is usually admitted. In turn patients may be prescribed unnecessary and potentially toxic antimicrobial drugs because commensal bacteria isolated from a badly taken specimen were considered significant and susceptibility results issued. Sometimes a great deal of effort and expense is put into treating colonizing organisms that are merely filling a vacuum left by the normal flora and would quietly disappear if antimicrobial chemotherapy were withheld.

Specimen collection

Clinical laboratories rely on the quality of the specimens they receive; none more so than microbiology departments where the final result may depend on the degree of care observed in taking the specimen. A single contaminating bacterium introduced into a blood culture during collection may result in a patient being incorrectly diagnosed as having bacteraemia. Similarly, extraneous nucleic acid contaminating a sample can cause a false positive result, for example in mid-stream samples from women tested for chlamydial or gonococcal infection. Such an error could have profound consequences.

Some of the more common problems are:

◆ *Inappropriate specimen*. Saliva is submitted instead of sputum; a superficial skin swab is taken instead of a swab of pus (a specimen of pus in a sterile bottle is always preferable to a swab when possible);

◆ *Inadequate specimen*. The specimen may be too small (especially fluids for culture for tubercle bacilli). Rectal swabs are not an adequate substitute for faeces. It is almost impossible to interpret the significance of microbes cultured in tracheal aspirate in a patient who is ventilated, because of the likely presence of colonizing upper respiratory tract flora. Deep respiratory specimens, such as broncho-alveolar lavage fluid, are highly preferable to make an accurate diagnosis of pneumonia in such critically ill patients;

◆ *Wrong timing*. Specimens taken after the start of chemotherapy, when the causative organism may no longer be demonstrable, or after the patient has recovered. It is not uncommon for the laboratory to receive rock-hard faeces from patients with 'diarrhoea'. Many laboratories will not process non-diarrhoeal faecal samples;

◆ *Wrong container.* Blood for culture put in a plain (sometimes non-sterile) bottle instead of the correct culture fluid; biopsies put into bactericidal fixatives such as formalin;

◆ *Clerical errors.* Incorrect labelling; incomplete or misleading information on request forms.

Specimen transport

Prompt specimen transport to the laboratory is essential. Material submitted for culture may contain living cells; any delay in reaching the optimal cultural conditions will result in loss of viability. With fastidious organisms such as gonococci or viruses this may result in failure to isolate the organism. Conversely, overgrowth of pathogens by fast-growing commensals also commonly occurs during the period between collection of the specimen and processing in the laboratory, potentially obscuring true pathogens or resulting in a false positive result. For example, urine that is left at room temperature will act as a culture medium; bacteria that may be present in only low numbers may multiply to levels above the quantitative threshold that is used to define a positive result.

Specimens from potential medical emergencies, such as bacterial meningitis or malaria, should be delivered to the laboratory as soon as possible after collection for immediate processing. For swabs, most laboratories recommend a form of suspended animation in which the specimen is placed in a special transport medium comprising soft, buffered agar containing charcoal to inactivate any toxic substances. The effect of transport delays on microbe survival can be minimized by inoculating culture media next to the patient and incubating them immediately. This may be achieved in special units with laboratories attached (for example, in some genito-urinary medicine clinics), but is not practicable in most situations. An exception is blood culture, where the counsel of perfection should apply.

Near patient tests

These are becoming more widely available, for example the detection of Group A streptococcal infection in patients presenting with pharyngitis, or the identification of respiratory syncytial virus infected infants presenting with bronchiolitis. Unfortunately, however, such rapid detection methods are sometimes less accurate or complete than the laboratory 'equivalent' tests, meaning that backup testing is required, so increasing costs. They often do not permit the assessment of the antimicrobial susceptibility of the pathogen, meaning that conventional culture may be required as a supplementary test.

There is likely to be an expansion in the number of molecular tests that can be performed close to the patient, as opposed to requiring transport to a diagnostic laboratory. Currently, it is possible to detect the presence of MRSA and *C. difficile* in nasal swabs and faecal specimens, respectively, using a simple to perform, PCR-based, near patient test. Such tests offer the opportunity of rapid diagnosis of colonization or infection, but demonstration of the cost-effectiveness of these types of tests, which are often considerable more expensive to purchase, hinders their uptake.

Specimen processing

The flow diagram (Fig. 12.1) outlines the main steps that occur when a specimen is submitted for bacteriological investigation: microscopy (especially for specimens from normally sterile sites), culture, identification, and antimicrobial susceptibility testing. Even with the most rapidly growing bacteria and with improved methods, results of culture and sensitivity often take 48–h. This may

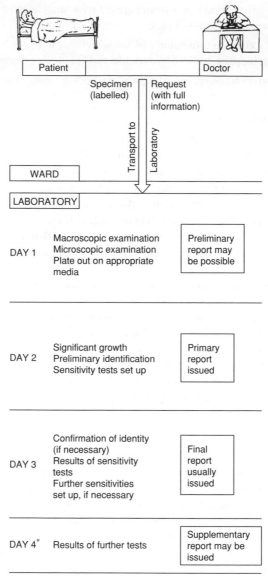

*N.B. isolation of *M. tuberculosis*, viruses, fungi, unusual organisms and special tests may take longer

Fig. 12.1 The various steps between obtaining a specimen from a patient and the issue of the final report. Note the importance of the period before the specimen arrives in the laboratory: unless the specimen is properly taken and transported it may be useless, and unless the request card is properly completed wrong tests may be done, and/or an incorrect interpretation of the result made.

be further delayed if there is a mixture of organisms or if slow-growing pathogens, such as *Mycobacterium tuberculosis*, obligate intracellar pathogens (e.g. chlamydiae), or viruses, are involved. Not all micro-organisms are readily cultivable and a report of 'sterile' or 'no growth' does not definitively mean that the specimen contained no organisms, but rather that the laboratory was unable to isolate a pathogen from the specimen. Conversely, many diagnostic specimens will grow microbes that would normally be expected to be found in particular anatomical sites, and it is important to distinguish these from pathogens; in practice this may be hard or impossible to achieve with certainty. A prime role of the medical microbiologist is to interpret such results, and advise on further testing and treatment as appropriate.

Because of the inevitable delay in obtaining culture results there is a need to inform clinicians of important preliminary findings before the complete results are known. Microscopy results are usually available on the same day as the specimen is received and in urgent cases can be reported within one hour or less. For example, a Gram-film of cerebrospinal fluid can be done very quickly and may give the physician a reliable guide to primary therapy (which may be life saving) while waiting for cultural confirmation of the result. Similarly, positive blood cultures and other findings serious to the individual patient or his immediate contacts are usually telephoned directly to the doctor. When the antibiotic sensitivity is predictable (e.g. *Streptococcus pyogenes* is always susceptible to penicillin) this advice may be given with the initial report. With many bacteria the report 'susceptibility to follow' is all that can be imparted before antimicrobial testing, although a 'best guess' based on known patterns of resistance in the hospital or community may be suggested.

Non-culture methods

Rapid advances in immunological and molecular techniques continue to provide new antigen and nucleic acid detection methods. These were initially used to make a diagnosis of infection where viruses or other difficult-to-culture pathogens were suspected. However, the diagnosis of some infections has been transformed by the availability of nucleic acid amplification tests. For example, detection of meningococcal-specific DNA in blood or cerebrospinal fluid makes specific diagnosis of a potentially life-threatening infection possible within hours. This approach can also identify the *Neisseria meningitidis* group and so detect early clusters of cases. One drawback of this approach is that without a viable pathogen it is not be possible to perform standard antimicrobial susceptibility tests (see below).

Detection of difficult to culture micro-organisms

Some micro-organisms are notoriously difficult, or indeed impossible, to culture *in vitro*. This applies to many viruses, *Chlamydia trachomatis*, a common sexually transmitted pathogen, and some very slow growing bacteria, e.g. *M. tuberculosis*. For these pathogens, culture techniques are being (e.g. *M. tuberculosis*) or have been (e.g. many viruses and *C. trachomatis*) replaced by other methods. For example, tests based on virus culture have shifted to the detection of anti-viral antibodies, usually using an enzyme immunoassay (EIA), and increasingly to direct detection of viral nucleic acid with or without quantification or typing.

Viral load measurements for the human immunodeficiency virus (HIV) are now routinely performed by a quantitative polymerase chain reaction method as part of HIV disease management. The results are used to assess patient prognosis and the effectiveness of antiretroviral therapy. Periodic monitoring of viral load can promptly identify treatment failure potentially due to the emergence of resistance to antiviral drugs. Hepatitis C virus (HCV) infection is detected initially by demonstration of anti-HCV antibodies (using an EIA). Also called 'Western blots', recombinant immunoblot assays are frequently used to confirm HCV antibody tests. Positive results are followed up by more specific tests that provided evidence of whether virus is circulating ('active') in the blood or quiescent. This is usually performed by a quantitative PCR test for HCV RNA. The next question in active HCV infection is which virus type is present, as some 'genotypes' are associated with poor response to anti-viral treatment. This is answered using a PCR test. Patients with genotypes 2 and 3, for example, are two to three times more likely to respond to interferon therapy than patients with genotype 1. Doctors typically prescribe a longer course of treatment, with higher doses of antiviral drugs, to patients infected with genotype 1.

Other molecular and mass spectroscopy tests

Micro-array technology is a method of DNA analysis that involves fixing potentially thousands of DNA probes on to a glass slide. After exposing the slide to a specimen containing pathogens, the DNA fragments that have bound to the probes are detected by chemiluminescence or fluorescence systems, the sensitivity of which may be increased using the polymerase chain reaction. This approach has been successfully applied to the detection of rifampicin-resistant strains of *M. tuberculosis*, so allowing informed choices to be made at the start of therapy. Such approaches offer an alternative source of antimicrobial susceptibility information. However, when many different mechanisms of resistance are possible, some of which may not be characterized by the presence of specific genes, then susceptibility testing by these approaches may not be possible. It is also possible that some genes although present may not be expressed *in vivo*.

Techniques based on micro-organism genotype (e.g. DNA fingerprint) rather than phenotype (e.g. whole cell protein and lipopolysaccharide profiles, antibiotic susceptibility profile, biochemical tests) are now used preferentially to determine the relatedness of clinical isolates. These techniques are useful in the investigation of outbreaks of infection, and in determining routes and sources of infection, including clusters of cases caused by antibiotic-resistant pathogens.

Even more powerful techniques for micro-organism detection and identification are starting to appear in some microbiology laboratories. Broad-range PCR is an alternative, cultivation-independent approach for identifying pathogens that recognizes conserved sequences of bacterial chromosomal genes encoding ribosomal RNA (rDNA). The resulting amplified rDNA fragments are sequences and compared with database results for known micro-organisms. Broad-range bacterial PCR has also been used to identify previously uncharacterized pathogens directly in clinical specimens.

Matrix-assisted laser desorption/ionization time of flight (MALDI/TOF) is a form of mass spectrometry, allowing the analysis of biomolecules (including proteins, peptides, and sugars). MALDI/TOF is increasingly used for the identification of micro-organisms such as bacteria or fungi. A colony of the micro-organism is smeared directly on the sample target and overlaid with matrix. The mass spectra generated are analyzed and compared with stored profiles. Micro-organism identification by this procedure is much faster, more accurate and cheaper than other procedures based on biochemical tests, which have hitherto dominated in clinical microbiology laboratories.

Antimicrobial susceptibility testing

Purpose of susceptibility testing

Since therapy of infection normally begins, quite properly, before laboratory results are available, antibiotic susceptibility testing primarily plays a supplementary role in confirming that the organism is susceptible to the agent that is being used. Sometimes it may enable the prescriber to change from a toxic to a less toxic agent, or from an expensive to a cheaper one.

Usually the laboratory report will influence treatment only if the patient is failing to respond. By this time, the laboratory should have succeeded in establishing the susceptibility pattern of the offending organism (if it is bacterial) and can advise the clinician as to how treatment might be modified. Susceptibility testing of non-bacterial pathogens is not usually possible, although limited antifungal testing is carried out in some centres. Antiviral susceptibility testing is available for certain viruses, for example HIV, cytomegalovirus, and herpes simplex; these tests require isolation of the virus and results are not usually available for a week or more.

Many laboratories record and disseminate data on the susceptibility patterns of common pathogens in the hospital and in the community to aid the choice of effective therapy. Patterns of bacterial susceptibility and resistance vary considerably from place to place and hospitals, or even wards, often have their own particular resistance problems so that the results need to be tailored to the individual circumstance. Regional, national, and international resistance trends are monitored by laboratory networks reporting to a central point.

Test methods

Most diagnostic microbiology laboratories test antibiotic susceptibility of bacteria by some form of agar diffusion test in which the organism under investigation is exposed to a diffusion gradient of antibiotic provided by an impregnated disc of filter paper. The disc diffusion method is flexible, simple, and cheap and a result can usually be obtained within a day with rapidly growing pathogens such as *Staphylococcus aureus, Pseudomonas aeruginosa*, and various enterobacteria; it is less suitable for fastidious or slow-growing bacteria such as anaerobes, streptococci, *Haemophilus* spp., and *Neisseria* spp., for which alternative procedures are preferable. *Mycobacterium tuberculosis* is very slow growing and needs special media for cultivation and susceptibility testing. These approaches are being replaced by semi-automated commercial devices, primarily when high throughput susceptibility testing is needed. Molecular methods that are able to detect DNA sequences associated with resistance traits (see above) are gradually becoming more common.

Minimum inhibitory and bactericidal concentrations

A more accurate estimate of the susceptibility of a bacterial isolate to antimicrobial agents can be obtained by titration in broth or on agar plates containing graded dilutions of antibiotics. The concentration that completely inhibits growth after a defined incubation period (usually overnight) is known as the minimum inhibitory concentration. The minimum inhibitory concentration can also be more easily (but more expensively) estimated by use of a commercial variant of the disc diffusion test, the 'Etest'.

If broth dilution procedures are used the minimum bactericidal concentration of antibiotic for the test strain may additionally be determined if so desired. The criterion for bactericidal activity is generally taken to be a one thousandfold reduction in the original inoculum after overnight incubation. This end-point is entirely arbitrary and takes no account of the rate of killing, which may be more important.

Estimation of bactericidal concentrations achieved in the patient's serum during therapy is sometimes used in infections (notably bacterial endocarditis) in which bactericidal activity is essential to a cure. The patient's serum, obtained one hour after a dose, is titrated against the organism responsible for the infection (so-called 'back titration'). The results are susceptible to methodological variation and their interpretation has been widely questioned; indeed recent guidelines do not recommend the use of these tests.

Clinical relevance of antibiotic sensitivity tests

A laboratory report of susceptibility or resistance by no means guarantees that the results will translate into clinical success or failure if the agent is used in therapy. Patients may fail to respond to antibiotics judged to be fully active against the offending microbe, or may recover despite the use of agents to which the organism is resistant. These situations arise because laboratory tests offer relatively crude estimates of susceptibility that fail to take into account many crucial features

Table 12.1 Some aspects of infection that may cause the results of *in vitro* tests not to be reflected during treatment

Micro-organism	Phenotype different *in vivo*
	Growth rate different *in vivo*
	May be adherent (e.g. device-related)
Location of infection	Intracellular versus extracellular
	Body compartment (CSF, lung, urine, etc.)
	May be associated with large collection of pus
	May be associated with foreign body
	May be within biofilm
Host immune response (and other defence mechanisms)	Contributes to recovery
	May be influenced by disease
	May be influenced by drugs (including antibiotics)
Pharmacology of drug	Pharmacokinetic behaviour
	Distribution (intracellular or extracellular)
	Metabolism *in vivo*
	Penetration to the site of infection (CSF, pus, sputum, etc.)

CSF, cerebrospinal fluid.

of the infection in the patient (Table 12.1). None the less, antibiotic sensitivity testing offers a generally reliable guide to therapy, particularly in the seriously ill patient in whom laboratory tests may provide an indispensable guide to patient care. The caveat here is that the timing of the start of antibiotic administration likely determines outcome in the very ill patient. Even delays of a few hours may reduce the clinical efficacy of antimicrobial treatment, despite the micro-organism being susceptible.

What the laboratory reports

The final report reaching the clinician must be self-explanatory, even dogmatic. It is not practicable, or desirable, to test each organism isolated against all antibiotics. A restricted range of antimicrobial agents is usually tested against isolates considered significant, with a different selection for Gram-positive and Gram-negative bacteria. Usually, only two or three of the susceptibilities tested are reported even if more are performed. Such restricted reporting has the important function of reinforcing local antibiotic policies and of discouraging clinicians from using inappropriate agents.

Primary testing is ordinarily restricted to a few old and well-tried agents that are perfectly adequate for most common infections (Table 12.2). More extensive (second-line) testing, particularly of expensive, broad-spectrum agents, is reserved for resistant isolates or bacteria from patients with serious infections that are presenting problems of management. Extended testing may also provide useful epidemiological information of trends of antimicrobial susceptibility and of clusters of multi-resistant bacteria, indicating cross-infection or spread from a common source.

Most infections are caused by a single organism, often a well-known pathogen. In these cases there is usually no problem in deciding what to test and report. However, some specimens (e.g. those from abdominal wounds) are often infected with mixtures of organisms and each must

Table 12.2 Examples of a restricted range of antimicrobial agents selected for primary susceptibility testing of some common pathogens

Organism	Antimicrobial agents tested
Staphylococcus aureus	Benzylpenicillin
	Flucloxacillin (meticillin)
	Erythromycin
	Vancomycin
Streptococcus pyogenes **(and other streptococci)**	Benzylpenicillin
	Erythromycin
Anaerobes	Benzylpenicillin
	Clindamycin
	Metronidazole
Escherichia coli **(and other enterobacteria)**	Ampicillin (amoxicillin)
	Cephalosporins[a]
	Trimethoprim
	Ciprofloxacin
	Gentamicin
Pseudomonas aeruginosa	Piperacillin–tazobactam (ticarcillin–clavulanate)
	Gentamicin (tobramycin)
	Ciprofloxacin (ofloxacin)
	Meropenem (imipenem)
Urinary isolates	Ampicillin (amoxicillin)
	Cephradine or an alternative oral cephalosporin
	Trimethoprim
	Nalidixic acid (ciprofloxacin)
	Nitrofurantoin

[a] A representative of the earlier (e.g. cefradine, cefalexin) and later (e.g. cefuroxime, cefotaxime) cephalosporins, is usually chosen for primary testing. Agents shown in brackets are examples of acceptable alternatives.

be individually identified and tested against appropriate antimicrobial agents. Laboratories usually restrict the reporting of such results to discourage a blanket therapy approach covering each and every micro-organism that is recovered from specimens taken from normally non-sterile sites.

The choice of antibiotic tested varies with the site of infection and the pharmacological properties of the drug. Some agents, such as nitrofurantoin and nalidixic acid, achieve therapeutic concentrations only in urine and are of no value in other infections. Information about the individual patient may alter drug testing:

◆ if the patient is allergic to penicillins alternatives will be sought in pregnancy, sulphonamides and trimethoprim should be avoided if possible because of the risk of folate deficiency;

◆ in a patient with worsening renal failure it may be preferable to avoid aminoglycoside therapy;

◆ tetracyclines should not be used in late pregnancy or in young children owing to deposition in teeth.

These limitations of susceptibility testing or reporting can be taken into account by the laboratory only if the appropriate information is given on the request card.

Restrictions imposed by the large number of available antibiotics may be approached in various ways. Some groups of agents, such as aminopenicillins (ampicillin, amoxicillin) or tetracyclines, are so similar in terms of their antibacterial spectrum that only one representative of each needs to be tested. With other drugs where there is differential susceptibility of bacteria to different members of the group, such a decision is less easy. An organism susceptible to cefalexin, one of the earliest cephalosporins, is also usually susceptible to all subsequent members of that group and this is often used as a screen for cephalosporin-susceptible bacteria. However, the converse is not true; an organism resistant to cefalexin may be susceptible to later cephalosporins and a definitive statement in this regard can be made only by testing the appropriate compound. The same principle applies to nalidixic acid and newer, more active quinolones.

Interpreting antimicrobial susceptibility reports

Consider a report on pus from an abscess that grew *Staph. aureus*, which was resistant to penicillin, but susceptible to erythromycin and cloxacillin. The statement 'this organism is resistant to penicillin' means that penicillin would not influence the outcome. The infection may well improve due to host defences or to adequate drainage of pus, but since penicillin-resistant staphylococci are invariably β-lactamase producers any penicillin that reached the abscess would be rapidly destroyed. Such a statement is based on sound laboratory and clinical evidence. If the *Staph. aureus* isolate was found to have relatively low-level resistance (i.e. where inhibition of growth is incomplete but less than that produced using a susceptible control organism) the likelihood of clinical resistance to penicillin is more difficult to determine; factors such as site of infection and drug penetration may be important in this respect. The laboratory will try to weigh up the evidence and score the result as 'susceptible' or 'resistant'; the term 'reduced (or intermediate) susceptibility' is sometimes used, but this is a less satisfactory alternative and leaves the clinician uncertain how to interpret the result.

The statement 'this organism is susceptible to cloxacillin' implies that use of this antibiotic (or a related β-lactamase-stable penicillin) would influence the outcome. This is more difficult to support than a statement about resistance. Treatment with the antibiotic may elicit little response in the patient because insufficient drug may have penetrated into a large collection of pus; the dosage prescribed and route of administration may be important here. More importantly (although unlikely in the present example, since *Staph. aureus* is commonly incriminated in infected wounds) the wrong organism (an innocent bystander) may have been tested. Host factors that may also influence therapeutic outcome are described in Chapter 13.

Conclusion

When in doubt, whether about the optimal specimen to submit, the interpretation of a test result or the most appropriate treatment, the laboratory should be consulted. For unusual diseases and problem cases it is often possible to seek help from specialized units such as tropical hospitals and institutes. In some countries reference laboratories are available that provide expertise in particular areas. In the UK many of these operate under the aegis of the Health Protection Agency. Worldwide, the Centers for Disease Control and Prevention, Atlanta, Georgia, USA, offer a service for the diagnosis and therapy of unusual infectious diseases.

Key points

- Supplying appropriate clinical details on request forms is crucial so that the correct tests and interpretations of results are made.

- An antibiotic susceptibility test result is relevant for a given pathogen recovered from a specific site and is not necessarily true for the same pathogen in a different site; this is because antibiotics generally penetrate some sites better than others.

- A report that a pathogen is antibiotic susceptible does not assure of treatment success; a pathogen that is reported as resistant to an antibiotic is very unlikely to respond to treatment with this agent.

- PCR-based tests are becoming the methods of choice for increasing numbers of infections, as they often offer increased sensitivity and more rapid results.

- PCR-based tests usually do not permit the assessment of antibiotic resistance, other than assays that detect specific genes/mutations associated with a resistant phenotype.

Further reading

Yang S, Rothman RE (2004), 'PCR-based diagnostics for infectious diseases: uses, limitations, and future applications in acute-care settings', *Lancet Infectious Diseases*, **4**: 337–348.

Fawley WN, Wilcox MH (2005), 'Molecular diagnostic techniques', *Medicine*, **33**: 26–32.

Mancini N, Carletti S, Ghidoli N, Cichero P, Burioni R, Clementi M (2010), 'The era of molecular and other non-culture-based methods in diagnosis of sepsis', *Clinical Microbiology Reviews*, **23**: 235–51.

Chapter 13

General principles of the treatment of infection

Antimicrobial agents are among the most commonly prescribed drugs. Their use has had a major impact on the control of most bacterial infections in man. More recently, effective antiviral drugs against herpes virus infections and HIV have revolutionized the treatment of these infections. Likewise, antifungal agents effective against invasive fungal disease are making an increasing impact. However, the repertoire of drugs to treat parasitic disease is still limited. At the same time, there are ever increasing concerns that the growing tide of drug resistance and unnecessary use are compromising their beneficial effect.

The principles governing the use of antimicrobial agents to be discussed in this chapter apply specifically to the management of bacterial infections, although the overall approach also applies when selecting treatment for other microbial diseases.

General issues

Antimicrobial therapy demands an initial clinical evaluation of the nature and extent of the infective process and knowledge of the likely causative pathogen(s). This assessment should be supported, whenever practicable, by laboratory investigation aimed at establishing the microbial aetiology and its susceptibility to antimicrobial agents appropriate for the treatment of the infection. The choice of drug, its dose, route, and frequency of administration are also dependent upon an appreciation of the pharmacological and pharmacokinetic features of a particular agent and evidence from clinical trials. Furthermore, the range and predictability of adverse reactions to a particular compound must be kept in mind and minimized whenever possible.

Clinical assessment

The clinical evaluation is critical to defining the anatomical location and severity of the infective process. The history and examination frequently determine such infective states as meningitis, arthritis, pneumonia, and cellulitis. Although such diseases may be caused by a wide variety of organisms, the range of pathogens is usually limited, and the pattern of susceptibility reasonably predictable on the basis of current microbiological, preferably local, information. This, therefore, permits a rational selection of chemotherapy in the initial management of such infections.

The anatomical location is not only critical from the point of view of the most likely pathogen and the most suitable choice of drug, but often determines the route of administration. Superficial infections of the skin, such as impetigo, which is caused by *Streptococcus pyogenes* or *Staphylococcus aureus*, or infection of the mucous membranes such as oral or vaginal candidiasis, caused by *Candida albicans*, respond well to topical application. However, if infection is caused by the microbial invasion of tissues or the bloodstream, adequate tissue concentrations of a drug may be achieved only by intravenous or intramuscular administration.

Other clues as to the nature of the infection are gleaned from epidemiological considerations such as the age, sex, and occupation of the patient. In tropical countries, diseases such as malaria, amoebiasis, and salmonellosis (including typhoid fever) are prime suspects in the investigation of fever and diarrhoea, and local knowledge about the prevalence of diseases such as filariasis, schistosomiasis, and trypanosomiasis, which are circumscribed in distribution, may be used to advantage. In countries free from these diseases as indigenous problems, a history of overseas travel should alert the physician to consider exotic infections.

Pre-existing medical problems may predispose to infection; such conditions include chronic lung disease, valvular heart disease, underlying malignancy, or the presence of prosthetic devices such as artificial hip joints, heart valves, or intravascular cannulae.

Under some circumstances the invading pathogen may be part of the host's normal flora. The normal host defences may be breached in a variety of ways. For example, the skin or mucous membranes, which are normally a most effective barrier against infection, may permit access of pathogenic organisms to the deeper tissues when traumatized by a surgical incision or by accident. Similarly, burns can denude large areas of the body with subsequent infection by bacteria, notably *Pseudomonas aeruginosa, Staphylococcus aureus*, and *Str. pyogenes*, which may be acquired from the host's normal flora or from contact with patients or staff within the hospital.

The host's inflammatory response includes circulating and tissue phagocytes, activation of the complement system and antibodies as well as the cytokine cascades, provide an important defence against infection. Therefore, an absolute or relative deficiency of circulating polymorphonuclear leucocytes is commonly associated with recurrent, frequently serious, infection. In patients with acute leukaemia, cytotoxic chemotherapy often depresses the circulating leucocytes to low levels for several days or weeks. Similar risks arise in relation to bone marrow transplantation. Such patients are extremely vulnerable to serious episodes of infection, particularly bloodstream invasion, which carries a high mortality if not properly treated.

Laboratory assessment

Few infective conditions present such a typical picture that a definitive clinical and microbiological diagnosis can be made without recourse to the laboratory. Therefore, whenever possible, a clinical diagnosis should be supported by appropriate laboratory investigations to confirm the microbiological nature of the infection. Such confirmation makes both the diagnosis and the management, in particular the selection of antimicrobial chemotherapy, more certain and allows for a more sound assessment of the likely prognosis. However, when infection is obvious or strongly suspected on clinical grounds, therapy should be commenced as soon as appropriate specimens for laboratory investigation have been taken. In some cases (e.g. pneumococcal or meningococcal meningitis) the patient's chances of survival are directly related to the promptness with which therapy is started. Furthermore, laboratory reports are not always contributory and several days may be lost trying to establish a microbiological diagnosis, during which time the patient's condition may deteriorate.

Serological tests that demonstrate antibody against specific microbial antigens are important in the diagnosis of more persistent infections such as syphilis, Lyme disease, and Q fever. Tests to demonstrate the presence of microbial antigens are also valuable in the diagnosis of selected infections. For example, fluorescent antibody reagents can detect *Pneumocystis jiroveci (carinii)* in sputum or bronchial lavage material, and pneumococcal antigen is often present in the urine of patients with pneumococcal pneumonia.

Assessment of sepsis and the systemic inflammatory response

Sepsis is defined as the combination of symptoms or signs of a localized primary site of infection plus evidence of a systemic inflammatory response. This systemic inflammatory response syndrome (SIRS) is often the first sign that infection is spreading from the primary site and that the patient may, for example, be bacteraemic (see Chapter 26).

Infection is not the only cause of systemic inflammatory response syndrome. Other causes include: accidental or elective trauma (it is a normal reaction to elective surgery); chronic inflammatory conditions (e.g. arteritis, systemic lupus erythematosus); and malignancy (especially lymphoma but also solid tumours). Also, the syndrome can be a response to infection by any type of pathogen, bacterial, fungal, protozoal, and viral. None the less, measurement of inflammatory response is a key part of the clinical assessment of bacterial infection. For example, if a woman presenting with dysuria plus frequency is found to have evidence of the systemic inflammatory response syndrome it means that she is likely to have more than a localized cystitis (Chapter 23), but that infection has spread into the kidney and possibly into the bloodstream.

Severe sepsis is characterized by hypotension, organ and tissue hypoperfusion leading to acute confusion, hypotension, oliguria, and hypoxia or lactic acidosis.

The greater the severity of infection and organ/tissue dysfunction, the higher the mortality associated with bacteraemia. On average this is 10–20%, but increases to 20–30% with systemic inflammatory response syndrome, 30–50% with severe sepsis, and 50–80% with septic shock.

Selection of antimicrobial chemotherapy

In vitro susceptibility

In vitro testing of drugs provides indirect evidence of the likely clinical response of a particular pathogen to a specific drug or drugs. Confirmation of clinical efficacy can be determined only *in vivo*; hence the importance of clinical evaluation of all new antimicrobial agents. Controlled experimental evidence gained from the treatment of artificial infections in animals provides indirect but often useful evidence of the likely clinical efficacy. Occasionally *in vitro* evidence of activity is not borne out by *in vivo* evidence of success. For example, *Salmonella enterica* serotype Typhi, the cause of enteric (typhoid) fever, is susceptible *in vitro* to many drugs active against Gram-negative bacilli, including gentamicin; however, typhoid fever responds clinically only to chloramphenicol, amoxicillin, co-trimoxazole, ciprofloxacin, ceftriaxone, and azithromycin. This may in part be due to the intracellular location of the pathogen in this disease.

Bacteristatic or bactericidal agents

Antibacterial agents are often separated into either bactericidal or bacteristatic agents according to their ability to kill or inhibit bacterial growth. Examples of bactericidal drugs include the β-lactam agents and fluoroquinolones; bacteristatic agents include the tetracyclines, sulphonamides, and chloramphenicol. This separation is somewhat artificial since some bacteristatic drugs may be bactericidal either in higher concentrations or against different bacterial species. Bacteristatic agents must rely on host defences, in particular the phagocytic cells, to finally eliminate the infection, since if the drug is withdrawn early, bacteria have the opportunity to recover. In the treatment of most mild to moderate infections, the choice between a bactericidal or a bacteristatic agent is not critical. This is not the case in the treatment of more serious infections such as infective endocarditis. Here bacteria are protected against phagocytic activity within the vegetations present on the deformed or prosthetic heart valve or adjacent endocardium. Under these circumstances it is important to use a bactericidal drug or combination of drugs that penetrate the vegetations and kill the infecting organism. Similarly, patients with neutropenia from cytotoxic chemotherapy or other causes of bone marrow aplasia are extremely vulnerable to infection. Bacteristatic drugs are inappropriate in these cases and bactericidal agents should be selected.

Pharmacokinetic factors

The aim of chemotherapy is to eliminate an infection as rapidly as possible. To achieve this, a sufficient concentration of the drug or drugs selected must reach the site of infection. The choice of agent is, therefore, as much dependent upon the pharmacological and pharmacokinetic features of the drugs, which determine absorption, distribution, metabolism, and excretion, as upon its antimicrobial properties. These aspects are discussed in more detail in Chapter 14.

In general, drugs are administered either topically, by mouth, or by intravenous or intramuscular injection. Oral absorption can be erratic. Drugs must first negotiate the acid condition of the stomach before being absorbed, usually from the proximal small bowel. This occurs most readily when the stomach is empty and it is generally advised that they be swallowed approximately 30 min before or four hours after a meal.

Absorption can be increased by protecting a drug from acid inactivation by a coating (so-called enteric coating), which subsequently breaks down once the tablet is beyond the stomach. Alternatively, the drug may be modified chemically to produce a more acid-stable formulation (see p. 156). For most minor infections, including skin, soft-tissue, respiratory tract, and lower urinary tract infection, oral therapy is quite appropriate.

In contrast to oral administration, intravenous administration avoids the vagaries of gastrointestinal absorption, and achieves rapid therapeutic blood and tissue concentrations. Intramuscular administration requires absorption through the tissue capillaries and is generally rapid except in conditions of cardiovascular collapse and shock, when tissue perfusion is impaired. It is little used in practice. Relatively avascular sites such as the aqueous, and in particular the vitreous humour of the eye, are difficult sites in which to achieve adequate concentrations of drugs. In contrast, the presence of inflammation increases the permeability of many natural barriers such as the meninges and in this situation allows higher concentrations of certain drugs, such as the penicillins, to be achieved within the cerebrospinal fluid. Other drugs, most notably chloramphenicol, are little affected by such inflammatory changes.

Choice of antimicrobial regimens

Drug dosing

There are no universally applicable guidelines for drug dosing. However, awareness of the relationship between the pharmacokinetic profile of a drug and the minimum inhibitory concentration (MIC) against a target pathogen has greatly assisted in improved definition of dosage regimens of some antibiotics. These provide a pharmacodynamic prediction of the optimum dosage regimen (Chapter 14). Other factors that influence drug dosing are tolerability and toxicity. Some agents, most notably the penicillins, have such a wide margin of safety that high doses can be safely prescribed. Only in a few cases (e.g. treatment of *Ps. aeruginosa* infection with piperacillin) does such antimicrobial overkill have a microbiologically rational basis. The ratio of peak plasma concentration (C_{max}) to the MIC, or area under the curve (AUC) to MIC is shown

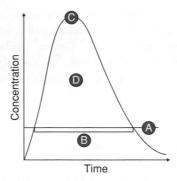

Fig. 13.1 Relationship between the pharmacokinetic profile of an antibiotic and the minimum inhibitory concentration against a hypothetical target microorganism. (A) Minimum inhibitory concentration; (B) time above minimum inhibitory concentration; (C) peak; (D) area under the curve >minimum inhibitory concentration. Redrawn from: Finch RG. Antimicrobial therapy: principles of use. *Medicine* 2009; **37**: 545–550 with permission from Elsevier.

in Fig. 13.1. This pharmacodynamics approach is often used to calculate the dose and frequency of administration to ensure the most effective drug concentrations. The C_{max}:MIC ratio is the best predictor of bacterial killing for the aminoglycosides and quinolones, while the AUC:MIC ratio is used to determine dosage schedules for β-lactam agents. In the case of bacterial meningitis much higher ratios are required to achieve therapeutic concentrations in the cerebrospinal fluid. However, for many earlier licensed agents, the dosages are based on experience gained from clinical trials of the treatment of a wide variety of infections and are included in the *Summary of Product Characteristics* (Data Sheets) of approved agents.

Length of therapy

Treatment should continue until all micro-organisms are eliminated from the tissues or the infection has been sufficiently controlled for the normal host defences to eradicate it. This end point is in general determined by clinical observation and evidence of the resolution of the inflammatory process such as the return of body temperature and white cell count to normal. Microbiological end points may be appropriate for some infections, such as urinary tract infections where repeat urine cultures can be obtained one week and four to six weeks after stopping therapy. These will indicate failed acute treatment and recurrent infection respectively. However, other outcomes include length of stay and time to discharge (for those in hospital), and time to return to former activities. These factors are important when determining the health economics of disease management.

Many infections come under control within a few days and five to seven days' treatment is often sufficient. Uncomplicated urinary tract infections usually respond very rapidly to short course (three day) therapy. Selection of the least dose compatible with complete resolution is desirable (see Chapter 23). In contrast, patients with pulmonary tuberculosis require six months' treatment with isoniazid and rifampicin after an initial two month three to four drug regimen if relapse is to be prevented (see Chapter 30). Furthermore, 10 days' penicillin treatment is necessary to eradicate *Str. pyogenes* from the throat in patients with streptococcal tonsillitis, although symptomatic improvement occurs within a few days. There is no universally 'correct' duration of chemotherapy and each problem should be judged on its merits based on the clinical response to treatment.

Adverse reactions

Antimicrobial agents, like all other therapeutic substances, have the potential to produce adverse reactions. These vary widely in their nature, frequency, and severity. Many reactions, such as gastrointestinal intolerance, are minor and short lived but others may be serious, life-threatening, and occasionally fatal. Drug reactions are unfortunately a common cause of prolonged stay in hospital or may precipitate hospital admission. Drug reactions may be predictable and dose-dependent, for example nephrotoxicity associated with the use of the antifungal agent amphotericin. However, many adverse reactions are unpredictable. The subject is discussed more fully in Chapter 17.

Combined therapy

In general, single-drug therapy of established infections is preferred, whenever possible. Such an approach is known to be effective and reduces the risks of adverse reactions and drug interactions that may accompany multidrug prescribing, as well as increasing the cost of treatment. None the less, for most commonly treated infections there are a few situations in which combined chemotherapy has definite advantages over single drug therapy (see below).

Initial therapy

In the management of acute and potentially life-threatening infections, combined chemotherapy covering all likely pathogens is often used until the cause of the infection is established. For example, it is common practice to combine a β-lactam (penicillin or cephalosporin) with an aminoglycoside, such as gentamicin, in the initial treatment of serious infections. If MRSA is a concern, vancomycin may be added. If there be evidence that the infection has arisen in association with mucosal surfaces, such as the gut or female genital tract, then metronidazole is frequently added to meet the possibility of a mixed anaerobic and aerobic bacterial infection. Once a definitive diagnosis is established, it is important to adjust the therapeutic regimen to one that is most appropriate.

Synergy, antagonism, and indifference

Under some circumstances, combined chemotherapy is selected for its known synergistic effect on a pathogenic organism. As such, the concentration of drug required to inhibit/kill the bacterium is significantly reduced in comparison with agents used alone. This increased ability to inhibit or kill the pathogen may speed resolution or reduce the risk of relapse when treating difficult infections. One of the commonest targets for synergistic therapy is the treatment of infective endocarditis caused by enterococci and occasionally by oral streptococci. The combination of two bactericidal drugs, penicillin and gentamicin (or streptomycin), is synergistic both *in vitro* and *in vivo* and is associated with a more favourable response to treatment than is single-drug therapy. Some drug combinations can be antagonistic such that the potency of the individual agents is reduced. Most combinations are simply additive, with no therapeutic advantage over a single drug therapy when targeting a particular pathogen. The *in vitro* effects of synergy, antagonism, and indifference against a target pathogen for various drug combinations are illustrated in Figure 13.2.

With regard to the potential for antagonistic effects of drugs in combination, one example recognized shortly after penicillin and tetracycline became available, was the fact that the two drugs together produced a worse clinical result in the treatment of pneumococcal meningitis

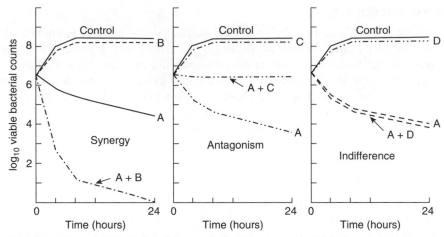

Fig. 13.2 *In vitro* bactericidal effects of drug A in combination with either drug B, C or D against a target organism to illustrate synergy, antagonism or indifference. Adapted from Lorian V. *Antibiotics in Laboratory Medicine*, 5th edition. Lippincott, Williams and Wilkins, 2005 with permission.

than did either drug alone. In this situation a bacteristatic agent (tetracycline) prevents penicillin from achieving its bactericidal effect on the bacterial cell wall, which is a function of bacterial growth.

Prevention of drug resistance

It is uncommon for a bacterial pathogen to become resistant during treatment, although some drugs—including rifampicin, fusidic acid, and nalidixic acid—encourage the rapid emergence of resistant bacteria. These bacteria do not develop resistance in response to treatment, but small numbers of pre-existing resistant mutants proliferate when the more numerous sensitive population is suppressed. Mutational resistance is more likely to arise in severe infections where the burden of infecting micro-organisms is high, such as accompanies severe multilobar pneumonia. In the treatment of tuberculosis combined chemotherapy is used specifically to prevent the emergence of resistant variants present in the tuberculous tissues (Chapter 30).

Cost

Antimicrobial drugs vary widely in their cost. In general, generic off-patent drugs cost less than proprietary preparations, and well-established, widely used agents tend to be less expensive. Injectable preparations are usually more expensive than oral preparations, and syrups and drops can be more expensive than tablets and capsules.

The use of very high dosage also escalates the cost. Sometimes this is unavoidable, as in the treatment of *Ps. aeruginosa* infections with large doses of expensive antipseudomonal agents. In general, high dosage regimens should not be used without justification.

Among the most expensive antimicrobial agents are the parenteral cephalosporins, macrolides, and quinolones, all antipseudomonal compounds, lipid formulations of amphotericin, and many antiviral agents, notably those used to treat HIV. It is, therefore, apparent that whenever drugs that are both equally effective and tolerated are available then it is reasonable to select the cheaper agent. This is a most important consideration in some developing countries where drug costs can place a disproportionate burden on an already meagre health budget. The *British National Formulary* provides a useful guide to the cost of individual drugs for prescribers in the UK.

In addition to the unit cost of a drug, other direct costs include the use of disposable materials for drug administration, staff time in preparation and administration, and assay costs to ensure adequate and safe dosaging. Comparative cure and relapse rates are also under constant scrutiny since the need for further treatment entails additional expense for the health service and more importantly risks for the patient. Economic evaluation is a key part of the assessment of healthcare but should not be limited to costs; a full economic evaluation must include measures of outcome for the patient and others such as family members or carers. The application of economic theory to evaluation of medicines is called pharmacoeconomics.

Failure of antimicrobial chemotherapy

Patients with established infection may fail to respond to antimicrobial therapy for a variety of reasons.

Choice of therapy

First, the choice of drug may be inappropriate for the infecting strain. This stresses the need to establish a microbiological diagnosis whenever possible so that the *in vitro* susceptibility of the pathogen can be confirmed. On the other hand, some infections are caused by intracellular pathogens, such as chlamydial disease, legionella infection, and typhoid fever. For treatment to be successful, sufficient antibiotic must penetrate the cell; this limits the number of agents that are clinically effective. Failure may also result if the drug is inadequately concentrated at the site of the infection; this may occur if the dose is insufficient or the route inappropriate. By changing to the parenteral route or increasing the dose, therapeutic success may follow.

The route of excretion also requires consideration. For instance, in renal failure, drugs normally excreted by the kidneys may fail to reach therapeutic concentrations in the urine so that treatment of a urinary tract infection with drugs such as nalidixic acid and nitrofurantoin may be unsuccessful.

Presence of necrotic material

Treatment may also fail because of the presence of necrotic material, an eschar, or abscess. Antibiotic penetration of such avascular material is poor, so surgical debridement of necrotic material or drainage of pus should be carried out early. Antibiotic treatment under these circumstances is an adjunct to such surgical management.

Presence of foreign material

Infection that occurs in association with bladder catheters, intravascular devices, hip prostheses, or inanimate foreign material, or that gains access to the tissues following surgical or traumatic injuries, may fail to respond to antimicrobial chemotherapy. Under these circumstances, total eradication of infection is rarely achieved until the foreign material is removed. This has serious implications for patients with prosthetic implants.

If antimicrobial therapy is to be successful, these drugs can only exhibit their full power as 'magic bullets' if used intelligently and if full recognition is paid to the need to individualize each course of treatment to both the patient and the pathogen.

Further reading

Finch RG (2009), 'Antimicrobial therapy: principles of use', *Medicine*, **37**: 545–550.

Lorian V (2005), *Antibiotics in Laboratory Medicine: Making a Difference* (5th edn). London: Lippincott, Williams & Wilkins.

Chapter 14

Pharmacokinetic and pharmacodynamic principles

Knowledge of the pharmacokinetic behaviour of a drug is key to defining its therapeutic role. Uniquely among drugs, antibiotics target infecting micro-organisms which may cause disease at either a single or at multiple body sites. Therefore, the ability to achieve sufficient concentrations at the site of infection, determines its therapeutic application. A number of pharmacokinetic factors are not only important in relation to determining infection-site drug concentrations, but also influence the safety profile of the agent. These factors are:

- Absorption
- Distribution
- Metabolism
- Elimination

Basis for therapeutic action

Absorption

When antibiotics are given systemically, the delivery and maintenance of effective concentrations at the site of infection is determined by the concentrations achieved in the blood. From serial measurements of the concentration of the agent in the serum—usually in healthy volunteers—it is possible to calculate both its rates of absorption and elimination and the volume in which the drug is distributed. The volume of distribution indicates whether it is largely confined within the vascular compartment or extends into the extracellular fluid—the site of most infections—or penetrates into cells where some organisms, (e.g. mycobacteria and legionella) multiply. The rates of transfer, volume of distribution, and other key properties can be given numerical values that provide succinct and quantitative statements of the drug pharmacokinetics. In this respect, antimicrobials do not differ from other drugs.

Many antibiotics do not produce adequate plasma levels when given by mouth and are available only as injectable preparations. In some countries injections are favoured over oral therapy, but this has more to do with cultural differences and traditions than with proven therapeutic benefit. In the UK antibiotics are usually given by mouth whenever possible, particularly in domiciliary practice, because of the convenience of the oral route.

The need for properties such as stability in solution means that pharmaceutical preparations (injections, capsules, tablets, syrups, etc.) can contain different derivatives of the drug, sometimes with distinct properties. However, in comparison with other drugs, information about intestinal elimination and distribution into tissues has special relevance for antimicrobial agents. Intestinal elimination determines the amount of an antimicrobial drug that reaches the colon, the impact on the normal flora at that site, and therefore the risk of adverse effects such as *C. difficile* colitis. Infections can occur in any tissue in the body and some pathogens survive within mammalian

Table 14.1 Bioavailability and intestinal elimination of some commonly prescribed antibacterial drugs after oral administration. Note that drugs that are well absorbed may still achieve high concentrations in the faeces because of secretion into bile or other enteral secretions. Similarly some drugs are eliminated in the intestine after parenteral administration (e.g. ceftriaxone)

Drug	Bioavailability (%)	Intestinal elimination
Amoxicillin	80–90	Concentrated up to 10-fold in bile
Cefalexin	80–100	Concentrated up to threefold in bile
Cefuroxime axetil	30–40	Bile concentrations up to 80% of serum
Ciprofloxacin	70–85	Concentrated up to 10-fold in bile; additional enteral secretion
Erythromycin	18–45	Concentrated up to 300-fold in bile
Metronidazole	80–95	Concentrations in bile similar to serum
Rifampicin	90–100	Concentrated up to 1000-fold in bile
Trimethoprim	80–90	Concentrated up to twofold in bile

cells; therefore, unlike other drugs the anatomical location of target receptors for antimicrobials is highly variable.

Oral administration

The fraction of a dose of an oral drug that is absorbed unchanged and available to interact with the target is known as its bioavailability. The degree to which antimicrobial compounds are absorbed when given orally differs greatly (Table 14.1). Absorption is one factor that determines the effect that an antimicrobial has on the normal flora of the colon but intestinal elimination is also important.

Antibiotic esters (pro-drugs)

Some drugs given orally are irregularly absorbed and often produce low plasma concentrations. Erythromycin is one example of this, and several derivatives have been produced in an attempt to overcome the difficulty. These include erythromycin estolate, which is microbiologically inactive, but is much more lipid soluble than the parent drug and much better absorbed in the small intestine, where non-specific esterases liberate the active erythromycin into the portal vein. Esterification as the means of improving the oral absorption of drugs has been fairly widely used, other examples being the esters of ampicillin, such as pivampicillin, and in the case of antivirals, aciclovir (valaciclovir). Such microbiologically inactive compounds that are converted *in vivo* to the active form are known as prodrugs. Esterification can also allow drugs such as cefuroxime axetil that must otherwise be administered by injection to be given orally. Others, like the erythromycin and ampicillin esters, increase the poor absorption of the native compound.

Parenteral administration

Intravenous injection

The most direct way of ensuring adequate concentrations of antibiotic in the blood is by intravenous injection. The highest instantaneous concentrations are, of course, achieved by a single rapid intravenous injection, but any benefit of this may be offset by rapid excretion, and many agents are given by infusion over 15–20 min. Sometimes slow infusion is necessary in order to minimize side effects (as with vancomycin, p. 177) or local reaction at the injection site.

Addition of antibiotics to drip infusions should be avoided if possible, since the slow rate of administration results in low plasma levels of the drug. Sometimes degradation of the drug in solution can occur over the prolonged period of administration, particularly if administration is combined with glucose. Certain combinations of β-lactam antibiotics and aminoglycosides mutually inactivate each other when mixed in intravenous solutions.

Intramuscular injection

When all the drug is delivered directly into the plasma, within a short time the plasma half-life is determined solely by the rate of elimination. When, however, uptake into the plasma is much slower, then the persistence of the drug will depend not only on the rate at which it is eliminated but also on the rate at which it is added. Absorption from intramuscular sites is usually rapid, but to maintain inhibitory levels of penicillin, special depot preparations, such as procaine penicillin, have been developed (p. 13). These allow slow release from the injection site so that the plasma concentration is prolonged. Intramuscular administration is now uncommon in UK practice.

Distribution

Protein binding

Compounds in the plasma generally reach the tissues by diffusion, although in some cases there is active secretion into, for example, saliva, bile, or urine. One important factor affecting the diffusibility of compounds is the degree to which they are bound to plasma proteins, mostly albumin. With some drugs, such as flucloxacillin, ceftriaxone, fusidic acid, or teicoplanin, more than 90% of the drug is bound and in this form is antibacterially inactive. Only the diffusible fraction of the drug reaches the tissues and only this fraction exerts any antimicrobial effect. As the unbound fraction diffuses away, more of the plasma-bound drug dissociates and the equilibrium between the bound and the free compound is maintained. Because of this effect in limiting the activity and diffusibility of the drug, high degrees of protein binding might be perceived as disadvantageous, notably in 'closed' sites such as joints.

However, two things have to be considered. The first is that, in order to be therapeutically effective, adequate concentrations of free drug must be achieved at the site of infection. That this occurs with the compounds mentioned, despite high degrees of protein binding, is clear from their clinical efficacy. The second is that bound drug will go wherever the protein goes and that includes the protein poured into the infected sites as a result of the inflammatory exudate. To this extent, protein-bound drug may be looked upon as a pro-drug with the valuable property of 'homing in' on to sites of inflammation. Once in the site, as far as is known, the concentration of free and active drug is still defined by the equilibrium between free and bound drug.

Another important aspect of protein binding is that drugs may compete for binding sites. It is possible for one drug to displace another of lower affinity, resulting in altered plasma concentrations and, possibly, toxicity of the liberated drug.

Tissue distribution

Infections occur in every tissue in the body, therefore information is required about distribution of antimicrobial drugs throughout the body. Most bacteria are located in the extracellular fluid. However, some bacteria (e.g. *Mycobacterium tuberculosis* and *Legionella pneumophila*) survive within cells and drugs that are used to treat these infections must be capable of entering into and functioning within mammalian cells. Viruses, chlamydiae, and malaria parasites are essentially intracellular organisms.

Distribution in extracellular fluid of non-specialized tissues

Most tissues are supplied by fenestrated capillaries, which allow the free diffusion of antimicrobial drugs from plasma to the extracellular fluid. In this case the average drug concentration in plasma is the same as in the extracellular fluid.

Plasma half-life

The time required for the concentration of drug in the plasma to fall by half is called the plasma half-life. Half-lives of different antibiotics vary considerably. That of benzylpenicillin, for example, is only 30 min, whereas that of the antimalarial mefloquine is about three weeks.

The concentration achieved in plasma while the drug is resident in the body can be measured relatively simply from serial blood samples, but the calculation of the true half-life must take into account the distribution phase (sometimes called α-phase) during which the compound is migrating from the plasma to the tissues. This is clearly influenced by the route of administration, since absorption from intestinal or intramuscular sites is not instantaneous (Fig. 14.1).

The half-life of a drug that is usually cited is that which follows distribution to the tissues and is designated the β-phase. Any metabolism of the drug, binding to plasma proteins, or alteration in the functional integrity of the organs of excretion (usually the kidney or the liver, or both) will affect the elimination of the drug and hence the plasma half-life.

Distribution of drugs into extracellular fluid of specialized tissues

In contrast to other tissues, the capillaries supplying the central nervous system, the posterior chamber of the eye, and the prostate are non-fenestrated. The tight junctions between the

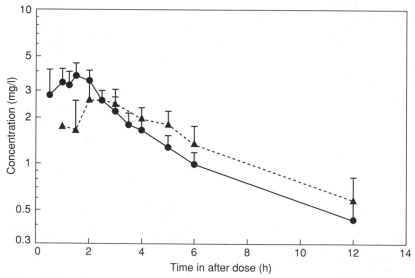

Fig. 14.1 Mean plasma (●) and inflammatory fluid (▲) concentrations following a single 750 mg oral dose of ciprofloxacin. The distribution (or α) phase lasts for two hours and is followed by the elimination (or β) phase. There is an even longer distribution phase in the inflammatory fluid where concentrations do not peak until about three hours after administration. There is a lag in diffusion of drug back into the plasma so that from three hours after administration tissue fluid concentrations are higher than plasma concentrations. Reproduced from Catchpole C, Andrews JM, Woodcock J and Wise R, 'The comparative pharmacokinetics and tissue penetration of single-dose ciprofloxacin 400 mg iv and 750 mg po' *Journal of Antimicrobial Chemotherapy*, **33**(1): 103–110, 1994 by permission of Oxford University Press.

endothelial cells of these capillaries can only be crossed by lipid-soluble drugs that are capable of passage through the cells. Concentrations of antimicrobial agents within these specialized sites cannot be predicted from knowledge of plasma concentrations. In addition to these naturally occurring specialized sites, infection may occur in sites with impaired blood supply because of trauma or because of collection of fibrin as in the cardiac vegetations that characterize bacterial endocarditis.

Intracellular fluid

Penetration of drugs into intracellular fluid depends on the lipid solubility of the drug. β-lactam antibiotics and aminoglycosides have poor lipid solubility and do not achieve high concentrations in cells. In contrast, lipid-soluble drugs such as macrolides and quinolones can achieve higher concentrations within cells than in the plasma or extracellular fluid.

Interpreting tissue distribution data

In most bacterial infections, the organisms are contained in the extracellular fluid (Table 14.2). For these infections it can be assumed that the average concentration in the plasma is a reasonable indication of the average drug concentration at the site of infection (Fig. 14.1) and knowledge of plasma kinetics is all that is required.

A drug's volume of distribution is an indicator of its tissue distribution. If the volume of distribution is between 10 and 20 litres, the drug distributes into extracellular compartments. If the volume of distribution is of the order of 25–40 litres, intracellular distribution is implied. In rare

Table 14.2 Kinetic requirements for treatment of bacterial infections at different anatomical sites

Anatomical site of infection	Natural barrier from blood to interstitial fluid?	Intracellular penetration desirable?	Penetration into luminal secretions required?
Biliary tract	No	None proven, causative organisms do not survive in cells	No conclusive evidence that antibiotics with high biliary concentrations are any more effective for treating cholecystitis
Central nervous system; meningitis	Yes, all infections	Only for listeria meningitis	Effective cerebrospinal fluid concentrations crucial
Respiratory tract	No	Essential for atypical pneumonia and tuberculosis but unnecessary for most common pathogens (*Str. pneumoniae* and *H. influenzae*)	High concentrations in bronchial secretions may be desirable when part of the aim of treatment is reduction of bacterial load in sputum (e.g. cystic fibrosis). Not essential in most pulmonary infections, including community acquired pneumonia
Skin and soft tissue	No	None proven, causative organisms do not survive in cells	Not relevant, organisms are only found in the extracellular fluid
Urinary tract	Only for prostatitis	Only for *Chlamydia trachomatis* (prostatitis/epididymo-orchitis); unnecessary for common causes of urinary tract infection	Effective urinary concentrations essential; drugs that achieve low concentrations in interstitial fluid (nitrofurantoin) are relatively ineffective in pyelonephritis

circumstances, distribution volumes may be measured in hundreds or even thousands of litres. These large volumes suggest extensive binding to intracellular protein or organelles.

Drug concentrations in tissue biopsies

Drug concentrations are measures in homogenized tissue samples; the result is therefore an average of the extracellular and intracellular concentrations. However, because cells make up about 70% of the volume of most tissue samples, the intracellular concentration has a dominant influence so that the result is not a good indicator of drug concentration in extracellular fluid, which is where most pathogens are located. For example, β-lactam antibiotics do not penetrate eukaryotic cells. Suppose that the concentration of a β-lactam in extracellular fluid is 10 mg/l: the concentration in a homogenized tissue biopsy would be only 3 mg/l because extracellular fluid accounts for only 30% of the biopsy.

Most intracellular bacterial infections occur in the lung where distribution of antibacterial drugs has been relatively well characterized. This information is of direct relevance to the management of infections caused by the obligate intracellular pathogens that cause pneumonia (*Legionella pneumophila, Chlamydophila pneumoniae, Mycobacterium tuberculosis*). Ability to penetrate eukaryotic cells is a prerequisite for drugs aimed at infections caused by these organisms. However, high lung tissue concentrations are of less certain relevance in most lung infections, which are caused by extracellular pathogens.

Drug accumulation

If large doses are given or the half-life of the drug is such that complete elimination has not occurred before the next dose is administered, the concentration of drug in the plasma will progressively rise. The excretion phase being logarithmic, the rate of elimination rises as the concentration of drug rises; eventually excretion proceeds as fast as the accumulation and the drug reaches a steady state (Fig. 14.2). In this example, the first dose results in plasma concentration that exceeds the minimum inhibitory concentration for the organism being treated but not throughout the dosing interval. If it is essential to reach higher concentrations immediately then a loading dose should be given, which is usually two to three times the maintenance dose.

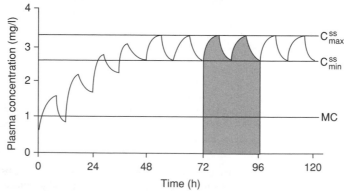

Fig. 14.2 Illustration of a drug dosed twice daily that takes five doses to reach steady state. The shaded area shows the area under the concentration-time curve at steady state over 24 h. C_{max}^{ss} is the maximum (or peak) concentration at steady state and C_{min}^{ss} is the minimum (or trough) concentration at steady state. MIC is the minimum inhibitory concentration for a target pathogen. Reproduced from 'Basis of Anti-Infective Therapy: Pharmacokinetic - Pharmacodynamic Criteria and Methodology for Dual Dosage Individualisation' by Sanchez-Navarro A and Sanchez Recio MM, *Clinical Pharmacokinetics*, 1999, **37**(4): 289–304, with permission from Wolters Kluwer Health.

The possibility of accumulation and its consequences must be considered when an agent with a long half-life is administered or the patient's capacity to eliminate the agent is known or thought likely to be impaired and the agent has dose-related side effects.

Metabolism

Many antibiotics are modified in the body; the resulting metabolites are important for several reasons. First, they are generally, though not always, microbiologically less active than the parent compound. Some metabolites show not only different degrees, but also different spectra, of activity. In addition, metabolites may differ from the parent compounds in toxicity. If they are relatively inactive and more toxic, conventional microbiological assay of the drug will give very poor guidance as to the toxic hazard. This is particularly true of allergy, which can be triggered by tiny concentrations of minor metabolites rather than the parent compound. Finally, the metabolites may display altered pharmacokinetic characteristics, so that the period for which they are present in the body and able to achieve an antibacterial (or toxic) effect may be longer, or shorter than that of the parent compound.

Occasionally, it is necessary to prevent metabolism from occurring. The carbapenem antibiotic imipenem is susceptible to a renal dehydropeptidase that opens the β-lactam ring. Consequently, imipenem is formulated with a dehydropeptidase inhibitor, cilastatin, which protects it from inactivation.

Antimicrobial agents that are metabolized are particularly liable to interact with other drugs. This is most likely to be a problem in intensive care, where patients are critically ill and receiving multiple drugs. Antimicrobial compounds that inhibit the metabolism of other drugs in the liver include macrolides, fluoroquinolones, and antifungal azoles. On the other hand, rifampicin is a non-specific inducer of hepatic metabolism and may therefore cause therapeutic failure of other co-administered drugs by increasing their clearance. Drugs frequently used in intensive care that are at risk of clinically relevant pharmacokinetic interactions with anti-infective agents include some benzodiazepines (especially midazolam and triazolam), immunosuppressive agents (cyclosporin, tacrolimus), anti-asthmatic agents (theophylline), opioid analgesics (alfentanil), anticonvulsants (phenytoin, carbamazepine), calcium antagonists (verapamil, nifedipine, felodipine), and anticoagulants (warfarin).

Elimination

Intestinal elimination

The human body harbours a large number of bacteria that have important functions, particularly in the gut. The adverse effects of antibiotics on the normal flora include emergence of resistant strains from among the normal flora and replacement of the normal flora by more harmful organisms, such as pathogenic fungi or *C. difficile*. Bioavailability of commonly prescribed antimicrobial drugs varies quite widely (Table 14.1). In general, poorly absorbed oral compounds have a more profound effect on the normal flora of the colon. However, after absorption from the gut, drugs may be eliminated from the body by secretion into bile or by secretion by enterocytes. Thus even intravenously administered antimicrobial agents may reach the gut in sufficient quantities to cause harmful effects on the normal flora.

Renal elimination

Most antibiotics are eliminated by the kidneys, so that very high concentrations may be achieved in urine. Excretion is by glomerular filtration or tubular secretion, and sometimes both.

The principal compounds excreted in the urine by active tubular secretion are the penicillins and cephalosporins. This process is so effective as to clear the blood of most of the drug during its passage through the kidney, and these compounds generally have a very short half-life of two hours or less. Increasing the frequency of administration can increase the period for which inhibitory levels of rapidly excreted agents are present in the blood. Alternatively, an agent that competes for the active transport mechanism may be used. The oral uricosuric agent probenecid shares the tubular route of excretion of penicillins and can be used to prolong the plasma half-life of these antibiotics.

Influence of infection

The vast majority of information about the pharmacokinetics of antimicrobial drugs comes from studies in normal volunteers. Infection is likely to change absorption, distribution, and elimination so plasma concentrations in patients may be profoundly different from those found in normal volunteers (Fig. 14.3).

Pharmacodynamics

In contrast to pharmacokinetics, which describes the way a drug is handled in the body, pharmacodynamics specifies the way the drug interacts with the microbial target in the conditions imposed by pharmacokinetic fluctuations (see Chapter 13 for an expanded discussion). This aspect of drug action is much more speculative, since it is not normally susceptible to direct measurement in situ, but is valuable insofar as it tries to define the dosing pattern likely to lead to the most efficient eradication of the offending microbe.

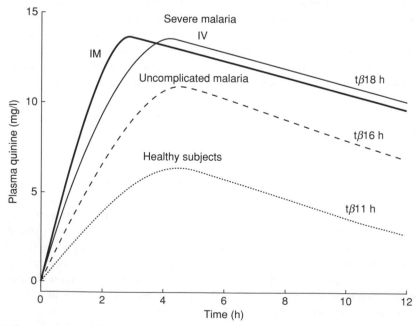

Fig. 14.3 Plasma concentrations of quinine in healthy subjects compared with patients with uncomplicated and severe malaria following administration of a loading dose of 20 mg (salt)/kg. Reproduced from White J, 'Antimalarial pharmacokinetics and treatment regimens'. *British Journal of Clinical Pharmacology* 1992; **34**: 1–10 with permission from Blackwell Publishing.

Among the factors to be considered are: whether the area under the concentration-time curve is more important than the peak level achieved; whether the regular replenishment of an inhibitory concentration for a short period is more, or less, efficacious than a continuously maintained inhibitory level; and whether antimicrobial activity is prolonged beyond the time for which an inhibitory concentration is achieved—the so-called post-antibiotic effect (p. 21).

Such judgements rely heavily on knowledge of how the micro-organism responds in laboratory-controlled conditions *in vitro* and models of varying degrees of elaboration are sometimes constructed to try to approximate more closely to the dynamic circumstances that exist in life. Extrapolation of these observations to the *in vivo* situation depends on the assumption that similar behaviour can be expected to occur in the complex, fluctuating conditions within an infected lesion and, indeed, on whether concentrations at the site of infection can be reliably predicted given individual variation.

Key points

◆ Supplying appropriate clinical details on request forms is crucial so that the correct tests and interpretations of results are made.

◆ An antibiotic susceptibility test result is relevant for a given pathogen recovered from a specific site and is not necessarily true for the same pathogen in a different site; this is because antibiotics generally penetrate some sites better than others.

◆ A report that a pathogen is antibiotic susceptible does not assure of treatment success; a pathogen that is reported as resistant to an antibiotic is very unlikely to respond to treatment with this agent.

◆ PCR-based tests are becoming the methods of choice for increasing numbers of infections, as they often offer increased sensitivity and more rapid results.

◆ PCR-based tests usually do not permit the assessment of antibiotic resistance, other than assays that detect specific genes/mutations associated with a resistant phenotype.

Further reading

Barger A, Fuhst C, Wiedemann B (2003), 'Pharmacological indices in antibiotic therapy', *Journal of Antimicrobial Chemotherapy*, **52**: 893–898.

Craig WA (1998), 'Pharmacokinetic/pharmacodynamic parameters: rationale for antibacterial dosing of mice and men', *Clinical Infectious Diseases*, **26**: 1–10.

Chapter 15

Prescribing in children and the elderly

Children should not be considered as small adults for the purposes of prescribing. The former practice of scaling down an adult dose on a weight basis often resulted in either sub-therapeutic or toxic concentrations and this is no longer acceptable. This applies to the prescribing of all drugs in childhood, not only antimicrobial agents. Similarly, the risks of adverse reactions increase significantly in elderly patients, especially if liver and kidney function is impaired by age or disease. The evaluation of new drugs in children and elderly people presents particular problems and is extremely important, since the pharmacological handling of the drugs and their unwanted effects may differ considerably in infants, young children, old people, and normal adults.

Paediatric prescribing

Age-related epidemiology of infections

When selecting antimicrobial therapy, knowledge of age-related infections is important in the initial management, before laboratory information is available. Many infections, although not entirely peculiar to infancy and childhood, are none the less much more frequently encountered in this age group. For example, respiratory syncytial virus infection of the lung and the classic viral exanthem of varicella are primarily diseases of childhood. Such age-related infections reflect the ready transmission of these agents and the susceptibility of a relatively non-immune population. Certain bacterial infections are also much more common in the very young. Neonatal meningitis is primarily caused by Group B streptococci and *Esch. coli*. Meningococcal infection is a disease of early childhood and young adulthood.

Upper respiratory tract infections are extremely common in childhood. Many are caused by viruses, but infection is often complicated by secondary bacterial invasion with *Streptococcus pneumoniae* or *Haemophilus influenzae*.

Cystic fibrosis is a disease that generally first becomes manifest in children, and through careful management many sufferers survive into adult life. A major complication of this disease is recurrent lower respiratory tract infection in which *Staphy. aureus* and *Pseudomonas* spp. predominate. Such infections are difficult to control and it is often impossible to eliminate *Pseudomonas* completely from the sputum.

Pharmacokinetic and pharmacodynamic considerations

In childhood, pharmacokinetic and pharmacodynamic factors often differ markedly from those in the adult (see Table 15.1), hence dosages may be adjusted according to surface area, which is more closely related than is body weight to the ability to metabolize drugs. This not only represents variation in the maturity of excretory organs (liver and kidneys) but also reflects differences in body water and fat. In infancy and early childhood the surface area is larger, relative to that of the older child and adult, and so there is a risk of overdosing when using such a system.

To arrive at a safe yet effective concentration of a drug is not without difficulties. In fact, for many drugs, the dosage regimens have not been accurately determined for every indication. In the case of new antimicrobial agents, until recently pharmacological and toxicological investigations

Table 15.1 Pharmacokinetic handling of drugs in childhood (compared with normal adult)

	Preterm	Neonate (0–4 weeks)	Infant (<1 year)	Early childhood (1–4 years)
Absorption	slightly reduced	no difference	no difference	no difference
Distribution				
body water	greatly increased	moderately increased	slightly increased	slightly increased
body fat	moderately reduced	slightly reduced	slightly reduced	no difference
plasma albumin	reduced	reduced	slightly reduced	no difference
Excretion (renal)				
glomerular filtration	moderately reduced	slightly reduced	slightly reduced[a]	no difference
tubular secretion	moderately reduced	slightly reduced	slightly reduced[a]	no difference

[a] First six months of life.

were more commonly carried out in an adult population, so that information in children and particularly in infants and neonates is often extremely limited. To derive the necessary information in childhood requires painstaking and careful observations in sick children, since pharmacokinetic information is not available from healthy children for ethical reasons. Lack of such information may preclude the widespread use of a potentially useful agent in childhood. Recent regulatory changes now actively encourage evaluation in childhood during drug development.

Paediatric prescribing recognizes the fact that growth and development, including organ function and metabolism, change in childhood. This is particularly so for the neonatal period in which chronological age, gestational age, and body weight are all important considerations. Furthermore, owing to physiological differences, information in the preterm or low-birthweight infant cannot necessarily be applied to heavier or full-term infants. Dosages of many drugs, including antimicrobial agents, vary on account of this state of flux of various physiological functions (Table 15.1).

Absorption

Gastric pH is neutral at birth, but falls to adult levels by age two to three years. Gastric emptying is also slower in the first three months of life. Acid-labile drugs, such as the oral penicillins, are absorbed more efficiently than in the older child or adult. However, in general, apart from pre-term neonates, intestinal absorption is not a major concern.

Transdermal absorption is markedly increased in infants and was formerly associated with hearing loss after the application of polymyxin, and with methaemoglobinaemia following topical mafenide acetate. Intramuscular absorption can be less reliable but is rarely used.

Distribution

Protein binding of drugs also varies with age, being lower in the neonate and infant and reflects the lower concentrations of serum albumin relative to adults. Reduced binding can increase the apparent volume of distribution of a drug, with an effect on peak and trough concentrations of certain agents. This is rarely of major therapeutic importance. However, variation in renal maturity, differences in the extracellular fluid volume, and the immaturity of various enzyme systems are important determinants of drug disposition and metabolism.

Metabolism

Many drugs, including antimicrobial agents, undergo metabolic biotransformation before their elimination from the body. Such transformation is effected by a variety of enzyme systems, many of which are present in the liver. In the neonate this organ and its enzymes are still maturing. Acetylation, oxidative, and conjugative phosphorylation are all less efficient in the first few weeks of life, particularly in the pre-term neonate. One example that led to the abandonment of its use is the inefficient glucuronidation of chloramphenicol in some neonates so that toxic blood and tissue concentrations may develop. This can result in hypotension, cardiovascular collapse, and death if unrecognized. The syndrome has been graphically described as the 'grey baby' syndrome.

Other problems of drug toxicity and drug interactions are not peculiar to childhood and are discussed in Chapter 13.

Excretion

In the neonate and especially the pre-term newborn, renal function is less efficient than in the older child since glomerular and tubular functions continue to mature. The creatinine clearance rate in the neonate is approximately one-third that of the older child. However, most infants achieve an adult glomerular filtration rate between six to 12 months of age. Hence, drugs excreted by the kidneys may require dose modification if toxicity is to be avoided.

Kidney function is not the only consideration. The volume of distribution of antibiotics is important in determining the dose that is necessary to achieve a therapeutic concentration at the site of infection. Agents that are essentially confined to the extracellular fluid compartment, such as the aminoglycosides, are affected by the proportionally larger extracellular fluid volume in the pre-term and full term neonate compared with the older child and adult. The extracellular fluid volume is approximately one-third of the body weight in the newborn.

To consider a specific example, the guidelines for prescribing the aminoglycoside gentamicin vary according to body weight, and also the chronological age, against which the drug's half-life varies inversely. This takes into consideration the immaturity of renal function, the different clearance rates, and the differing volumes of distribution. Thus the mean half-life of gentamicin in neonates less than a week old is about four to five hours, whereas for infants older than one month the half-life decreases to two to five hours. In order to ensure safe, yet therapeutic, drug concentrations in pre-term and term newborns, the dosages of gentamicin are adjusted for: premature neonate <1000 g 3.5 mg/kg every 24 h; term newborn 5–7 days postnatal 2.5 mg/kg every 12 h; term newborn 4–7 days postnatal and >2000 g 2.5 mg/kg every eight hours.

Materno-fetal prescribing

Drugs, including antibiotics, are frequently prescribed to pregnant women. Antimicrobial agents are most commonly prescribed in pregnancy for maternal urinary and respiratory tract infections. They may also be prescribed to treat intrauterine infections such as amnionitis.

Pregnancy frequently alters the pharmacokinetic handling of drugs, including anti-infective agents. Plasma concentrations of ampicillin are 50% of those observed in the non-pregnant state, as a result of increased plasma clearance. The same applies to many cephalosporins.

Any decision to prescribe drugs during pregnancy, including antibiotics, should only be taken after careful assessment of the risks and benefits, in order to avoid unnecessary exposure of the developing fetus.

Placental passage of antimicrobial agents

The placenta is not only an important defence against fetal infection, but also largely determines the concentration of a drug in fetal tissues. The transplacental passage of drugs may be by simple diffusion, or by an active transport system. As in other membrane situations, molecular weight, protein binding, ionizability, lipid solubility, and blood flow are all important considerations. In addition, the placenta is able to metabolize drugs through oxidation, conjugation, reduction, and hydrolysis. Drugs of low molecular weight (<1 kDa) tend to cross readily.

Antimicrobial agents that achieve good concentrations in fetal tissues include ampicillin, penicillin G, sulphonamides, metronidazole, and nitrofurantoin. The aminoglycosides cross moderately well and have occasionally been associated with fetal ototoxicity. The cephalosporins and clindamycin cross less readily, and erythromycin is particularly poor in this respect.

The general caution restricting all unnecessary prescribing in pregnancy, in particular during the first three months when organogenesis is maximal, also applies to antimicrobial drugs. For example, the antifolate properties of trimethoprim and the sulphonamides carry a theoretical risk of inducing fetal abnormalities. However, of more importance is the complication of hyperbilirubinaemia that can result should sulphonamides be prescribed in the latter few weeks of pregnancy or during the neonatal period. Displacement of protein-bound bilirubin by sulphonamide may result in toxic concentrations of bilirubin in the basal ganglia of the brain with the resultant risk of kernicterus.

Excretion of antimicrobial agents into breast milk

In common with other drugs, antimicrobial agents can enter human breast milk and therefore may potentially affect the suckling infant.

The secretory process may either be active or passive and the final concentration is determined by factors such as molecular weight, lipid or water solubility, the degree of protein binding and, of course, maternal serum concentrations. Breast milk has a neutral pH, which will affect the ionization of drugs.

Few antimicrobial drugs pass readily into breast milk to achieve concentrations similar to those in maternal blood. However, isoniazid and some sulphonamides do so. Tetracyclines achieve moderate concentrations and could possibly cause discoloration of primary dentition and enamel hypoplasia and hence its contra-indication in early childhood. Erythromycin is found in concentrations approximately half those present in maternal blood. Metronidazole achieves concentrations comparable with maternal serum levels. The penicillins and cephalosporins are generally poorly excreted into human breast milk.

In general, such concentrations are of more theoretical than of practical significance. There have been occasional reports of dapsone and nalidixic acid associated drug toxicity in children with glucose-6-phosphate dehydrogenase deficiency. Disturbance of the bowel flora has been reported with ampicillin; use of clindamycin has resulted in bloody diarrhoea. Under most circumstances, the short-term administration of antimicrobial agents to lactating mothers need not interfere with breast feeding.

Compliance in children

Of particular importance in paediatric prescribing is the acceptability of the medication to the patient. Injections are understandably unpopular with children and their anxious parents; oral preparations are preferred whenever possible provided their use does not compromise the likely success of therapy. In some cases antibiotics that are otherwise poorly absorbed when given by the oral route are available as esters or salts that exhibit greatly improved oral absorption, as for example with erythromycin. The need to make preparations palatable with syrup and flavourings is important if compliance is to be observed. Children generally find tablet and capsule preparations difficult to swallow—hence the popularity of flavoured syrup suspensions. A word of caution is necessary, since some preparations contain high concentrations of sucrose, which may encourage dental caries. This applies essentially to children on long-term preparations, which for the most part will be drugs other than antimicrobial agents.

In addition to palatability, compliance is increased by making the prescribing instructions clear and least disruptive to the normal daily routine. Unnecessary disturbance of sleep patterns is a sure way to reduce compliance.

An important aspect of all prescribing, particularly with paediatric formulations, which may be attractively coloured and sweet tasting, is the need to warn parents that any residual medication should be discarded. Drugs should not be stored in anticipation of using them for a future infection. The shelf-life of antibiotics is limited and prolonged storage is associated with loss of potency. It is important to emphasize that accidental self-poisoning in childhood may occasionally be life threatening.

Prescribing for the elderly

As with most therapeutic agents, use of antibiotics is greatest in old age. This reflects the increased susceptibility to microbial disease as a result of degenerative, neoplastic, and metabolic disorders. Furthermore, the host response to infection is often impaired owing to involution or the immunosuppressive effects of disease or drugs. The inflammatory response is often dampened and this may lead to more serious infective states, which can have a profound effect on major organ function and thus modify response to antimicrobial therapy.

Age-related infection

Infection is an important cause of morbidity and mortality in elderly people. The classic infections of childhood have little impact in old age, whereas infections of the respiratory tract, urinary tract, and skin structures become more common as one grows older. For example, the lower respiratory tract, often compromised by life-long exposure to cigarette smoke and atmospheric pollution, is an important target for infections that require medical consultation, hospital admission, and the administration of antibiotics.

Urinary tract infections increase substantially beyond the age of 50. In men this is largely related to benign or malignant enlargement of the prostate; in women it may have various causes, including sphincter disturbance, uterine prolapse, pelvic neoplasms, and poor hygiene compounded by periods of immobility.

Intra-abdominal infection may complicate gall bladder disease, diverticulosis, and malignancy of the bowel; metabolic disorders, notably diabetes mellitus, predispose to infection of the urinary tract and septicaemia, as well as infected ischaemic or neuropathic ulcers of the feet.

Pharmacokinetic and pharmacodynamic changes in elderly people

Elderly people are the least homogeneous population in relation to drug prescribing. Morbidities can be multiple and are compounded by the involution of many physiological systems.

Gastric acid output often falls, with a rise in gastric pH; reduced blood flow to the gut and liver may lower first-pass extraction leading to increased oral bioavailability. Changes in lean body mass and body water may lower the apparent volume of distribution. Of greatest significance are changes in the functional integrity of the kidneys and liver, which can substantially alter drug disposition and elimination; superimposed disease can further aggravate the natural decline in function.

These changes may have the advantage of allowing higher concentrations of drug to be achieved, but the risk of toxicity may also increase. Loss of glomerular function is a normal concomitant of advancing years and may not be clinically apparent. For this reason all drugs should be used with caution in old people, especially those compounds for which the route of excretion is primarily renal. Use of aminoglycosides in elderly patients requires careful attention to dosage and monitoring of serum concentrations to ensure therapeutic, yet non-toxic, levels that may further impair renal, auditory, or vestibular function.

Adverse reactions

Unwanted effects of drugs are more common in elderly people. It is estimated that 10% of hospital admissions in the UK are caused solely, or in part, by adverse drug reactions. Some of these will be due to antimicrobial drugs. While some are idiosyncratic, others are related to dose or dose duration. This partly follows from the increased frequency of drug prescribing in this group, as well as the impaired efficiency of the excretory organs. However, certain drug reactions cannot be explained by such considerations as, for example, the increased frequency and severity of serious adverse reactions to co-trimoxazole seen in the elderly such as rashes, including the Stevens–Johnson syndrome with extensive skin and mucous membrane ulceration, and major blood dyscrasias. The effect is almost certainly related to the sulphonamide component of this drug.

Old people are often prescribed multiple drugs. Such polypharmacy raises important issues of drug interactions that may affect pharmacological activity, as well as increasing the risks of side effects. Examples include the chelation of tetracyclines by antacids and the effect of H_2-antagonists on the absorption of drugs such as the quinolones that are affected by alterations in pH. Likewise, the co-administration of theophyllines and quinolones, such as ciprofloxacin, or macrolides, such as erythromycin, can result in toxic concentrations of the former leading to agitation, confusion, and even seizures.

Poor compliance with medication may be the result of cognitive or visual impairment. Compliance with complex polypharmaceutical regimens can be assisted by daily 'dosette' containers and supported by written instructions for the patient or carer. Much can be done to mitigate the present high rate of adverse effects of medication.

Conclusion

The principles of antimicrobial prescribing are common to all age groups, but greater attention to issues of drug distribution, excretion, and potential for adverse reactions is necessary in patients at the extremes of age. The burden of infection falls most heavily on the very young and the very old and antibiotic prescribing is correspondingly more common in these age groups. In the treatment of infection in children and the elderly it is essential to choose the safest and most effective agent, and to use it in appropriate dosage for the shortest time necessary.

Key points

+ Children and the elderly are the target of most antibiotic prescribing.
+ Immaturity or involution of many physiological systems alters the pharmacokinetics of drug handling and increases the risks of drug toxicity.
+ Dose adjustment is necessary for many drugs, particularly in the premature and newborn infant. Caution is necessary when prescribing drugs in pregnancy.

Further reading

Remington JS, Klein JO, Wilson CB, Nizet V, Maldonado Y (2011), *Infectious Diseases of the Fetus and Newborn Infant.* (7th edn). London: Elsevier.

Chapter 16

Outpatient parenteral antimicrobial therapy (OPAT)

Outside hospitals antibiotics are generally administered by the oral route. However, over the past 20 years there has been increasing development of services for administration of intravenous antibiotics to patients in the community. Various terms have been used to describe this, including community-based parenteral anti-infective therapy, hospital in the home therapy and non-inpatient parenteral antimicrobial therapy. However, OPAT is the term most commonly used (Table 16.1, http://www.e-opat.com/).

In the USA over 250 000 patients receive OPAT annually. Establishment of OPAT has been slower in other countries, probably because of differences in healthcare financing. In the USA hospitals are reimbursed for each patient treated so there is a clear financial incentive to treat as many patients as possible and to minimize the duration of hospitalization. In contrast, in most other countries hospitals are reimbursed for delivering treatment to populations and geographic regions. However, OPAT is becoming increasingly common in Australia and Europe.

Indications for OPAT

OPAT was first developed for children with cystic fibrosis, who had recurrent pulmonary infections and subsequently for adult patients with osteomyelitis. Initially carers or patients were trained to administer parenteral antibiotics at home but increasingly services were developed for parenteral administration by health professionals, either in patients' homes or in outpatient clinics. Infections that require prolonged parenteral therapy (endocarditis, prosthetic device infections, and bone and joint infections) are still amongst the commonest indications for OPAT. However, short-term OPAT treatment for skin and soft tissue, pyelonephritis, and other infections is increasingly common.

The most important determinants of suitability for OPAT therapy are the patient and their carers (Table 16.1). Patients must be clinically stable and have home circumstances that support OPAT, including effective communication with healthcare professionals. Consequently, although pneumonia is the commonest indication for parenteral antibiotics in hospital it is not amongst the commonest indications for OPAT because most patients with pneumonia require other support from hospitals during the time that they need parenteral therapy. In contrast many patients with skin and soft tissue infection are suitable for OPAT.

Requirements for OPAT

The first requirement for OPAT is a multidisciplinary team capable of delivering the treatment and all the necessary support services (Table 16.2). Delivery of OPAT needs to be supported by guidelines for patient selection, support, and monitoring (Table 16.2). Recording of outcomes is essential and can be supported by a freely accessible online database (http://www.e-opat.com/).

In addition to a clinical database the development of OPAT services requires a strong business case to ensure the necessary support services (http://www.e-opat.com/). This is particularly

Table 16.1 Specific considerations in evaluating patients for outpatient parenteral antimicrobial therapy (OPAT)

Reproduced with permission from Tice AD, Rehm SJ, Dalovisio JR, Bradley JS, Martinelli LP, Graham DR, Gainer RB, Kunkel MJ, Yancey RW, Williams DN (2004) Practice guidelines for outpatient parenteral antimicrobial therapy. IDSA guidelines. *Clinical Infectious Diseases* **38**(12): 1651–1672.

1. Is parenteral antimicrobial therapy needed?

2. Do the patient's medical care needs exceed resources available at the proposed site of care?

3. Is the home or outpatient environment safe and adequate to support care?

4. Are the patient and/or caregiver willing to participate and able to safely, effectively, and reliably deliver parenteral antimicrobial therapy?

5. Are mechanisms for rapid and reliable communications about problems and for monitoring of therapy in place between members of the OPAT team?

6. Do the patient and caregiver understand the benefits, risks, and economic considerations involved in OPAT?

7. Does informed consent need to be documented?

important for hospitals that are not reimbursed on a per-patient basis. In these systems reducing length of hospital stay does not necessarily increase hospital income or reduce operational costs. It is more important to emphasise the benefits to patients, which include reduction in risk of healthcare associated infections, particularly *C difficile* infection. OPAT should be seen as the best standard of care and not simply a method for cost containment.

Technology for OPAT

Standard peripheral IV cannulas are not suitable for most patients with OPAT because they require to be changed every two to three days. Peripherally inserted central catheters (PICC) provide a more durable alternative that can be inserted or removed in the outpatient setting and have a low infection rate. Because of their central positioning, they are suitable for administration of concentrated antibiotics solutions.

Intravenous injection over five to 10 minutes is the most convenient method for administration of OPAT for patients and staff. Intravenous infusion at home is technically possible through compact, battery-operated, computerized infusion pumps. However, these generally are expensive to purchase and can be difficult for patients to manage.

Antibiotics for OPAT

The most suitable antibiotics are those that can be administered once daily by a short intravenous injection, for example, ceftriaxone and teicoplanin. Although gentamicin fits these requirements it is rarely used for OPAT because of the need for therapeutic drug monitoring. OPAT is rarely used to deliver antiviral drugs because most are available in oral formulations and patients who require parenteral therapy usually have other clinical problems that require hospitalization. The antifungal drug caspofungin has been used for OPAT in patients with endocarditis.

In the USA ceftriaxone and vancomycin are the drugs most commonly used for OPAT (Fig. 16.1). Teicoplanin is not licensed for use in the USA but is used instead of vancomycin in Australia and Europe. Penicillins are rarely used for OPAT because they require continuous infusion or administration at least three times daily.

Table 16.2 Key elements required for an outpatient parenteral antimicrobial therapy (OPAT) program

Reproduced with permission from Tice AD, Rehm SJ, Dalovisio JR, Bradley JS, Martinelli LP, Graham DR, Gainer RB, Kunkel MJ, Yancey RW, Williams DN (2004) Practice guidelines for outpatient parenteral antimicrobial therapy. IDSA guidelines. *Clinical Infectious Disesases* **38**(12): 1651–1672.

1. Health care team

    A. An infectious diseases specialist or physician knowledgeable about infectious diseases and the use of antimicrobials in OPAT

    B. Primary care or referring physicians available to participate in care

    C. Nurse expert in intravenous therapy, access devices, and OPAT

    D. Pharmacist knowledgeable about OPAT

    E. Case manager and billing staff knowledgeable about therapeutic issues and third party reimbursements

    F. Access to other health care professionals, including a physical therapist, a dietitian, an occupational therapist, and a social worker

2. Communications

    A. Physician, nurse, and pharmacist available 24 h per day

    B. System in place for rapid communication between patient and team members

    C. Patient education information for common problems, side effects, precautions, and contact lists

3. Outline of guidelines for follow-up of patients with laboratory testing and intervention as needed

4. Written policies and procedures

    A. Outline of responsibilities of team members

    B. Patient intake information

    C. Patient selection criteria

    D. Patient education materials

5. Outcomes monitoring

    A. Patient response

    B. Complications of disease, treatment, or program

    C. Patient satisfaction

Monitoring of OPAT

Although the home environment has many advantages for the patient, the careful regular monitoring that occurs in hospitals is not possible at home. Patients receiving OPAT need to be seen at least weekly, either in their home or in an outpatient setting. Specific factors to assess on review include response to therapy, evidence of drug adverse effects and other complications such as infection related to the venous cannula. It is important that there are clear policies for monitoring of specific drugs. In addition to prevention of side effects, measurement of serum drug concentrations is used to ensure effective therapy. This is particularly important for achieving optimum dosing frequency. For example, with teicoplanin most patients can maintain effective concentrations for treatment of bone and joint infections with three times weekly administration. This is much more convenient than daily administration for patients and does not require weekend services for OPAT. However, it is critical to ensure that effective serum concentrations can be maintained.

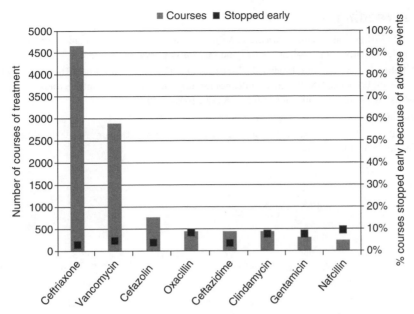

Fig. 16.1 Number of OPAT courses and % of courses that were stopped early because of adverse events in an OPAT registry. Drawn from data in Tice AD, Rehm SJ, Dalovisio JR, Bradley JS, Martinelli LP, Graham DR, Gainer RB, Kunkel MJ, Yancey RW, Williams DN (2004) Practice guidelines for outpatient parenteral antimicrobial therapy. IDSA guidelines. *Clinical Infectious Diseases* **38**(12): 1651–1672.

Adverse events that are serious enough to stop treatment occur in about 4% of patients (Fig. 16.1). However, serious adverse events are more common with penicillins and gentamicin than with cephalosporins or glycopeptides (Fig. 16.1). This is probably due to the fact that penicillins and gentamicin are more difficult to administer safely in an outpatient environment because of the need for multiple injections or continuous infusion (penicillins) or therapeutic drug monitoring (gentamicin).

Key points

♦ Over the past 20 years there has been increasing development of services for administering IV antibiotics to patients in the community. This practice is most common in the USA but is now increasingly common in Australia and Europe.

♦ The most important determinants of suitability for OPAT are the patient and their carers. Patients must be capable of self-management and clinically stable. The commonest indications for OPAT are infections that require long or repeated courses of IV treatment and skin or soft tissue infections.

♦ Patients must be supported by a multidisciplinary team capable of delivering the treatment and all the necessary support services.

♦ Standard peripheral IV cannulas are not suitable for most patients with OPAT, who usually require peripherally inserted central catheters. The most convenient antibiotics for OPAT are given once daily by short intravenous injection.

♦ Patients receiving OPAT need to be seen at least weekly, either in their home or in the outpatient setting.

Further reading

Nathwani, D (2010), 'Non-Inpatient Parenteral Antimicrobial Therapy (NIPAT)', in *Infectious Diseases*, Cohen, J, Powderly, WG, Opal, SM (eds) London: Mosby/Elsevier, 1333–1339.

Tice, AD, Rehm, SJ, Dalovisio, JR, Bradley, JS, Martinelli, LP, Graham, DR, Gainer, RB, Kunkel, MJ, Yancey, RW, Williams, DN, 'Practice guidelines for outpatient parenteral antimicrobial therapy. IDSA guidelines', *Clinical Infectious Disease* 2004; **38** (12): 1651–1672.

OPAT database and business case. Available at:http://www.e-opat.com/.

Prudent Antibiotic User, Vignette 21 Outpatient Parenteral Antibiotic Therapy. Available at: http://www. pause-online.org.uk.

Chapter 17

Adverse drug reactions

No antimicrobial agent is totally free from unwanted side effects. About 5% of patients prescribed antimicrobial therapy will develop an adverse reaction of some sort. Most are trivial; some merely inconvenient. Others may require admission to hospital for specialist management, but a few are life threatening or fatal. Adverse drug reactions are not unique to antimicrobial agents and may have major implications for the patient and add to the costs of healthcare delivery. Due caution should always be exercised before a patient is placed on antimicrobial therapy, to see whether there is an identifiable contraindication to the use of the agent. Unnecessary or inappropriate prescribing is to be deplored for several reasons, but in particular for unjustifiably running the risk of avoidable adverse reactions.

Adverse reactions range from the allergic to the toxic. Others are unpredictable and defined as idiosyncratic. Alterations to the microbial flora can also occur and result in complicating disease. However, it is important to keep a proper perspective on the relative frequency of adverse events (Table 17.1) so that a realistic risk–benefit judgement can be made before prescribing.

Determinants of toxicity

Genetic

A few adverse reactions are genetically determined. For example, patients deficient in the enzyme glucose-6-phosphate dehydrogenase are at risk of developing acute haemolysis when prescribed sulphonamides, nitrofurantoin, or the antimalarial primaquine. Occasionally, the use of chloramphenicol, or nalidixic acid, may be similarly complicated. This reaction may be avoided by screening for this X-linked erythrocyte enzyme defect, which is more common among people of Mediterranean, Far Eastern, or African stock. Similarly, the ability to acetylate the antituberculosis drug isoniazid is genetically determined; there is a risk of isoniazid toxicity in slow acetylators.

Chemical

Many intravenously administered drugs, including antimicrobial agents, produce local irritation which may lead to frank phlebitis. To overcome this, the pH of an intravenous infusion can be adjusted by suitable buffering. Similarly, pain may accompany the intramuscular injection of a drug. Many drugs may produce gastrointestinal symptoms due to a local chemical irritation of the gastric and intestinal mucosa. Here again, suitable buffering, enteric coating, or slow-release formulations can diminish these symptoms and increase the acceptability of a drug.

Metabolic

Drug accumulation

Drugs usually undergo oxidation, reduction, hydrolysis, or conjugation to a greater or lesser degree before excretion. The liver is the major site of this metabolism, although other organs such as the kidneys are also involved. When disease impairs renal or hepatic function there is the

Table 17.1 Relative frequency of selected adverse reactions to antimicrobial agents (the more serious or important adverse drug reactions are shown in bold type). Source: Davey P, 'Antimicrobial Chemotherapy' in DJ Weatherall, JGG Ledidngham, and DA Warrell (eds.) *Oxford Textbook of Medicine*, (3rd edn), Vol. 1 (1996).

Antimicrobial agent	Infrequent	Frequent
Aminoglycosides	Rashes	Ototoxicity
		Nephrotoxicity
Cephalosporins	Anaphylaxis	Hypersensitivity rashes
	Haematological toxicity	*Candida* overgrowth
Chloramphenicol	Aplastic anaemia	Dose-related marrow toxicity
	Grey baby syndrome	
	Optic neuritis	
Clindamycin	Hepatitis	Rash
	Pseudomembranous colitis	Diarrhoea
Co-trimoxazole and sulphonamides	Haematological toxicity	Rashes (sulphonamide)
	Megaloblastic anaemia	
Erythromycin	Cholestatic jaundice	Gastrointestinal intolerance
	Deafness	
Fusidic acid	Hepatotoxicity (intravenous)	Gastrointestinal intolerance (oral)
Nalidixic acid and other quinolones	Confusion/convulsions	Gastrointestinal intolerance
	Photosensitivity	Rashes
Nitrofurantoin	Hypersensitivity pneumonitis	Gastrointestinal intolerance
	Haemolysis	
	Peripheral neuropathy	
	Rashes	
Penicillins	Anaphylaxis	Hypersensitivity reactions—mainly rashes
	Haematological toxicity	
	Encephalopathy	
	Interstitial nephritis	
Rifampicin	Hypersensitivity	Hepatotoxicity
	'Influenza syndrome' (intermittent treatment)	Liver enzyme induction
	Haematological toxicity	
Tetracyclines	Photosensitivity	Gastrointestinal intolerance
	Nephrotoxicity	Candidiasis
		Dental staining and hypoplasia in childhood
Vancomycin	Nephrotoxicity	'Red man' syndrome

risk of accumulation of the drug, or a metabolite, which may reach toxic concentrations in the tissues.

Similarly, in the premature or full-term neonate both renal and hepatic functions are physiologically immature so that some adjustments of dosaging may have to be made (see Chapter 15).

Enzyme induction

Certain drugs may cause hepatic enzyme induction or the synthesis of a new enzyme. Rifampicin is a powerful enzyme inducer, decreasing the half-lives of many drugs such as prednisone, warfarin, digoxin, ketoconazole, and the sulphonylureas. Women simultaneously prescribed rifampicin and the contraceptive pill may conceive owing to inadequate circulating hormone concentrations resulting from rifampicin induction of hepatic enzymes. Likewise, simultaneous administration of certain quinolones (e.g. ciprofloxacin) can result in the accumulation of toxic concentrations of theophyllines.

Histamine release

Too-rapid infusion of vancomycin can result in the release of histamine, which in turn, can produce acute flushing, tachycardia, and hypotension—a reaction descriptively known as 'red man' syndrome. This can be avoided by extending infusion rates per dose to two hours.

Drug interactions

Drugs may interact with other agents *in vitro* when mixed before administration, or *in vivo* once the drugs are ingested or injected. The study of drug interactions has become increasingly important and complex as new therapeutic agents become available. In general, incompatibilities can be avoided by mixing the agents separately and administering them by a different route or at different times.

In vitro incompatibilities

Table 17.2 indicates the variety of *in vitro* incompatibilities associated with antimicrobial agents. This list is far from complete. Pharmaceutical advice should be sought or the relevant section of the *British National Formulary* consulted.

In vivo interactions

In vivo drug interactions include competition for plasma protein-binding sites and inhibition or induction of liver enzymes, thus interfering with or potentiating other therapeutic effects. Table 17.3 indicates the variety of effects that have been described. Among the more important is interference with anticoagulant drugs, a problem that is commonly, but not exclusively, caused by

Table 17.2 *In vitro* incompatibilities of selected antimicrobial agents

Antimicrobial agent	Agents with which incompatibility exists
Penicillin G	Metronidazole, tetracyclines, vancomycin, amphotericin
Flucloxacillin	Blood products; aminoglycosides if mixed
Cefuroxime	Aminoglycosides if mixed
Clindamycin	Ampicillin, phenytoin, ranitidine
Vancomycin	Hydrocortisone, heparin
Gentamicin	Penicillins, cephalosporins, erythromycin, heparin

Table 17.3 *In vivo* incompatibilities of selected antimicrobial agents

Antibiotic(s)	Interacting agent(s)	Adverse reaction
Aminoglycosides	Non-depolarizing muscle relaxants	Neuromuscular blockade
Chloramphenicol	Phenytoin	Phenytoin toxicity
Metronidazole		
Isoniazid		
Ciprofloxacin	Theophylline	Agitation, convulsions
Clarithromycin		
Erythromycin		
Fluconazole	Warfarin	Increased anticoagulation
Griseofulvin	Warfarin	Decreased anticoagulation
Ketoconazole	Oral antacids and H_2 antagonists	Decreased absorption of antifungal
Aminoglycosides	Cyclosporin A	Cyclosporin nephrotoxicity
Ketoconazole		
Quinolones		
Metronidazole	Alcohol	Nausea and vomiting (disulfiram effect)
Rifampicin	Oral contraceptives	Decreased contraceptive efficacy
Co-trimoxazole	Anticoagulants	Increased anticoagulation
Sulphonamides		
Tetracyclines	Oral antacid preparations and oral iron	Decreased tetracycline absorption

antimicrobial agents. For example, rifampicin and griseofulvin impair anticoagulation by enzyme induction, whereas sulphonamides, co-trimoxazole, erythromycin, metronidazole, and the azole antifungals increase anticoagulation by enzyme inhibition, so that bleeding may occur.

Hypersensitivity

Among the antibiotics the β-lactam compounds have the greatest potential to produce hypersensitivity reactions. Because of the similar structure of the penicillins, hypersensitivity to one agent is usually accompanied by hypersensitivity to the whole group. Moreover, structural similarities between cephalosporins and penicillins are accompanied by a degree of cross-hypersensitivity: about 10% of patients who are hypersensitive to penicillins show cross-hypersensitivity to cephalosporins. This is much more likely to occur in patients who have experienced a previous anaphylactic response to a penicillin, when the subsequent use of all β-lactam antibiotics (see Chapter 1) must be avoided. The monobactam agent aztreonam is less allergenic and may be given to patients with a history of hypersensitivity to other β-lactam antibiotics. This suggests that the sensitizing moiety of these drugs lies in a site other than the β-lactam ring.

Immediate reactions

Immediate hypersensitivity reactions to penicillins and cephalosporins can, within minutes, produce nausea, vomiting, pruritus, urticaria, wheezing, laryngeal oedema, and cardiovascular collapse. In extreme cases the patient may die unless the attack is controlled with adrenaline and attention to the integrity of the airways. The estimated frequency for anaphylaxis is one to five for every 10 000 courses of penicillin prescribed. It is more common in parenteral administration.

Delayed reactions

Delayed hypersensitivity reactions include drug fever, erythema nodosum, and a serum-sickness-like syndrome. Hypersensitivity rashes are particularly common with semisynthetic penicillins such as ampicillin and its analogues and to a lesser degree, cephalosporins. The rashes are usually maculopapular and pruritic but may also be vesicular, bullous, urticarial, or scarlatiniform.

The use of ampicillin is associated with a generalized maculopapular eruption in more than 90% of patients suffering from infectious mononucleosis (glandular fever) and, less frequently, in association with cytomegalovirus infection. The exact reason for these hypersensitivity rashes is uncertain, although both infections are characterized by intense polyclonal antibody responses. The response is short lived and does not reflect long-lasting penicillin hypersensitivity, so that future cautious use of penicillins is possible in these patients.

Other antimicrobial agents that commonly produce hypersensitivity drug rashes are the sulphonamides, clindamycin and a number of drugs used to treat HIV/AIDS, notably nevirapine and abacavir. The sulphonamides and co-trimoxazole are responsible for a wide variety of eruptions that range from urticarial to maculopapular to erythema multiforme and its more severe variant, the Stevens–Johnson syndrome in which there is both cutaneous and mucous membrane involvement and a significant mortality rate.

Hypersensitivity reactions may also involve individual organs. For example, the penicillins occasionally produce an interstitial nephritis. Nitrofurantoin may affect the lungs, and erythromycin estolate is associated with hypersensitivity cholestasis. Haemolytic anaemia, neutropenia, and thrombocytopenia may occasionally occur with the penicillins, cephalosporins, and sulphonamides.

Predicting hypersensitivity

This is difficult. Some individuals have a strong family history of drug allergy or of allergic disease such as asthma or atopic eczema. Skin testing is occasionally carried out, but is unfortunately poorly predictive. It is therefore imperative to inquire about any previous episodes of hypersensitivity. When reactions occur they should be carefully documented and explained to the patient, so that serious hypersensitivity reactions can be avoided in the future.

Altered microbial flora

Antimicrobial drugs cannot distinguish between pathogenic organisms and those that make up the normal flora of the host. Even so-called 'narrow-spectrum' antibiotics such as penicillin have a profound effect on the normal flora of the mouth and gut to eliminate or suppress penicillin-sensitive strains of streptococci and anaerobic bacteria. As a rule this alteration of the normal flora is without clinical consequence and is rapidly reversed on stopping treatment.

Some agents have a greater potential to suppress the normal flora, which may be complicated by the overgrowth of drug-resistant organisms, which in turn may give rise to superinfection. In general, the worst culprits are broad-spectrum antibiotics such as the tetracyclines, aminopenicillins (ampicillin, amoxicillin), and cephalosporins. Their use is occasionally associated with the overgrowth of yeasts, particularly within the oral cavity or in the vagina, where they may result in candidiasis (thrush).

Of greater importance is the syndrome of antibiotic-associated colitis caused by toxin-producing strains of *Clostridium difficile*. This may follow the use of various agents, although clindamycin, ampicillin, cephalosporins and the quinolones are most commonly incriminated. It is thought, but not proven, that antibiotic use selectively favours proliferation of the causative organism. The colitis caused by the toxin may be severe, even life threatening. Outbreaks of *C. difficile* colitis in hospitals are frequent. Oral metronidazole or vancomycin are successfully used to control the condition when it arises.

Finally, patients treated with antimicrobial agents are at risk of acquiring organisms from the environment. Because of the intensive selection pressure operating in many hospital units, organisms acquired in hospital are often more virulent and frequently exhibit resistance to a variety of antibiotics, putting the patient at increased risk.

Tissue- and organ-specific toxicity

Gastrointestinal tract

Antimicrobial agents are commonly administered orally provided that absorption from the bowel is satisfactory. It is scarcely surprising, therefore, that a variety of gastrointestinal side effects are associated with their use. Nausea, vomiting, and increased bowel movement, sometimes amounting to diarrhoea, are common, but are generally of minor inconvenience and do not interrupt treatment. Diarrhoea occurs in about 5–10% of patients taking oral ampicillin or clindamycin. However, the most serious gastrointestinal complications are overgrowth of *Candida* spp. or toxigenic strains of *C. difficile* (see above).

Skin

Skin rashes are among the more frequent adverse reactions caused by antimicrobial drugs. Most reactions are caused by hypersensitivity, but a wide variety of other eruptions may occur, including maculopapular, vesicular, and bullous eruptions, exfoliation, and erythema multiforme. Delayed hypersensitivity reactions with sulphonamides may result in erythema nodosum, which may be part of a serum-sickness-like syndrome with drug fever and arthralgia.

Photosensitivity occurs with long-acting sulphonamides, tetracyclines (particularly demeclocycline), and quinolones. The skin becomes red, oedematous, and vesicular. This is more common in hot climates.

Dental staining

Tetracyclines are taken up by developing bones and teeth. In the former this causes no significant long-term complications, but staining of the teeth is unsightly and ranges from patchy cream to extensive brown discolouration. Enamel hypoplasia may also result. The ability to cause dental staining varies among the tetracyclines, being least with oxytetracycline. However, avoidance of all tetracyclines in children under 12 years of age will prevent staining of the permanent dentition.

Respiratory tract

Hypersensitivity manifested by bronchial asthma and pulmonary eosinophilia can occur in sensitized individuals. Asthmatic reactions are most likely in people with an underlying bronchospastic tendency. Nitrofurantoin, sulphonamides, and β-lactam agents may cause such reactions. Long-term use of nitrofurantoin has also been associated with a chronic interstitial pneumonitis progressing to fibrosis. The changes may be only partially reversible on stopping the drugs.

An indirect side effect of antibiotic therapy is opportunistic lung infection following modification of the normal flora. This usually occurs in patients with underlying malignant disease and those receiving cytotoxic or immunosuppressive therapy. Patients who are artificially ventilated are particularly vulnerable.

Liver

Antibiotics may affect the liver to produce an acute hepatitis or cholestasis. Such reactions are often unpredictable, although pre-existing liver disease suggests caution in prescribing potentially hepatotoxic drugs.

Several antimicrobial drugs, including cephalosporins, clindamycin, and intravenously administered fusidic acid, may produce minor elevations of liver enzymes which uncommonly progress to a frank hepatitis with nausea, vomiting, and a tender enlarged liver. Cholestasis may be seen in association with nitrofurantoin, erythromycin derivatives, and prolonged use of flucloxacillin, especially in the elderly.

Isoniazid is a frequent cause of hepatitis, which is uncommon below the age of 20 years, but increases significantly in people of middle age and beyond. Symptoms usually develop within the first two months of treatment and subside on stopping treatment. Transient asymptomatic elevation of liver enzymes is common but of little significance. Routine testing of liver function is not justified for those treated for tuberculosis unless symptoms develop.

Rifampicin may also produce elevation of liver enzymes, although when used in combination with isoniazid—as it may be in the treatment of tuberculosis—clinical hepatotoxicity appears to be no more frequent than when isoniazid is used alone.

A more serious variety of liver toxicity may follow the use of intravenous tetracycline in patients with pre-existing liver disease or during pregnancy. Under these circumstances liver necrosis may prove fatal.

Neurological system

Central nervous system

Ototoxicity is an important side effect of aminoglycoside antibiotics. However, their individual potential for either vestibulotoxicity or cochleotoxicity varies and is least for tobramycin. Vestibulotoxicity is recognized by unsteadiness of gait and nystagmus; cochleotoxicity is recognized by a hearing loss that initially affects high frequencies that may only be detected by audiography. Deafness may also occasionally complicate the use of intravenous erythromycin.

Although penicillins are (setting aside penicillin allergy) the least toxic of antibiotics, encephalitic reactions may complicate massive parenteral doses of penicillin G (12 g or more per day). Such heroic doses are rarely indicated.

Other β-lactam antibiotics such as the cephalosporins and imipenem may also be associated with convulsions and encephalopathy when given in high doses. High dose quinolones are proconvulsant. The phenomenon of benign intracranial hypertension may follow the use of nalidixic acid, tetracycline, and, occasionally, penicillin. This is reversible on stopping treatment. Optic neuritis is a rare complication of the use of chloramphenicol; ethambutol is also associated with dose-related optic nerve damage and retinopathy.

Peripheral nervous system

Several agents may cause a peripheral neuropathy, although the mechanisms are not well understood. Isoniazid is known to interfere with pyridoxine metabolism. Nitrofurantoin competes with thiamine pyrophosphate and thus interferes with pyruvate oxidation. Metronidazole may produce a reversible peripheral neuropathy with prolonged use. The nucleoside analogues used in the treatment of HIV disease are all associated with peripheral neuropathy.

Neuromuscular blockade, although rare, is potentially serious and occurs in association with the use of aminoglycosides and tetracyclines. The aminoglycosides produce neuromuscular blockade by a curare-like anticholinesterase effect and by competing with calcium; this is more likely to be seen following the use of non-depolarising muscle relaxants during anaesthesia. They should be avoided in patients with myasthenia gravis.

Kidneys

Since the kidneys are the major route of drug excretion, it is not surprising that nephrotoxicity is relatively frequent. It is often dose related and is more common either in those with pre-existing renal failure or in those receiving other nephrotoxic agents.

Haematological toxicity

Bone marrow toxicity may be selective and affect one cell line, or be unselective and produce pancytopenia and marrow aplasia. Immune-mediated haemolysis, in which Coombs' antibodies are detected, may also occur. Bleeding may occur from platelet dysfunction or from thrombocytopenia. Eosinophilia may represent a hypersensitivity reaction.

Sulphonamides

Some early sulphonamides, which were rapidly excreted and poorly soluble, were prone to deposit crystals within the urinary tract, sometimes causing tubular damage and ureteric obstruction. This is uncommon with later sulphonamides, which are generally more soluble and more slowly excreted. It may complicate high dose co-trimoxazole used in the treatment of pneumocystis pneumonia. A similar complication has been linked to the protease inhibitors indinavir and ritonavir, used in the treatment of HIV infection.

Tetracyclines

These may occasionally be nephrotoxic, particularly in patients with pre-existing renal insufficiency and older people with physiological renal impairment. The degree of renal failure varies, but is usually reversible. An explanation of the phenomenon may lie in the anti-anabolic effect of tetracyclines among which doxycycline is unique in being devoid of nephrotoxicity, reflecting its primary hepatobiliary route of excretion.

A specific effect of demeclocycline is the production of nephrogenic diabetes insipidus, a phenomenon that has been put to therapeutic advantage in the management of the syndrome of inappropriate antidiuretic hormone secretion.

Adverse reactions by class of drug

Aminoglycosides

These are the antibiotics most frequently associated with renal toxicity. Their nephrotoxic potential varies and occurs in decreasing order of frequency with gentamicin, tobramycin, amikacin, and netilmicin. Nephrotoxicity is potentiated by pre-existing renal disease, prolonged or repeated courses of treatment, or the simultaneous administration of other nephrotoxic agents. It is more common in the elderly. Renal damage is often reversible, although permanent impairment including renal failure does occur.

Amphotericin

Nephrotoxicity is the leading complication of the use of amphotericin. This results from a combination of a reduction in glomerular filtration, renal tubular acidosis, and decreased concentrating ability. Careful monitoring of renal function is a prerequisite to the use of this agent. Lipid formulations of amphotericin (p. 76) are less nephrotoxic.

β-Lactam antibiotics

The penicillins may rarely produce a primary haemolytic anaemia and Coombs' antibody-positive disease. Selective white cell depression has been described with ampicillin and flucloxacillin. Similarly, the cephalosporins may be associated with a positive Coombs' test, although frank haemolysis is uncommon. Eosinophilia occurs with variable frequency, as does the selective depression of white cells, and occasionally platelets, following the development of platelet antibodies. A vitamin K-dependent bleeding disorder has been associated with early cephalosporins possessing a thiotetrazole side chain, such as cefamandole, cefotetan, and cefoperazone. In many countries these are no longer available. Although uncommon, bleeding occurs in elderly or malnourished patients undergoing major surgery. It is both treated and prevented by the administration of vitamin K.

Sulphonamides

Among the more important groups of agents to produce haematological side effects are the sulphonamides and sulphonamide-containing mixtures such as co-trimoxazole. Marrow toxicity may result in aplastic anaemia, or a selective neutropenia, or thrombocytopenia. In addition, haemolysis may be either primary or related to glucose-6-phosphate dehydrogenase deficiency. Co-trimoxazole may produce megaloblastic bone marrow changes or, less commonly, a peripheral megaloblastic anaemia. This tends to occur with prolonged therapy and is related to the joint antifolate action of the two components of co-trimoxazole.

Chloramphenicol

This has achieved notoriety for inducing marrow depression, which is manifested in two ways. The more common dose-related bone marrow depression is seen when the daily dose exceeds 4 g. There is a progressive anaemia, neutropenia, and sometimes thrombocytopenia, which is reversible on either discontinuing treatment or reducing the dosage. A more serious reaction is that of total bone marrow depression and aplastic anaemia. This is unpredictable but is estimated to occur with a frequency of one in 24 000 to one in 40 000 treatment courses. Mortality from aplastic anaemia is in excess of 50%. Thiamphenicol, a derivative of chloramphenicol available in some parts of the world, appears to be devoid of the irreversible toxic effects on the bone marrow although still produces a dose-dependent reversible depression of haemopoiesis.

Adverse reactions to antiviral drugs

The past decade has seen the licensing of many new antiviral drugs, largely for the treatment of herpesviruses and HIV infections. Inevitably this has led to the recognition of a range of adverse reactions, some of which are unique to this class of agents.

Antiherpesvirus agents

Aciclovir has proved remarkably free from serious toxicity. However, if administered in high dosage crystal deposition in the renal tubules can occur, occasionally leading to renal failure, unless patients are kept adequately hydrated. Neurotoxicity manifested by tremor, ataxia, and seizures can also complicate high dosage treatment or administration to patients with renal impairment. These side effects usually resolve on stopping treatment.

Ganciclovir, in contrast to aciclovir, is a more toxic drug. The major complication of use is bone marrow suppression, particularly neutropenia. This can prove difficult to manage since the drug is often required to treat cytomegalovirus infection in bone marrow and organ transplanted patients. Such patients are already extremely immunosuppressed and any additional drug-induced bone marrow suppression is undesirable. Foscarnet is an alternative to ganciclovir for the treatment of cytomegalovirus infections. While it is not associated with bone marrow suppression, its major adverse effect is dose-related renal impairment. This requires careful monitoring of renal function during treatment, with dose reduction and sometimes cessation of therapy. An unusual complication is genital ulceration.

Antiretroviral agents

This group of agents has expanded rapidly over the past two years. The clinical trials programme has often been accelerated resulting in early licensing before the full range of adverse reactions has been defined. Furthermore, the potential for interaction both between these agents and between other classes of drugs, is high and they therefore require considerable caution and expertise in their use. A selection of side effects to commonly used agents is provided.

Nucleoside reverse transcriptase inhibitors

Zidovudine (AZT) was the first antiretroviral drug to be approved and is still in widespread use. Bone marrow suppression primarily causing mild to moderate anaemia is the most common side effect. This tends to be macrocytic in nature since the drug is less suppressive to early immature forms of erythrocytes, than the mature red cell. Other side effects include myopathy, hepatotoxicity, and pigmentation of the nails.

Didanosine and stavudine can both cause a sensory neuropathy, often starting in the feet. Unless detected early, it can progress to produce severe paraesthesiae and sensory loss. Another unusual yet serious adverse effect of these drugs is acute pancreatitis. Careful monitoring and measurement of serum amylase can avoid this complication. Bone marrow toxicity may also occur.

Lipodystrophy is another relatively common side effect of long-term treatment with nucleoside analogues, particularly when used in combination with protease inhibitors. This may manifest as both increased deposition of fat as well as lipoatrophy and mitochondrial dysfunction.

Abacavir is a potent drug but may cause a severe hypersensitivity reaction, which precludes continued use. Skin rashes can also be troublesome.

Lamivudine is widely prescribed and generally safe. Pancreatitis occurs rarely.

Non-nucleoside reverse transcriptase inhibitors

Nevirapine is most commonly linked to early onset skin rashes. These occur in approximately 20% of patients within the first month of treatment and in a small number are severe and life threatening especially causing the Stevens–Johnson syndrome. Nevirapine is a potent inducer of the cytochrome P-450 enzymes; drugs such as rifampicin and rifabutin require dose adjustment if co-administered.

Efavirenz frequently causes mild to moderate neuropsychiatric side effects in the first few weeks of treatment. These include anxiety, insomnia, vivid dreams, depression and, rarely, a suicidal response.

Protease inhibitors

Saquinavir is generally well tolerated but notorious for interactions with other agents. It increases the plasma concentrations of terfenamide and astemizole, while other drugs either reduce plasma concentrations of saquinavir (rifampicin, rifabutin) or increase them (ketoconazole, ritonavir). The interaction with ritonavir has been exploited pharmaceutically, since it is often co-marketed in fixed dose formulations of other protease inhibitors (e.g. lopinavir + ritonavir) to boost their plasma concentrations to therapeutic advantage.

Nelfinavir is associated with dose-related mild to moderate diarrhoea.

Prevention of adverse reactions

There are major difficulties in preventing adverse drug reactions. Patients frequently respond idiosyncratically to antimicrobial agents, as to other drugs; the chief problem, especially with the rarer side effects, is their unpredictability. Awareness of the possibility of adverse effects is obviously important, and a close working relationship with either a clinical pharmacist or a specialist in the use of antimicrobial agents will help to overcome problems as they arise.

When toxic effects develop or are suspected, the decision has to be made whether to stop or change the patient's treatment. The drug may often be continued provided the dose is adjusted by reducing each individual dose or by prolonging the interval between doses.

Antibiotic assays are important in determining whether dosage adjustment is necessary, particularly in the case of aminoglycosides, in which the leeway between effective and toxic levels is small.

Finally, the reporting of adverse drug reactions, whether caused by antimicrobial agents or other drugs, remains the responsibility of all practising doctors. In the UK the Medicines and Healthcare Products Regulatory Agency operates a voluntary adverse reactions reporting system (see Postscript, p. 373).

Key points

- Adverse drug reactions are common, often avoidable.
- Assessment of the risk to benefit of a drug is the basis of safe prescribing practice.
- Metabolic and excretory organ impairment often require adjustment of dosage regimens to avoid drug toxicity.
- Subtherapeutic or toxic concentrations complicate multidrug prescribing; such drug interactions are often avoidable.
- ADR which are unusual, severe, or caused by recently licensed agents should be reported to the regulatory authorities (MHRA).

Further reading

Davey P (1996), 'Antimicrobial Chemotherapy', in Weatherall DJ, Ledingham JGG, and Warrell DA (eds) *Oxford Textbook of Medicine*, (3rd edn) Vol 1, Oxford: Oxford University Press.

Rawlins M, Vale JA (2009), 'Drug therapy and poisoning', in Kumar P, Clark M (eds) *Clinical Medicine*, (7th edn), London: Saunders Elsevier, 923–952.

Chapter 18

Chemoprophylaxis and immunization

Chemoprophylaxis

Chemoprophylaxis is the prevention of infection by the administration of antimicrobial agents as distinct from prevention by immunization. Individuals who require prophylaxis differ from the normal population in that they are known to be exposed to a particular infectious hazard or their ability to respond to infection is impaired.

Prophylaxis should be confined to those periods for which the risk is greatest, so that the problems of disturbance of the normal flora, superinfection with resistant organisms, untoward reactions, and cost will be minimized. The benefits and risks of chemoprophylaxis depend on:

◆ the likelihood of infection in the absence of prophylaxis;

◆ the potential severity of the consequences of infection;

◆ the effectiveness of prophylaxis in reducing the likelihood of infection and the severity of the consequences;

◆ the likelihood and consequences of adverse effects from prophylaxis.

Prevention strategies for infectious disease can be characterized by the traditional concepts of primary, secondary, and tertiary prevention. *Primary prevention* can be defined as the prevention of infection. *Secondary prevention* includes measures for the detection of early infection and effective intervention before symptoms occur or recur. *Tertiary prevention* consists of measures to reduce or eliminate the long-term impairment and disabilities caused by established infection.

Failure to consider fully the risks of prophylaxis or to be realistic about the benefits has made unnecessary chemoprophylaxis one of the commonest forms of antibiotic misuse. None the less it is important to recognize that the judgement about what is and is not necessary chemoprophylaxis may require complex decisions about the balance of benefits and risks to individual patients and to the population. The example of prevention of neonatal infection by Group B Streptococci (see below) shows how national guidelines committees can produce different recommendations based on their risk assessment of the same evidence.

Primary chemoprophylaxis

Most indications for primary chemoprophylaxis involve starting prophylaxis before a period of defined risk (e.g. elective surgery or travel to regions with endemic malaria or intrapartum exposure of neonates to maternal infections) or following exposure to a patient who is known to have a contagious, dangerous infection (e.g. meningococcal meningitis).

Prophylaxis in surgery

Reducing the risk of surgical infection is probably the most common indication for chemoprophylaxis and accounts for up to a third of total antibiotic use in an acute hospital. There is no doubt that prophylaxis can reduce the risk of surgical infection, but at best it is only one component of effective infection control and unnecessary use or duration of prophylaxis puts patients at risk

Table 18.1 American Society of Anesthesiologists classification of physical status

ASA score	Physical status
1	Normal healthy patient
2	Patient with a mild systemic disease
3	Patient with a severe systemic disease that limits activity, but is not incapacitating
4	Patient with an incapacitating systemic disease that is a constant threat to life
5	Moribund patient not expected to survive 24 hours with or without operation

Adapted from American Society of Anesthesiologists. New classification of physical status. *Anesthesiology* 1963; **24**: 111.

of infection by *Clostridium difficile* or antimicrobial-resistant bacteria with no compensating benefit.

Classification of operations by risk of infection

The aim of chemoprophylaxis is to reduce the risk of surgical site infection, meaning infection in any part of the operative field from the superficial wound down to the deepest tissues involved in the operation. Post-operative infections can occur at other sites (e.g. the respiratory or urinary tract) but chemoprophylaxis is targeted at surgical site infection.

The US Centers for Disease Control's (CDC) NNIS (National Nosocomial Infections Surveillance) risk index is an internationally recognized method for infection risk adjustment. Risk adjustment is based on three major risk factors:

◆ the American Society of Anesthesiologists (ASA) score, reflecting the patient's state of health before surgery (Table 18.1);

◆ wound class, reflecting the state of contamination of the wound (Table 18.2);

◆ duration of operation, reflecting technical aspects of the surgery.

Primary prevention by chemoprophylaxis is only achievable for clean, clean-contaminated, or contaminated wounds because the process of infection has started pre-operatively in dirty wounds. The risk of infection rises progressively according to the NNIS score (Fig. 18.1). The relative weightings of the elements in this score mean, for example, that a prolonged operation with a clean wound in a patient with co-morbidities carries approximately a 5% risk of wound infection, which is markedly higher than the 3.5% risk for a contaminated wound in a patient with no co-morbidities and a short operation. Such data underscore the risk associated with the underlying fitness of the patient at the time of surgery.

In addition to the probability that an infection will occur, it is important to consider the consequences of infection for the patient and the health service. Surgical site infection following colon surgery is associated with substantially increased risk of mortality and prophylaxis significantly reduces death within 30 days of surgery. An increasing proportion of surgical procedures involve the implantation of devices such as prostheses (e.g. artificial joints) or cardiac pacemakers. Post-operative infection can rarely be controlled without removal of these devices, resulting in long-term morbidity, which can be reduced through surgical prophylaxis. Because of these dire consequences, even small reductions in the risk of surgical site infection by prophylaxis may be justifiable.

Principles of surgical prophylaxis

The key to successful surgical prophylaxis is to achieve effective antimicrobial concentrations in the wound before bacterial contamination occurs (Fig. 18.2). Prophylaxis can still be effective if it

Table 18.2 Classification of surgical operations according to risk of contamination of the wound by bacteria

Class	Conditions of operation
Clean	No inflammation is encountered and the respiratory, alimentary or genito-urinary tracts are not entered. There is no break in aseptic operating theatre technique
Clean-contaminated	The respiratory, alimentary or genito-urinary tracts are entered but without significant spillage
Contaminated	Acute inflammation (without pus) is encountered, or there is visible contamination of the wound. Examples include: gross spillage from a hollow viscus during the operation; compound injuries operated on within four hours
Dirty	Presence of pus, a previously perforated hollow viscus, or compound injuries more than four hours old

From: Culver DH, Horan TC, Gaynes RP, Martone WJ, Jarvis WR, Emori TG, et al. 'Surgical wound infection rates by wound class, operative procedure, and patient risk index. National Nosocomial Infections Surveillance System', *American Journal of Medicine* 1991; **91**(3B): 152S–7S.

is administered within two hours after the start of the operation but later administration is much less effective. However, prophylaxis should not be administered too early before the start of the operation or antibiotic concentrations in the surgical site will have declined below effective levels before bacterial contamination occurs. The ideal time to administer intravenous prophylaxis is in the anaesthetic room no more than 30 min before the start of surgery and before any tourniquet is applied to reduce blood supply to the surgical site. For drugs with a short half-life (two hours or less) additional doses may be required during the operation if it is prolonged or if there is substantial blood loss (1500 ml or more) or haemodilution by 15 ml/kg or more.

It follows that there is no value in administering additional doses of prophylaxis once the wound has been closed. For most operations a single dose of prophylaxis is all that is required. There is still some controversy about the benefits and risks of extending prophylaxis for up to

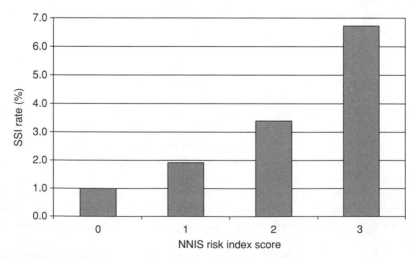

Fig. 18.1 Surgical site infection rate according to NNIS risk index score.
(From Culver DH, Horan TC, Gaynes RP, Martone WJ, Jarvis WR, Emori TG et al. 'Surgical wound infection rates by wound class, operative procedure, and patient risk index. National Nosocomial Infections Surveillance System'. *Americal Journal of Medicine* 1991; **91**(3B):152S–7S.

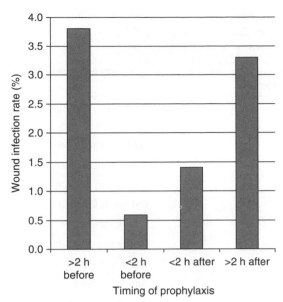

Fig. 18.2 Risk of wound infection by time of administration of antibiotic prophylaxis. Data from a prospective study of 2847 patients undergoing elective clean or clean-contaminated surgery who received prophylactic antibiotics. The timing of prophylaxis refers to the time of administration of the first dose in relation to the start of the operation. From Classen DC, Evans RS, Pestotnik SL, Horn SD, Menlove RL, Burke JP, 'The timing of prophylactic administration of antibiotics and the risk of surgical-wound infection'. *New England Journal of Medicine* 1992; **326**: 281–286.

24 h post-operatively, the argument in favour being that wounds are insufficiently sealed to prevent bacterial contamination. However, there is absolutely no doubt that prophylaxis should not continue for more than 24 h after surgery. Extended antibiotic 'prophylaxis' risks selecting for antibiotic resistant bacteria, or complications such as *C. difficile* infection and other drug related adverse events.

Guidelines for surgical prophylaxis

Unequivocal evidence for the effectiveness of antibiotic prophylaxis comes from controlled clinical trials with a 'no treatment' or placebo arm. Once effectiveness has been established for a specific operation it may be considered unethical to do placebo-controlled trials in similar operations. For example, the recommendation to give prophylaxis before total knee replacement is based on expert opinion that the strong evidence supporting prophylaxis for total hip replacement supports prophylaxis for all total joint replacements. Guidelines should be explicit about the expected standard of care by distinguishing between: operations for which prophylaxis should be the rule; those for which local policy makers or surgeons may identify exceptions; and operations for which prophylaxis should not be given at all (Table 18.3). This judgement is based on a combination of the evidence about effectiveness of prophylaxis and estimates of the consequences of surgical site infection for the patient.

However effective prophylaxis is at reducing the risk of surgical site infection there must be a point when the risk of infection is so low without prophylaxis that the benefits are questionable. The number of patients that must receive prophylaxis to prevent one surgical site infection rises exponentially as the risk of infection diminishes (Fig. 18.3). For clean wound surgery in a patient with no other risk factors the probability of surgical site infection is only 1%. If prophylaxis halves

Table 18.3 Examples of recommendations for surgical prophylaxis in a national guideline. Adapted from Scottish Intercollegiate Guidelines Network (SIGN), Guideline 104. Antibiotic Prophylaxis in Surgery, 2008. http://www.sign.ac.uk/pdf/sign104.pdf

Recommended: prophylaxis reduces risk of major morbidity and is likely to decrease overall consumption of antibiotics

Cardiothoracic surgery	Cardiac pacemaker insertion
	Open heart surgery
	Pulmonary resection
ENT surgery	Clean-contaminated head and neck surgery
Neurosurgery	Craniotomy
	CSF shunt insertion
Orthopaedic surgery	Total joint replacement at any site
	Fracture fixation with internal fixation
	Spinal surgery
General surgery	Appendicectomy
	Colorectal surgery
	Gastro-duodenal or small bowel surgery
	Oesophageal surgery
Obstetrics and gynaecology	Caesarean section
	Abdominal hysterectomy
	Vaginal hysterectomy
	Induced abortion
Urology	Shock wave lithotripsy
	Transurethral resection of prostate
	Transrectal prostate biopsy
Vascular surgery	Lower limb amputation
	Abdominal or lower limb vascular surgery with graft

Should be considered but local policy makers and surgeons may identify exceptions: prophylaxis may increase overall consumption of antibiotics if given to low-risk patients

Abdominal therapeutic endoscopic procedures (endoscopic retrograde cholangiopancreatography and percutaneous endoscopic gastrostomy)	Consider in high risk patients
General surgery	Biliary surgery
	Breast surgery
Urology	Cystoscopy (if evidence of UTI, prophylaxis is recommended)
Obstetrics	Manual removal of placenta

Table 18.3 (continued) Examples of recommendations for surgical prophylaxis in a national guideline. Adapted from: *Antibiotic Prophylaxis in Surgery*. Scottish Intercollegiate Guidelines Network

Not recommended: prophylaxis is likely to increase hospital antibiotic consumption for little clinical benefit	
ENT surgery	Clean ear surgery
	Clean head or neck surgery (should be considered for malignant surgery or neck dissection)
	Nose or sinus surgery
	Tonsillectomy
	Adenoidectomy *(by curettage)*
Orthopaedic surgery	Orthopaedic surgery without implanted device
General surgery	Laparoscopic cholecystectomy
	Hernia repair
Urology	Transurethral resection of bladder tumours

ENT, ear, nose, and throat; CSF, cerebrospinal fluid.

the risk of infection that means that 200 patients must receive prophylaxis in order to prevent one surgical site infection. The balance between benefits and risks of prophylaxis therefore depends on how a surgical site infection will be managed if it occurs. An infected hip prosthesis may require two months or more of antibiotic treatment (over 200 doses of flucloxacillin); consequently, administration of single doses of prophylaxis to 200 patients is still likely to reduce total antibiotic use in the hospital if it prevents one infection.

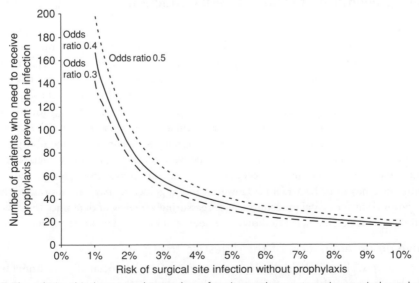

Fig. 18.3 The relationship between the number of patients who must receive surgical prophylaxis to prevent one surgical site infection and the risk of infection without prophylaxis. The three lines show results for operations in which the odds ratio of infection with prophylaxis versus no prophylaxis is 0.3 (– · –), 0.4 (—) and 0.5 (....).

The choice of agents for chemoprophylaxis should be guided by local sensitivities and antibiotic policies. The only requirement is that the regimen covers the common pathogens that cause infection at the surgical site. The single dose for prophylactic use is in most circumstances the same as would be used therapeutically.

Prophylaxis for travellers

Malaria

Protecting travellers to areas where malaria is common fulfils all of the criteria for successful chemoprophylaxis. The chances of acquiring the disease are high, the results can be grave, and the period at risk is well defined: from arrival in the area until 4 weeks after departure—the time taken for any parasites that may have been acquired to be finally eliminated. Although resistance is an increasing problem in malaria it is still possible to identify a drug that is suitable for prophylaxis for most travellers (see p. 359). Failure to take chemoprophylaxis or to continue for four weeks after leaving a region of endemic malaria are the commonest reasons for malaria presenting in countries where malaria is not endemic.

As in surgery, chemoprophylaxis for malaria should be seen as only one component of risk reduction. They should also do all that they can to avoid contact with malaria vectors: use of protective clothing; window netting; insect repellants; and sleeping under insecticide-impregnated bed netting.

Apart from transient visitors to endemic regions the only other clear candidates for antimalarial chemoprophylaxis are resident women during pregnancy.

Other prophylaxis for travellers

Chemoprophylaxis can reduce the risk of traveller's diarrhoea but early treatment of symptomatic cases is highly effective and is preferable.

Primary prevention of other bacterial infections

Endocarditis

Prevention of bacterial endocarditis in people with abnormal heart valves or other endocardial disease is similar in principle to surgical prophylaxis. The aim is to achieve effective plasma concentrations of antimicrobial drugs before the start of a procedure that carries substantial risk of causing bacteraemia and therefore contamination of the endocardium. The logic behind routine prophylaxis for dental procedures is that bacteria from the normal oral flora account for a substantial proportion of cases of endocarditis and that recent dental treatment is a known risk factor. Having said that, there is little direct evidence on the reduction in risk achieved by chemoprophylaxis for dental procedures, and even less for endoscopy of the gastrointestinal or urinary tract. National and local guidelines used to recommend prophylaxis for patients at risk undergoing a wide range of procedures that may cause bacteraemia. However, recent guidelines have not supported the use of routine prophylaxis for dental procedures, and, reassuringly, review of data since the new recommendations were issued has failed to show any evidence of increased incidence of endocarditis.

Selective decontamination of the digestive tract

Chemoprophylaxis has a role in the prevention of ventilator-associated pneumonia but once again, only as part of a risk reduction strategy that includes other effective measures. Selective decontamination of the digestive tract, started at the time of intubation and targeted at Gram-negative aerobic bacilli and fungi, reduces the risk of ventilator-associated pneumonia, especially in trauma victims. However, adoption of such prophylaxis is very variable across the world, largely because of ongoing controversy about long-term outcome and specifically whether mortality is affected. Concern about antibiotic resistance selection also remains a concern.

Another example of selective decontamination of the digestive tract is oral administration of co-trimoxazole or quinolones to afebrile neutropenic patients. However, this is no longer recommended practice in most national guidelines because the risks from selection of drug-resistant bacteria are thought to outweigh any clinical benefit. Again, evidence that mortality is reduced by this approach is lacking.

Neonatal infection with Group B streptococci

Colonization of the vagina or rectum with Group B streptococci (*Streptococcus agalactiae*) is very common in pregnancy (prevalence 20–30%). It does not usually cause morbidity in mothers but can cause serious neonatal infections (10% overall mortality but 23% mortality in premature infants of less than 35 weeks' gestation). However, routine intrapartum chemoprophylaxis does not significantly reduce neonatal mortality and most guidelines recommend targeted intrapartum prophylaxis. There are three different approaches, each advocated by at least one set of national guidelines:

- **Risk-based assessment:** intrapartum prophylaxis with penicillin is offered to women with known risk factors (e.g. previous baby with neonatal Group B streptococcal disease; Group B streptococcal bacteriuria during pregnancy; premature delivery) or intrapartum fever. The UK Royal College of Obstetricians and Gynaecologists (2006 guidelines) currently advocate this approach.

- **Bacteriological screening:** vaginal and rectal swabs are taken from all women between 35 and 37 weeks of gestation and intrapartum prophylaxis is offered to those with positive swabs. Prophylaxis is also offered to women who go into labour before swabs have been taken or cultured. This approach is currently advocated by the Centers for Disease Control and Prevention in the USA.

- **Bacteriological screening with targeted prophylaxis:** the screening process is the same as in option 2 (bacteriological screening) but intrapartum prophylaxis is offered only to women who also have one of the risk factors outlined in option 1 (risk-based assessment).

In 2007 the UK Royal College of Obstetricians and Gynaecologists reviewed practice on Group B streptococcal intrapartum antibiotic prophylaxis in 13 countries. Seven guidelines recommended universal bacteriological screening, four guidelines promoted a risk-based strategy, one recommended universal bacteriological screening but women would only be offered prophylaxis if they had a positive streptococcal culture and another risk factor, and one gave no strong preference. The arguments for and against are based on estimation of the benefits, costs, and risks of each strategy. The reason that the UK guidelines do not favour routine bacteriological screening is that they estimate that at least 24 000 women would need to be screened and about 700 women receive intrapartum prophylaxis to prevent one neonatal infection, whereas with risk-based assessment the number of women who must be treated to prevent one neonatal infection is about 200. The risk assessments and decisions made by the national guideline groups will have been heavily influenced by the different legal systems in the UK and North America, and differences in disease epidemiology according to ethnicity and social status.

Post-exposure prophylaxis of bacterial infections

Examples of primary post-exposure chemoprophylaxis for bacterial infection include:

- exposure to *Neisseria meningitidis*;
- exposure of vulnerable, unvaccinated children to *Bordetella pertussis*;

- prevention of ophthalmia neonatorum in babies born to mothers with gonorrhoeal or chlamydial infection;
- prophylaxis following sexual assault.

For *N. meningitidis* there are two distinct situations. The first is prophylaxis of contacts of sporadic cases, which is confined to close contacts (e.g. household or mouth-kissing contacts) and healthcare workers who have been heavily exposed to respiratory droplets or secretions). The second is in epidemic situations, where chemoprophylaxis may be used to supplement vaccination strategies for Group A or C strains and for epidemics caused by Group B strains. Sulphonamides are no longer effective for prophylaxis of meningococcal infection because of drug resistance; the current agents of choice are rifampicin or ciprofloxacin.

Primary prevention of recurrent bacterial infections

All of the previous examples involve short-term risk reduction but there are a few situations where risk reduction has to be continued for prolonged periods; for example, prevention of bacterial infection following splenectomy or rheumatic carditis, or prevention of recurrent infections.

For recurrent infections it may be possible to identify repeated short periods of risk. For example, some women with recurrent urinary tract infection may be able to achieve satisfactory control by taking a single dose of antibiotics following sexual intercourse, which is really repeated post-exposure prophylaxis.

Primary prevention of viral infections by chemotherapy

An example of prophylaxis before exposure is intrapartum treatment of mothers who are known to be HIV positive in order to reduce the risk of perinatal infection. The principles of prophylaxis here are the same as for neonatal Group B streptococcal infection.

Examples of post-exposure antiviral chemoprophylaxis include exposure to influenza A virus (amantadine, rimantadine), influenza A or B virus (zanamivir or oseltamivir), and HIV (antiretroviral drugs). There are two common indications for post-exposure prophylaxis against HIV: after occupational or environmental exposure, and after sexual exposure.

Secondary chemoprophylaxis

Secondary prevention strategies involve the identification of early or asymptomatic infection with subsequent treatment so that such infections are eradicated and sequelae are prevented. Although most secondary prevention programmes involve intervention at the individual level through the use of chemoprophylaxis, they may also operate within the context of a population-based or institution-based screening effort. Routine screening programmes for sexually transmitted diseases such as *Chlamydia* infection are examples of secondary prevention strategies. Contact investigations for partners of persons with sexually transmitted diseases are also part of a secondary prevention strategy focused on those with known exposure. Another example of a secondary prevention programme that uses chemoprophylaxis is the screening of high-risk populations for tuberculosis infection and subsequent therapy with an antimicrobial drug such as isoniazid to prevent active disease.

Tertiary prophylaxis

Tertiary prevention efforts are measures to eliminate long-term impairment and disability that may result from an existing condition. Because most infectious diseases are treatable, tertiary prevention activities are less common than those used with chronic diseases such as hypertension, diabetes, and coronary artery disease. However, this concept is still applicable to the control of infectious diseases; for example, some chronic viral infections cannot be eradicated and there are a number of latent infections that cause symptoms only in immunosuppressed patients.

Treatment of HIV infection now relies on highly active antiretroviral therapy (HAART) with combinations of drugs that reduce viral load to undetectable levels and restore counts of CD4 lymphocytes to > 200/mm^3. Provided that the patient can tolerate the treatment and there is no major resistance to antiviral drugs in the infecting strain of HIV, this treatment can maintain normal immunity for many years and prevent recurrence of latent opportunistic infections (see Chapter 33). However, once the CD4 lymphocyte count falls below 200/mm^3 the cumulative risk for developing an AIDS-defining opportunistic infection is 33% by year 1 and 58% by year 2, so chemoprophylaxis must be considered.

Latent infection means that many patients are already infected with these organisms before they become immunosuppressed. With normal immunity the infections may have been asymptomatic from the start or may have caused a transient illness but then remain dormant for very long periods. *Pneumocystis carinii* rarely if ever causes symptomatic infection in people with normal immunity, whereas herpes simplex does cause recurrent symptoms even with normal immunity. However, in immunosuppressed people the frequency and consequences of symptomatic infection are greatly increased. Other indications for tertiary prophylaxis of latent infection include:

- primary immunodeficiency;
- severe malnutrition;
- after organ transplantation;
- cytotoxic or immunosuppressive treatment of cancer, connective tissue disorders, and other diseases, including long-term corticosteroids.

The general principles of chemoprophylaxis are the same for long-term suppression of latent infection as for short-term primary or secondary prevention. However, with long-term prophylaxis the issues of inducing resistance, risk of adverse effects, and cost-effectiveness are even more important.

Resistance or cross-resistance has become increasingly common with prophylaxis for the *Mycobacterium avium* complex, fungal infections, and *P. carinii*. For example, following prophylaxis with clarithromycin for *M. avium* complex infections over half the infections that occur are caused by strains that are resistant to clarithromycin, delaying clinical recovery and requiring treatment with alternative less effective or more toxic agents. Prophylactic regimens may also lead to the development of cross-resistance against more common pathogens. For example, rifabutin used for prophylaxis of infections with opportunistic mycobacteria may result in the emergence of rifampicin-resistant strains of *M. tuberculosis* and use of antibiotics, such as clarithromycin, azithromycin, or co-trimoxazole may lead to the development of resistance among organisms such as pneumococci that were not the primary targets of prophylaxis.

Patients with HIV infection are particularly vulnerable to adverse reactions to drugs. The reason is probably a combination of immunomodulation or other HIV-related idiosyncrasy, pre-existing organ damage in late stage disease, and interaction between the large number of potentially toxic drugs that these patients require.

The balance of risks and benefits of taking long-term prophylaxis versus treating symptomatic infections when they occur determine cost-effectiveness. The issue is not purely financial: the costs of prophylaxis include the inconvenience to the patient of having to take large numbers of medicines all the time and their negative impact on quality of life. In general long-term prophylaxis is cost-effective for *P. carinii* or opportunistic mycobacteria but not for fungal infection or cytomegalovirus.

Immunization

The contribution of immunization to reducing the morbidity and mortality due to infectious diseases is enormous. For example, the introduction of vaccines (initially separately and then in a combined product) against measles, mumps, and rubella (MMR) was followed by dramatic reductions in the incidences of these diseases. In the 1950s and 1960s approximately half a million recorded cases of measles occurred each year in England and Wales. Routine measles vaccination was introduced in 1968, and by the time that the combined MMR vaccine followed in 1988 the annual incidence of measles had fallen fivefold to approximately 100 000 cases. A decade later there were 56 confirmed cases of measles in the UK. After (subsequently unfounded) controversy about the safety of MMR vaccination began, compliance dropped sharply in the UK from 92% in 1996 to 84% in 2002. In some parts of London, compliance was as low as 61% in 2003, which was far below the rate needed to avoid an epidemic of measles. Depressingly, in 2008 there were 1370 confirmed cases of measles. The incidence is now starting to fall again, coincident with enhanced population vaccination rates as the safety concerns have been refuted.

A full review of immunization is beyond the scope of this text, but it should be noted that the complexity of immunization schedules continues to increase markedly as new vaccines are

Table 18.4a UK Immunization schedule 2011

AGE	Immunization (Vaccine Given)
2 months	**DTaP/IPV(polio)/Hib** (diphtheria, tetanus, pertussis (whooping cough), polio, and *Haemophilus influenzae* type b)—all-in-one injection, plus:
	PCV (pneumococcal conjugate vaccine)—in a separate injection.
3 months	**DTaP/IPV(polio)/Hib** (2nd dose), plus:
	MenC (meningitis C)—in a separate injection.
4 months	**DTaP/IPV(polio)/Hib** (3rd dose), plus:
	MenC (2nd dose)—in a separate injection, plus:
	PCV (2nd dose)—in a separate injection.
Between 12 and 13 months	**Hib/MenC** (combined as one injection—4th dose of Hib and 3rd dose of MenC) plus:
	MMR (measles, mumps, and rubella—combined as one injection), plus:
	PCV (3rd dose)—in a separate injection.
Around 3 years and four months	Pre-school booster of:
	DTaP/IPV(polio) (diphtheria, tetanus, pertussis (whooping cough), and polio), plus:
	MMR (second dose)—in a separate injection.
Around 12–13 years (girls)	**HPV** (human papillomavirus)—**three injections** The second injection is given 1–2 months after the first one. The third is given about six months after the first one.
Around 13–18 years	**Td/IPV(polio) booster** (a combined injection of tetanus, low-dose diphtheria, and polio).
Adults	**Influenza and PCV** if you are aged 65 or over or in a high-risk group.
	Td/IPV(polio)—at any age if you were not fully immunized as a child.

From http://www.patient.co.uk/health/Immunisation-Usual-UK-Schedule.htm.

Table 18.4b UK Immunization schedule 1996

Age	Vaccine
2 months	D/Ta/P, PV and Hib 1st dose
3 months	D/Ta/P, PV and Hib 2nd dose
4 months	D/Ta/P, PV and Hib 3rd dose
12–15 months	MMR
3–5 years	Booster D/Ta and PV, MMR second dose
10–14 years or infancy	BCG
13–18 years	Booster D/Ta and PV

From http://www.dh.gov.uk/dr_consum_dh/groups/dh_digitalassets/@dh/@en/documents/digitalasset/dh_4073001.pdf.

discovered and new age groups are included (for example, the elderly now routinely receive pneumococcal and influenza vaccines). This can be seen, for example, by comparing the recommended UK immunization schedules in 1996 and 2011 (Tables 18.4a and b). New recent additions include extended coverage pneumococcal conjugate and human papilloma virus vaccines. It is very likely that further vaccines will be introduced given the substantial health benefits (and profits) achieved to-date.

Key points

- The patient's state of health before surgery, type of wound (clean, contaminated, dirty) and duration of operation are key determinants of infection risk.

- Antibiotic prophylaxis should be preferably be given just before (e.g. in the 30 minutes before) surgery starts.

- Antibiotic prophylaxis is indicated in many but importantly not all surgical operations, as a way of reducing infection risk and overall antibiotic consumption.

- Practice varies considerably concerning intrapartum antibiotic prophylaxis against Group B streptococcal infection.

- Immunization coverage (compliance) in the at risk population is crucial in determining the overall effectiveness of a vaccine.

Further reading

Royal College of Obstetricians and Gynaecologists and London School of Hygiene and Tropical Medicine (2007), The Prevention of Early-onset Neonatal Group B Streptococcal Disease in UK Obstetric Units. An audit of reported practice in England, Scotland, Wales and Northern Ireland. Available at: http://www.rcog.org.uk/files/rcog-corp/uploaded-files/neonatal_summary_050207a.pdf.

Scottish Intercollegiate Guidelines Network (2008), Guideline 104: *Antibiotic prophylaxis in surgery*. Available at: http://www.sign.ac.uk/pdf/sign104.pdf.

UK Department of Health. *Immunisation against infectious disease—'The Green Book'*. Available at: *http://www.dh.gov.uk/en/Publicationsandstatistics/Publications/PublicationsPolicyAndGuidance/ DH_079917.*

Chapter 19

Guidelines, formularies, and antimicrobial policies

The discovery of antibiotics undoubtedly transformed the outcome of severe bacterial infection. However, a less comfortable aspect of the antibiotic revolution was that within 10 years over 80% of patients with acute bronchitis were receiving antibiotics without any evidence of clinical benefit A link between antimicrobial prescribing and resistance has been clear from the start of the therapeutic use of sulphonamides and penicillin. Collateral damage to the normal bacterial flora also results in infection by other pathogens such as *Clostridium difficile* and fungi. Logic dictates that antimicrobial drugs should only be prescribed when benefit outweighs risk and that unnecessary use should be avoided. Consequently antibiotic stewardship has two aims:

1 Ensure that patients with bacterial infections receive prompt, effective treatment;

2 Minimise the risk of collateral damage by selecting the right drug and duration of treatment for those with infection and avoiding unnecessary treatment of patients who will not benefit.

Definition of terms

The terms guidelines, formularies, and policies are often used interchangeably but they are separate, complementary components of a strategy for prudent antimicrobial use.

◆ **Guidelines** provide advice about what drug should be prescribed for a specific clinical condition. They may take the form of a care pathway or flow chart outlining processes of care including investigations and therapies other than just antimicrobial compounds (e.g. use of fluid replacement and oxygenation in a pneumonia guideline).

◆ A **formulary** is a limited list of drugs available for prescription. It may include information about available formulations (by route of administration), dosing instructions, and advice about drug safety or interactions but it does not include detailed guidance for use.

◆ An **antimicrobial policy** is a set of statements about an organization's strategy for promoting prudent antimicrobial prescribing. This can include a limited list of antimicrobial agents that are generally available to all prescribers—in other words an antimicrobial formulary. However, an antimicrobial policy should also contain guidelines about treatment of specific conditions.

  • **Restrictive policies.** In addition to guidance, antimicrobial policies may include enforcement strategies such as requiring authorization of initial prescription or automatic stop orders (e.g. orders for intravenous vancomycin will be stopped after three days unless authorization for continued use is obtained from a consultant microbiologist).

  • **Persuasive policies.** This term is used to distinguish policies that do not include enforcement strategies and rely on persuading professionals to follow the policy. This term is preferred to educational because most restrictive policies have an educational component.

An antimicrobial management team is a multidisciplinary team in which each member is given specific roles and which collectively takes responsibility for implementation of local policies (Fig. 19.1). To be effective the team must have full support from hospital leadership and provide

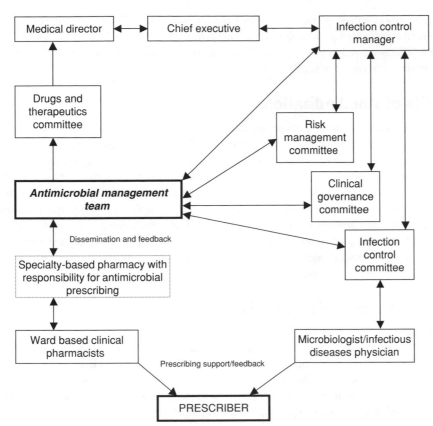

Fig. 19.1 Model pathway for implementing improvements in antimicrobial prescribing practice in hospitals. The antimicrobial management team has a central coordinating role in feedback of information to individual prescribers, clinical teams, and senior management. Reproduced from Dilip Nathwani and The Scottish Executive Health Department Healthcare Associated Infection Task Force on behalf of Scottish Medicines Consortium (SMC) Short Life Working Group (2006), 'Antimicrobial prescribing policy and practice in Scotland: recommendations for good antimicrobial practice in acute hospitals'. *Journal of Antimicrobial Chemotherapy* :dk1137, 2006 by permission of Oxford University Press.

regular feedback to individual clinicians and clinical teams about their compliance with policies. This rule applies equally to primary care and to hospital care; the key point is that guidelines, formularies, and policies will not change practice unless they are actively implemented.

National policies and laws

Self-medication with antimicrobial drugs is the norm in countries where they are freely available over the counter; self-medication is estimated to account for over 90% of all antimicrobial drug use in the Philippines. There are undoubtedly some potential advantages to increasing the availability of antibacterial agents without prescription, such as convenience for the patient, faster initiation of treatment, and reduction in primary care workload. However, in the European Union and North America the risks of increasing access are thought to outweigh these benefits. The degree of control of supply of antimicrobial compounds is highly variable between countries. In the most conservative countries free sale is banned, professional limits are placed on prescription practices by law and there is statutory control of advertising. No advertising is allowed to the lay public and the content of professional advertising is limited by law. To be effective these comprehensive restrictions need to be backed up by tightly controlled availability of antimicrobial drugs and rigorous enforcement of regulations.

Benefits of standardization

Antimicrobial formularies and policies should be seen as part of more general efforts to promote rational prescribing. In any therapeutic area there are likely to be several drugs that have similar effectiveness for specific conditions and there are advantages to standardizing which of the options is chosen for common indications. There are additional benefits to standardizing the range of antimicrobial drugs used (Table 19.1). At the same time there may be concerns that continuous use of a limited range of antimicrobial compounds will promote the development of resistance by focusing the selection pressure on to a narrow range of drugs. Although this sounds logical several lines of evidence indicate that use of a restricted range of antimicrobial agents is strongly associated with lower total use. Prudent antimicrobial prescribers are conservative about who they give these drugs to as well as the range of compounds that they use.

Prudent antimicrobial prescribing

Prudent antimicrobial prescribing has been defined as:

The use of antimicrobial drugs in the most appropriate way for the treatment, or prevention, of human infectious diseases having regard to the diagnosis (or presumed diagnosis), evidence of clinical effectiveness, likely benefits, safety, cost (in comparison with relevant alternative choices), and propensity for the emergence of resistance. The most appropriate way implies that the indication and, if needed, choice of drug, route, dosage, frequency, and duration of administration have been rigorously determined.

This definition of prudent prescribing can be broken down into two principal components:

1 Evidence that needs to be included in decision making:
   - the diagnosis (or presumed diagnosis);
   - evidence of clinical effectiveness;
   - likely benefits;
   - safety;
   - cost (in comparison with relevant alternative choices);
   - propensity for collateral damage.
2 Decisions that need to be made:
   - does the patient need antimicrobial therapy?
   - if needed, what is the most appropriate drug, route, dosage and frequency of administration?
   - when should response to treatment be reviewed?
   - when should treatment be stopped?

Content of antimicrobial policies

Antimicrobial policies should promote prudent prescribing by ensuring that an effective range of antimicrobial drugs is maintained. They should define effective treatment (including appropriate dosages), avoid unnecessary treatment, reduce the emergence of antimicrobial resistance, promote

Table 19.1 General and specific benefits of limiting the range of drugs used for conditions through guidelines, formularies, and policies. Reprinted from Davey PG, Nathwani D and Rubinstein E (2010), 'Antimicrobial Policies', in *Antimicrobial and Chemotherapy* Finch RG, Greenwood D, and Norrby R (eds) London: Elsevier 126–143, with permission from Elsevier

Category	Benefits
Knowledge	*General*:
	Promotes awareness of benefits, risks and cost of prescribing
	Focuses learning about safety and drug interactions on a limited range of drugs
	Reduces the impact of aggressive marketing by the pharmaceutical industry
	Encourages rational use of drugs based on analysis of pharmacology, clinical effectiveness, safety, and cost
	Specific to antimicrobial agents:
	Targets education about local epidemiology of pathogens towards knowledge of their susceptibility to a limited range of compounds
	Promotes awareness of the strengths and weaknesses of specific antimicrobial drugs
Attitudes	*General*:
	Acceptance by clinicians of the importance of setting standards of care and prescribing
	Acceptance of peer review and audit of prescribing
	Specific to antimicrobial agents:
	Recognition of the complex issues underlying antimicrobial chemotherapy
	Recognition of the importance of the special expertise required for full evaluation of antimicrobial chemotherapy
	Diagnostic microbiology
	Epidemiology and infection control
	Clinical diagnosis and recognition of other diseases mimicking infection
	Pharmacokinetics and pharmacodynamics of antimicrobial agents
Behaviour	*General*:
	Increased compliance with guidelines and treatment policies
	Reduction of medical practice variation
	Specific to antimicrobial agents:
	Improved liaison between clinicians, pharmacists, microbiologists, and the infection control team
Outcome	*General*:
	Standardization is a key strategy for improving patient safety.
	Improved efficiency of prescribing by increasing sensitivity (patients who can benefit receive treatment) and specificity (treatment is not prescribed to patients who will not benefit:
	Improved clinical outcome
	Reduces medicolegal liability
	Specific to antimicrobial agents:
	Limits emergence and spread of drug resistant strains

good practice, and contain costs. Contact details should be given for further advice (e.g. about public health and infection control issues or about therapeutic drug monitoring). Policies should be dated and state when the document will be revised. In the UK, the National Audit Office recommends at least annual revision of hospital policies.

Ideally policy recommendations should be linked to evidence. This can be relatively easy to achieve if the local policy is adapted from a national document based on systematic review of evidence. However, it is unreasonable to expect individual primary or secondary care organizations to conduct their own systematic reviews of evidence. This would involve massive duplication of effort and it is highly unlikely that all have the necessary skills. National and international organizations should take responsibility for regular review of evidence to support development of antimicrobial policies. National templates are an efficient method for defining the core evidence for antimicrobial policies, while still leaving a lot of decision making to local policy makers, who can select a range of effective antimicrobial agents based on local information about susceptibility patterns and drug costs.

It is debatable whether local policies should include detailed information about dosing, side effects, and contraindications. While it saves prescribers having to look up multiple documents, the information is readily available in national formularies or similar documents and inclusion makes local policies less easy to use.

Recommendations about treatment of specific conditions should include advice about withholding therapy. Antimicrobial treatment should not be prescribed, for example, for patients with asymptomatic bacteriuria (except in pregnancy; see Chapter 23) or for most patients with upper respiratory symptoms (see Chapter 21).

Advice should be given about methods for assessment of severity of infections. These can either be generic (e.g. diagnosis of sepsis, severe sepsis, and septic shock) or disease specific (e.g. the CURB-65 score for assessment of severity of community acquired pneumonia described in Chapter 21). Advice about chemoprophylaxis (see Chapter 18) should be included in addition to treatment of infection. Hospital policies should include guidance on criteria for intravenous administration and for switching patients from intravenous to oral formulations.

Policies in primary and secondary care

In North America and Europe there are numerous examples of recommendations from government agencies and professional societies that hospitals and primary care organizations should have antimicrobial policies in place. Moreover most of these recommendations extend to measurement of practice against policy recommendations with feedback of information to individual prescribers. National surveys show that most (but not all) organizations have local policies in place or refer prescribers to national policies. However, surveys in the UK and USA show that only a minority of hospitals regularly measure practice against policy recommendations.

Implementation of policies

There is increasing emphasis on the need for antimicrobial management teams, who work closely with infection control teams (Fig. 19.1, see also Chapter 20). The core skills of the team should include diagnosis of infection, assessment of severity, surveillance of prescribing and resistance, pharmacokinetics, and pharmacodynamics. It is critical that the team has the full support of senior management and good communication with risk management and clinical governance teams. There are potential risks to reducing antimicrobial use and it is unlikely that the antimicrobial management team has all the skills necessary to assess these risks or to devise a balanced set of measures that will reassure everybody that change in prescribing is an improvement.

Antimicrobial management teams are becoming well established in hospitals and the same model can be adapted to primary care. The need to interact with infection control, risk management, and clinical governance is just as pressing, especially in residential care and nursing homes. Multidisciplinary involvement in prescribing is increasingly common in primary care.

Do antimicrobial policies work?

It is very easy to be too ambitious in setting aims. The first aim should be to change medical practice, which may have a variety of secondary aims (e.g. improving quality of prescribing, limiting drug resistance, reducing unnecessary prescribing costs). Antimicrobial policies should be seen as part of an overall plan for prescribing quality improvement (see Key points at end of this chapter).

There is a lot of evidence about the effectiveness of interventions to change antimicrobial prescribing but unfortunately much of it is unreliable. The Cochrane Library contains two reviews on interventions to improve antimicrobial prescribing in primary and hospital care. Over half of the studies in primary care and hospitals were rejected because the articles reported uncontrolled evaluations. It is impossible to assess the impact of an intervention without some information on what would have happened in its absence. This does not mean that randomized controlled trials are the only acceptable method for evaluation; much simpler designs can be used. These include controlled before-and-after studies (Table 19.2) and interrupted time series (Fig. 19.2).

There are striking differences in the methods that have been used to change antimicrobial prescribing in primary and hospital care. Less than 10% of the interventions in primary care were restrictive whereas nearly half of the hospital interventions included some form of restriction. This difference arises from the very different structures of primary and hospital care. First, practitioners in primary care are more likely to be independent rather than salaried employees of an organization. Second, it is much easier to restrict supply of drugs in a single hospital than in a primary care organization that may include tens or even hundreds of offices in different locations. A further difference is that 31% of the primary care interventions targeted patients, either alone or alongside interventions on professionals. Again this reflects the very different context, because shared decision making between patients and professionals is the norm in primary care, whereas it is still uncommon in hospitals, especially during inpatient care of acute illness. Taken together the Cochrane reviews evaluated eight different persuasive and five different restrictive strategies and found that all are supported by at least one successful study. Consequently there is a lot of evidence about the changes that can be made to prescribing. More importantly there is increasing

Table 19.2 Example of a controlled before-and-after study that showed a large reduction in primary care antimicrobial drug prescribing for acute bronchitis with no adverse effect on rates of repeat consultation for bronchitis or pneumonia

	Antimicrobial prescribing (%)		Repeat consultations (%)	
	Before	After	Before	After
Control (no intervention)	82	77	6	7
Partial intervention[a]	78	76	4	4
Full intervention[b]	74	48	6	5

[a] Supply of patient information leaflets to doctors' offices.

[b] Supply of leaflets plus information targeted at households at the start of the winter as well as a clinician intervention consisting of group education, practice-profiling, and one-to-one education of individual prescribers.

Data from Gonzales R, Steiner JF, Lum A, Barrett PH (1999) 'Decreasing antimicrobial use in ambulatory practice: impact of a multidimensional intervention on the treatment of uncomplicated acute bronchitis in adults', *Journal of the American Medical Association* **281**: 1512–1519.

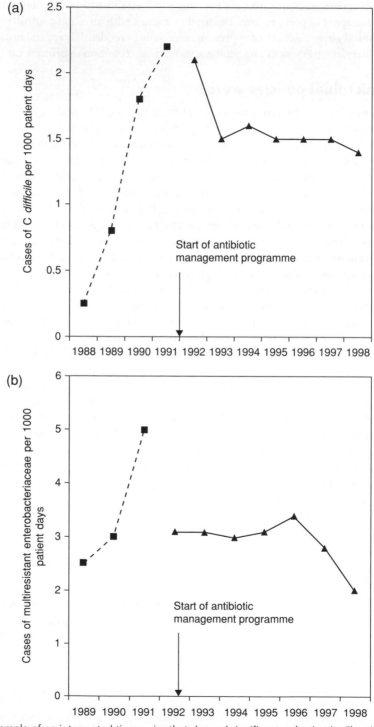

Fig. 19.2 Example of an interrupted time series that showed significant reduction in *Clostridium difficile* associated diarrhoea (a) and infections with multiresistant Enterobacteriaceae (b) after introduction of an antimicrobial management programme in one hospital. Drawn with data from: Carling P, Fung T, Killion A, Terrin N, Barza M (2003) 'Favourable impact of a multidisciplinary antimicrobial management program conducted during 7 years', *Infection Control and Hospital Epidemiology* **24**: 699–706.

evidence to show that change in prescribing results in improvement to both clinical and microbial outcomes (see Key points at end of this chapter). The hospital studies provide the most convincing evidence that changing antimicrobial prescribing can improve microbial outcomes such as *Clostridium difficile*-associated diarrhoea and infection with multiresistant bacteria.

Which antimicrobial policies work best?

The answer to this question depends on what we are trying to accomplish. It is reasonable to restrict the aim to achieving a reduction in prescribing if it is clear that this is likely to result in improvements in microbial outcome without risks to clinical outcome. Examples include aiming for a 50% reduction in unnecessary use of antimicrobial drugs for acute bronchitis in primary care or in surgical prophylaxis lasting more than 24 h in hospitals. In both cases the intervention is supported by evidence that change will be an improvement. Having answered the first two questions about quality improvement (see Key points at end of this chapter) it is relatively easy to answer the third: what changes can we make that will result in improvement?

The most successful guidelines and policies involve the professionals who are the targets for change in development, dissemination, and implementation. Involvement in implementation is best accomplished by concurrent feedback of information about practice in comparison with agreed standards. Concurrent feedback means that prescribers receive information about patients that they are actively treating, rather than retrospective information about patients that they treated last week, month, or year. However, this approach may require considerable investment of time by both the professionals carrying out the intervention and those who are its targets, plus information systems that are capable of providing concurrent, patient-specific feedback. Simply providing prescribers with educational information can be successful, requires much less resource, and may be more cost-effective than a complex multifaceted intervention. As in most areas of medicine, the most complex and effective intervention available is not necessarily the most appropriate.

In hospitals restrictive interventions do have a much greater immediate impact on prescribing than persuasive ones, so restriction is justified when there is a need for rapid change in prescribing. However, restrictions do have unintended consequences. Clinicians may be very resentful about having restrictions imposed on their practice, in which case they will find ways to overcome them. Hospitals that have tried to limit vancomycin prescribing by restriction to 'documented cases of MRSA infection' have experienced pseudo-epidemics of MRSA infection because prescribers write on the compulsory order form whatever they have to in order to get vancomycin for their patient. Unless there is a very clear justification for needing an immediate impact on prescribing (e.g. an outbreak of infections caused by multiresistant bacteria) then it may be more effective in the long term to use a slower, persuasive strategy.

In primary care multifaceted interventions that aim to influence patients as well as professionals have generally produced much greater changes in prescribing than interventions that are aimed only at patients or professionals. Delayed prescriptions have been consistently successful in reducing prescribing for respiratory tract infections. The doctor says to the patient or parent that in their opinion there is no need to prescribe an antimicrobial drug; they provide an information sheet explaining how the symptoms will resolve without treatment but they also say that they will leave an antimicrobial prescription at reception to be collected if required. Between 50 and 70% of these delayed prescriptions are never collected.

Antibiotic stewardship at the population level

The principles of antibiotic stewardship are described in Chapter 20. The European Commission prepared a comprehensive Community strategy against antimicrobial resistance in 2001. At that

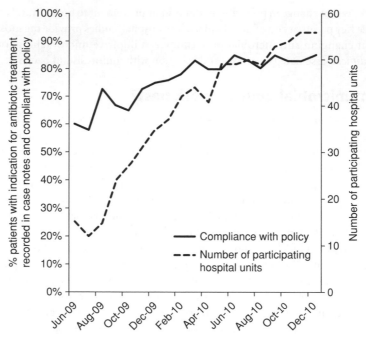

Fig. 19.3 Improvement in compliance with hospital antibiotic policy in hospitals in Scotland. Hospitals collect data monthly from acute medical and surgical admissions unit. By December 2010 all 56 hospital units in 14 Health Boards were collecting data and compliance had improved from 60% to 85%.

time only six European countries had a national action plan to contain antimicrobial resistance. By 2003, 16 countries had developed a national strategy to contain antimicrobial resistance and by 2008, 23 (85%) of 27 countries had an action plan for management of antimicrobial resistance. There is evidence of success in reduction of infections caused by MRSA and *C, difficile* in European countries. European Surveillance of Antimicrobial Consumption (ESAC) has developed methods for sustainable measurement of prescribing and indicators of prescribing quality. In Scotland the ESAC indicators were adopted in 2009 as national targets to support reduction in *C, difficile* infection. In hospitals there has been a steady increase in the number of participating hospital units and in their compliance with local antibiotic policies (Fig. 19.3) and in primary care there has been a 20% reduction in use of antibiotics associated with *C, difficile* infection (Fig. 19.4) since 2009. These changes in prescribing were associated with 42% reduction in *C, difficile* infection in persons aged 65 and over between October 2008–September 2009 and October 2009–September 2010 (http://www.hps.scot.nhs.uk/haiic/sshaip/wrdetail.aspx?id=46771&wrtype=6).

Implications for research and practice

The most important deficiency to address is in the quality of the research evidence. The criteria for reliable evidence are simple and readily accessible through the ORION guidelines for transparent reporting of **O**utbreak **R**eports and **I**ntervention studies **O**f **N**osocomial infection (see http://www.idrn.org/orion.php). All that remains is for sponsors of research and journal editors to refuse to support collection and publication of poor quality evidence.

There is ample research evidence about changing antimicrobial prescribing and prescribing in general. The focus needs to move towards how to increase prudent antimicrobial prescribing.

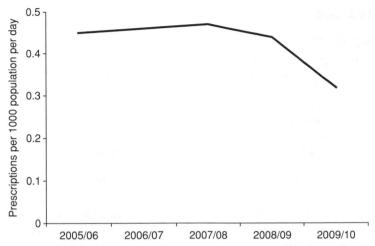

Fig 19.4 Reduction in use of antibiotics associated with *C. difficile* infection (ciprofloxacin and other quinolones, cephalosporins, clindamycin and co-amoxiclav) in primary care in Scotland after introduction of national target for reduction in *C. difficile* in 2009. Redrawn from data in Scottish Antimicrobial Prescribing Group (2010) *Primary Care Prescribing Indicators.* Available at http://www.isdscotland.org/isd/6463.html (24th February 2011, date last accessed).

This means that future research studies should capture clinical and microbial outcomes, not just prescribing outcomes (Fig. 19.3, and Table 20.6). This should not deter antimicrobial management teams from implementing policies based on the evidence that already exists and using prescribing outcomes as a measure of success in their organization.

Measurement of antimicrobial prescribing, surveillance of important microbial outcomes, and balancing measures of clinical outcome should be part of routine practice in primary and hospital care. Antimicrobial resistance is a key public health problem so measures of prudent prescribing are important for patient safety.

Key questions for quality improvement

◆ What are we trying to accomplish?

◆ How will we know that change is an improvement?

◆ What changes can we make that will result in improvement?

Box 19.1 Key points for testing change through PDSA (Plan Do Study Act) cycles

◆ **Plan**—the change to be tested or implemented. Define the objective, questions (who? what? where? when?) and predictions. Plan data collection to answer the questions.

◆ **Do**—carry out the test or change and collect data and answers to the questions.

◆ **Study**—data before and after the change, compare the data with predictions. Summarize and reflect on what was learned.

◆ **Act**—decide whether the change can be implemented. If not, plan the next change cycle. If so, plan full implementation and spread.

Further reading

Antibiotic policies

Arnold SR, Straus SE. (2005), 'Interventions to improve antibiotic prescribing practices in ambulatory care', *The Cochrane Database of Systematic Reviews*, Issue 4. Art. No.: CD003539. DOI: 10.1002/14651858.CD003539.pub2.

Davey PG, Nathwani D, Rubinstein E. (2010), 'Antimicrobial Policies', in *Antibiotic and Chemotherapy. Anti-infective agents and their use in therapy*. Finch RG, Greenwood D, Norrby SR. (eds). London: Churchill Elsevier 126–143.

Davey P, Brown E, Fenelon L, Finch R, Gould I, Hartman G, Holmes A, Ramsay C, Taylor E, Wilcox M, Wiffen P. (2005), 'Interventions to improve antibiotic prescribing practices for hospital inpatients', *The Cochrane Database of Systematic Reviews*, Issue 4. Art. No.: CD003543. DOI: 10.1002/14651858. CD003543.pub2.

European Commission: Key documents on antimicrobial resistance. Available at http://ec.europa.eu/ health/antimicrobial_resistance/key_documents/index_en.htm (24th February 2011 data last accessed).

Nathwani D, Sneddon J, Malcolm W, Wiuff C, Patton A, Hurding S, Eastaway A, Seaton A, Watson E, Gillies E, Davey P, Bennie M. Scottish Antimicrobial Prescribing Group (SAPG) (2011), *Development and impact of the Scottish National Antimicrobial Stewardship Programme International Journal of Antimicrobial Agents*.

Scottish Antimicrobial Prescribing Group. Policies and guidance. Available at http://www.scottishmedicines. org.uk/SAPG/Policies_and_Guidance (24th February 2011 data last accessed).

Improvement methods

IHI (Institute for Healthcare Improvement) Open School of Health Professions online courses. These are free to students, trainees and faculty. Available at: http://www.ihi.org/IHI/Programs/IHIOpenSchool.

NHS Institute for Innovation and Change guide to Plan Do Study Act cycles. Available at:http://www. institute.nhs.uk/quality_and_service_improvement_tools/quality_and_service_improvement_tools/ plan_do_study_act.html.

Chapter 20

Antibiotic stewardship and the multi-professional antimicrobial management team

Stewardship is responsible caretaking; the concept is based on the premise that we don't own resources, but are managers of resources and are responsible to future generations for their condition. The twin goals of antibiotic stewardship are first to ensure effective, timely treatment of infection, and second to minimize collateral damage from unnecessary use. Hence antibiotic stewardship needs to balance the priorities of individual and societal needs. The World Health Organization (WHO) strongly recommends that governments focus control and prevention efforts in four main areas:

♦ Surveillance for antimicrobial resistance;

♦ Rational antibiotic use, including education of healthcare workers and the public;

♦ Introducing or enforcing legislation related to stopping the selling of antibiotics without prescription;

♦ Strict adherence to infection prevention and control measures, including the use of hand-washing measures.

There needs to be clear definition of responsibilities for antibiotic stewardship at all levels of a healthcare organization with regular audit and feedback of information about antimicrobial use and compliance with policies (Table 20.1).

Antimicrobial prescribers

Medical prescribers

Doctors are responsible for most antimicrobial prescriptions and most doctors prescribe antimicrobials regularly. However, each doctor is only likely to be responsible for management of a narrow range of infections. Existing guidance on the management of some infections may be too long and complex for many doctors to have time to absorb, so it is important to help busy doctors identify what is most important for them in their routine clinical practice (Table 20.2). The aim should be to help doctors use antibiotics safely while protecting their patients and public health. Doctors are ideally placed to take the lead on managing infection control promoting best practice, sharing knowledge and ensuring that the understanding of infection and antibiotic prescribing are a mandatory part of training. There is also a need to develop 'antibiotic officers', physicians trained in antibiotic stewardship who will support change within clinical teams.

The first priority must be to ensure that patients with life-threatening infection receive effective antibiotic treatment immediately (Table 20.2). However, assessment of appropriateness of antibiotic treatment of common infection in hospital usually reveals evidence of under-treatment of severe infection in addition to unnecessary over-treatment of less severe infection (Table 29.1).

Table 20.1 Key domains for healthcare organizations to assess their antibiotic stewardship. (Adapted from Cooke J, Alexander K, Charani E et al. Antimicrobial stewardship: an evidence-based, antimicrobial self-assessment toolkit (ASAT) for acute hospitals. *Journal Antimicrobial Chemotherapy* 2010; **65**: 2669–73)

1. Antimicrobial management within the organization

- Structures and lines of responsibility and accountability are clearly defined
- There is high level notification of reports on antibiotic stewardship to the Board and its non-executive directors
- There is an Antimicrobial Management Committee with regular, documented meetings and action lists with clear lines of reporting to infection control, drug and therapeutics committees and to clinical groups.

2. Operational delivery of an antimicrobial strategy

- Antimicrobial management policies in place
- Restricted access to selected antimicrobials
- Evidence-based guidelines for treatment of common infections
- Frequent (at least two yearly) review of all policies and guidelines
- Availability of electronic versions through networked computers
- Availability of an easily accessible printed summary to all wards and prescribers (e.g. pocket guide)
- Selection for the guidelines is informed by local microbiological sensitivity patterns with selective reporting of results by microbiology laboratory in line with formulary choices
- There is a policy stipulating that indication should be recorded before antimicrobials are prescribed
- The policy stipulates that course length or review date is recorded on the prescription chart at time of prescribing
- The policy stipulates that prescriptions for antimicrobials be reviewed at least every 48 hours
- The policy stipulates that appropriate de-escalation of therapy takes place and includes IV to oral switch guidelines
- The policy provides guidance on choice, dose, route, IV switch, and typical duration of treatment for each indication
- There are antimicrobial ward rounds
- Advice from a medical microbiologist/ID physician is available by telephone.

3. Risk assessment for antimicrobial chemotherapy

- Guidelines include advice on managing the following risks:
  - Managing patients with allergies to antimicrobials
  - Safe administration of IV antimicrobials
  - Dosing optimization for antimicrobials with a narrow therapeutic index
  - Therapeutic drug monitoring for high risk antimicrobials
- Safety of antimicrobials is linked to incident reporting with feedback and action plans
- Incident reports are sent to the antimicrobial management committee.

4. Clinical governance assurance

- There is a programme for audit of the antimicrobial policy, treatment, and prophylaxis guidelines with feedback of results to each clinical group at least once a year
- Total antimicrobial consumption is monitored
- Total antimicrobial consumption is reported to clinical groups
- Attendance at audit feedback meetings is recorded
- Action plans by clinical groups are recorded and shared with the antimicrobial management committee.

Table 20.1 (continued)

---

5. Education and training

- There is an antimicrobial education and training Strategy
- All antimicrobial prescribers receive printed information about antimicrobial prescribing, formulary, and guidelines at induction
- All pharmacists receive printed information about antimicrobial prescribing, formulary, and guidelines at induction
- An annual update on safe and effective antimicrobial prescribing is available for all prescribers, pharmacists, and staff who administer antimicrobials
- The proportion of trainee doctors and senior doctors who attend training on safe and effective antimicrobial prescribing is recorded
- The proportion of staff attending training on safe and effective antimicrobial prescribing is recorded
- Competency assessment is carried out for antimicrobial prescribers.

6. Antimicrobial pharmacist

- There is a substantive antimicrobial pharmacist post in place
- The lead antimicrobial pharmacist has a higher qualification than first degree (e.g. Diploma/MSc)
- The lead antimicrobial pharmacist has specialist training in infection management and antimicrobial use
- The lead antimicrobial pharmacist has written objectives with an annual appraisal.

7. Patients, carers, and the public

- There is a policy for providing information on antimicrobials to patients
- Patients or their legal guardian are informed that they have been prescribed an antimicrobial, the reason why this is necessary and the risks and side effects associated with antimicrobial treatment
- Patients who are taking antimicrobials at home are informed about the course length, the importance of finishing the course, and what to do if side effects develop at home.

In this cohort study of the management of skin and soft tissue infection, 12 (6%) of 189 patients had severe sepsis with 33% mortality at 30 days, but 11 of them received inadequate initial therapy (two received oral treatment and nine received treatment that would not be effective against all potential pathogens). Evidence about the management of severe sepsis shows that prompt administration of effective antibiotics saves lives and that mortality increases with every hour of delay in the initiation of antibiotic treatment (Chapter 26).

Unnecessary over-treatment is the commonest error made by medical prescribers in primary and secondary care. In primary care the commonest problem is unnecessary antibiotic treatment of upper respiratory infections (Chapter 21). In hospitals the commonest problems are unnecessary use of broad-spectrum antibiotics and intravenous administration for patients without evidence of sepsis (Table 29.1).

Non-medical prescribers

Non-medical prescribing is being implemented increasingly. Most of the literature is about nurse prescribing but in the UK legislation allows nurses, optometrists, pharmacists, physiotherapists, podiatrists, and radiographers to train as prescribers. Independent prescribing means that the non-medical prescriber can prescribe without direction from another profession (Table 20.3). Supplementary prescribing means that the prescriber is working within a written plan for an

Table 20.2 Role of the doctor in effective antibiotic prescribing as defined by the Royal College of Physicians Healthcare Associated Infections Working Group (http://www.rcplondon.ac.uk/resources/top-ten-tips-series)

Effective Antibiotic Prescribing

Antibiotics are essential to modern medicine and may be life-saving, but their abuse leads to resistance. All physicians who prescribe antibiotics have a responsibility to their patients and for public health to prescribe optimally

Top Ten Tips

◆ Institute antibiotic treatment immediately in patients with life-threatening infection

◆ Prescribe in accordance with local policies & guidelines avoiding broad spectrum agents

◆ Document in clinical notes indication(s) for antibiotic prescription

◆ Send appropriate specimens to the microbiology lab draining pus and removing foreign bodies if indicated

◆ Use antimicrobial susceptibility data to de-escalate/substitute/add agents and to switch from intravenous to oral therapy

◆ Prescribe the shortest antibiotic course likely to be effective

◆ Always select agents to minimise collateral damage (i.e selection of multi-resistant bacteria/*C. difficile*)

◆ Monitor antibiotic drug levels when relevant (e.g. vancomycin)

◆ Use single dose antibiotic prophylaxis wherever possible

◆ Consult your local infection experts

Royal College of Physicians Healthcare Associated Infections Working Group (More detailed advice can be found on the RCP website *www.rcplondon.ac.uk*)

individual patient or defined groups of patients (Table 20.3). In the UK, legislation to increase the number of non-medical, independent prescribers was passed in 2006 with the following aims:

◆ Improve patient care without compromising patient safety;

◆ Make it easier for patients to get the medicines they need;

◆ Increase patient choice in accessing medicines;

◆ Make better use of the skills of healthcare professionals;

◆ Contribute to the introduction of more flexible team working across the National Health Service.

A systematic review in 2008 identified 23 studies with direct comparison of nurse prescribers with physicians (Table 20.4). Seven of the studies involved independent nurse prescribing, one study involved supplementary nurse prescribing, five studies described a mix of independent and supplementary prescribing, and five studies looked at prescribing by group protocols. The studies were conducted in the UK (n=11), USA (n=7), Netherlands (n=3), Canada (n=1) and Colombia (n=1). Sixteen studies were conducted in primary care and seven in secondary care. Overall the results showed that in comparison with physicians, nurses prescribed to a similar number of patients, with similar clinical outcomes but greater patient satisfaction (Table 20.4). Four studies (all in primary care) were about antibiotic prescribing for upper respiratory infections with strikingly different results (Table 20.5). In one study antibiotics were prescribed to 7% of patients seen by a nurse compared with 93% patients seen by a doctor. However, in the other three studies nurses prescribed antibiotics as often (two studies) or significantly more often than doctors. All of these studies focused on upper respiratory infections for which antibiotics should not have been prescribed. Two small, single practice studies from the UK do provide some evidence about

Table 20.3 Terms used to describe non-medical prescribing

Independent prescribing	This term is applied to any prescriber who is legally permitted and qualified to prescribe who is accountable for the clinical assessment of the patient, establishing a diagnosis and the clinical management required. In the UK nurses or pharmacists trained as independent prescribers are fully responsible for their own prescribing decisions and are able to prescribe any licensed medicine from the British National Formulary, for any medical condition with the exception of some controlled drugs.
	In addition District Nurses and Health Visitors can be trained to prescribe only from the Nurse Prescribers Formulary for Community Practitioners and other professions (e.g. optometrists, podiatrists) can be independent prescribers for selected sections of the BNF.
Supplementary prescribing	Supplementary prescribing, formerly referred to as 'dependent prescribing' is defined as a voluntary partnership between an independent prescriber and a supplementary prescriber to implement an agreed patient-specific Clinical Management Plan or Patient Group Directive (see below). The key principles of supplementary prescribing emphasize the importance of communication between the prescribing partners, the need for access to shared patient records and that the patient is treated as a partner in their care. Current UK legislation allows six professions to be supplementary prescribers: nurses, pharmacists, chiropodists/podiatrists, physiotherapists, and radiographers. The supervising independent prescriber must be a doctor or a dentist. The supplementary prescriber can work in hospital or community care and can use any of the relevant prescribing documents.
Clinical Management Plan (CMP)	CMPs are the foundation for supplementary prescribing to specific patients. Before supplementary prescribing can take place, it is obligatory for an agreed CMP to be in place (written or electronic) relating to a named patient and to that patient's specific condition(s) which will be managed by the supplementary prescriber.
Patient Group Direction (PGD)	A PGD is a written instruction for the sale, supply, and/or administration of a named medicine in an identified clinical situation. It applies to a group of patients who may not be individually identified before presenting for treatment. So, a health care professional could supply (e.g. provide an inhaler or tablets) and/or administer a medicine (e.g. give an injection or a suppository) directly to a patient without the need for a prescription or an instruction from a prescriber. PGDs allow the supply and administration of specified medicines to patients who fall into a group defined in the PGD; using a PGD is not a form of prescribing. Unlike nurse and pharmacist prescribing, health care professionals entitled to work with a PGD require no additional formal qualification. However, for a PGD to be valid, certain criteria must be met both in terms of the patient group that the PGD can be used for, and in how the PGD itself is drawn up

the positive aspects of nurse prescribing, for example increasing patient satisfaction and self-care through patient-centred consultation (Table 20.5). Overall the evidence suggests that simply increasing the number of non-medical prescribers of antibiotics will increase unnecessary prescribing.

However, nurses with additional training in patient-centred consultation have the potential to reduce antibiotic prescribing. Further evidence is required about the positive effects of non-medical prescribing of antibiotics, in particular about facilitating patient access to necessary treatment.

In the UK Department of Health guidance suggests that particular caution should be used when deciding whether to use a Patient Group Directive (PGD) for an antimicrobial medicine. Antimicrobial resistance is a public health issue of great concern and care should be taken to ensure that the PGD would not jeopardize any strategy to control increasing resistance. A PGD should not allow the supply and/or administration of a medicine for minor viral diseases that are

Table 20.4 Difference in outcomes between nurse and physician prescribers. From data in Van Ruth LM, Mistiaen P, Francke AL 'Effects of nurse prescribing of medication: a systematic review'. *The Internet Journal of Healthcare Administration* 2008, **5** http://www.ispub.com/ostia/index. php?xmlFilePath=journals/ijhca/vol5n2/nurse.xml) (1st May 2011, date last accessed)

Outcome	Studies	Country	Difference		
			None	Nurses > physicians	Physicians > nurses
Number of patients prescribed treatment	11	UK, USA	7	2	2
Clinical outcome	9	UK, Canada, Colombia, Netherlands	6	2	1
Patient satisfaction	8	UK, Canada, Netherlands	3	5	0

unaffected by antibiotics, for example, to treat sore throats in the absence of good evidence of bacterial infection. A local microbiologist or public health specialist with appropriate expertise should be involved in drawing up the PGD. Local drug and therapeutics/medicines management committees or area prescribing committees should ensure that any PGD is consistent with local policies and subject to regular audit. Patient Group Directives can be used to enable pharmacists to manage complex prescribing decisions in patients with chronic conditions (e.g. HIV or cystic fibrosis) and could also be used to enable pharmacists to prevent antibiotic prophylaxis for surgical patients exceeding 24 hours.

In summary, non-medical prescribing is increasing but with a limited evidence base about the advantages and disadvantages. Current legislation in the UK allows nurses and pharmacists to become independent prescribers after a 26 day course and 12 days of learning in practice. Concerns have been expressed about nurses' lack of pharmacological knowledge and pharmacists' lack of diagnostic and examinations skills. However, these concerns could be addressed by integration of non-medical prescribing training into the undergraduate curricula of these professions. Non-medical prescribing is unlikely to have much impact on antibiotic use in secondary care. The limited evidence about antibiotic prescribing in primary care is inconsistent and there are legitimate concerns that increasing the number of prescribers will increase antibiotic use for clinical problems that do not benefit from antibiotic treatment.

Measurement of antimicrobial use

In order to achieve the WHO's aim of rational antibiotic use, information is required about current use and about the impact of interventions to change use. Ideally all healthcare organizations should be able to measure the number of patients treated, the indication for treatment and the details of therapy, including drug, dose, route, and duration. In reality this level of detail is only available in research databases (e.g. Fig. 21.1). The only routine information that is available in most countries is about the total amount of antibiotic used. In order to compare between countries or organizations a standardized method is required for estimating the number of people treated, adjusted for population size.

Longitudinal surveillance

Estimating the number of people treated with antimicrobials

The origins of the WHO ATC/DDD method for surveillance of drug use can be traced to a symposium in Oslo in 1969 entitled *The Consumption of Drugs*, where it was agreed that an internationally

Table 20.5 Comparisons of nurse and doctor prescribing for respiratory tract infections in ambulatory care identified by a systematic review (Van Ruth 2008). References to the studies are given in further reading

Study	Problem	Country	Period	Population	Results
Butler 2001	URTI	UK	1999	Single general practice, 365 patients	132 consulted the nurse, 234 consulted doctors. The nurse had additional training in examination and patient-centred consultation skills. The nurse referred patients to the doctor if she thought antibiotics were indicated. Patients seen by the nurse were younger but there were no other differences between patient groups.
					Antibiotics were prescribed to 7% of patients seen by the nurse vs 93% of patients seen by doctors (p<0.001). Reconsultation rates within two weeks were not significantly different: 17% vs 10%.
Cox 2000	Sore throat	UK	1997	Single general practice, 435 patients	435 patients, 247 consulted the doctor, 188 consulted the nurse. The nurse treated 137 patients and referred 51 patients to the doctor.
					Overall antibiotic prescription was 55% for patients seen by the nurse and 57% for patients seen by the doctor. Antibiotics were prescribed to 42% patients seen entirely by the nurse and 88% of patients referred by the nurse to the doctor.
					At follow up, patients who consulted the nurse were significantly more likely to recall advice about home remedies (76% vs 54%, p<0.001) and had shorter median duration of symptoms (4 days vs 5 days, p=0.02).
Ladd 2005	URTI, pharyngitis, and bronchitis	USA	1997–2001	National surveys, 14 194 patients	506 nurse practitioner and 13,692 medical doctor visits. Rates of prescribing were similar for any antibiotic (50% vs 53%) and for broad-spectrum antibiotics (37% vs 33%)
Roumie 2005	Respiratory diagnoses	USA	1995–2000	National survey, 2.18 billion patients	2.13 billion consultations by practicing physicians and 51 million by nurse practitioners or physician assistants. Results were subdivided by place of visit. Nurse practitioners were consistently more likely to prescribe antibiotics for respiratory diagnoses in which antibiotics are rarely indicated in office practice (52% vs 39%), emergency departments (71% vs 65%), and hospital practice (46% vs 33%). In contrast prescribing rates were similar for respiratory diagnoses for which antibiotics are often indicated.

accepted classification system for drug consumption studies was needed. In order to measure drug use, it is important to have both a classification system and a unit of measurement. Norwegian researchers developed a system known as the Anatomical Therapeutic Chemical (ATC) classification and a technical unit of measurement called the Defined Daily Dose (DDD). The Nordic Council on Medicines was established in 1975 and the Nordic Statistics on Medicines using the ATC/DDD methodology was published for the first time in 1976.

In 1981, the WHO Regional Office for Europe recommended the ATC/DDD system for drug utilization studies and in 1996 WHO recognized the need to develop use of the ATC/DDD system as an international standard. The aim was to support WHO's initiatives to achieve universal access to needed drugs and rational use of drugs particularly in developing countries. Access to standardized and validated information on drug use is essential to allow audit of patterns of drug utilization, identification of problems, educational or other interventions, and monitoring of the outcomes of the interventions.

It is important to recognize that the classification of a substance in the ATC/DDD system is not a recommendation for use, nor does it imply any judgements about efficacy or relative efficacy of drugs and groups of drugs.

The European Surveillance of Antimicrobial Consumption (ESAC) project was established in 2001 and uses the WHO ATC/DDD system to provide publicly accessible information about antimicrobial consumption in European countries. National data come from two principal sources: wholesale supply of drugs or national systems for reimbursement of patients or healthcare professionals for the cost of dispensing drugs from community pharmacies or doctors' offices. Data about consumption of antimicrobials in ambulatory care are available for 30 countries whereas hospital data are only available for 19 countries. The ESAC hospital care data come from national wholesale suppliers and only give an indication of total consumption at the national level. It is not possible to identify consumption by individual hospitals. In contrast many countries can provide detailed regional data about consumption in ambulatory care, adjusted for regional population size. Consequently most of the ESAC publications and reports about national consumption focus on ambulatory care.

Some countries record the number of prescriptions for antimicrobials (Fig. 11.3). For antimicrobials this is a good indicator of the number of people treated because most patients only receive a single prescription for each course of treatment. In the USA most hospitals have electronic records of treatment dispensed to individual patients and can provide information about actual days of treatment.

Estimating population size

In ambulatory care antibiotic use is usually adjusted for number of inhabitants (e.g. DDD per 1000 inhabitants or prescriptions per 1000 inhabitants). In hospitals estimation of population size is more complicated. The WHO recommends that antimicrobial use is expressed per 1000 occupied bed days. However, the denominator (occupied bed days) is a product of number of admissions and length of stay. In many hospitals changes in the healthcare system such as laparascopic surgery have led to increased admissions with decreased length of stay. In these hospitals expression of antibiotic use as DDD per 1000 admissions would decrease over time whereas DDD per 1000 occupied bed days would be stable. ESAC has established a standardized method for hospitals to compare their antibiotic use, which suggests that determination of changes in antibiotic exposure of hospital patients over a period of time is unreliable if only one clinical activity variable (such as occupied bed days) is used as the denominator. ESAC recommends inclusion of admissions, occupied bed days, and length of stay in statistical, time series analysis of antibiotic use in hospitals.

Point prevalence surveys

In hospitals, point prevalence surveys have been used to estimate the prevalence of healthcare associated infection and antimicrobial use. This provides additional information about indication for treatment, daily dose, and route of administration. The basic method is to collect data from every patient who is in the hospital on one day. Depending on the size of hospital and the amount of data to be collected from each patient, the survey may be completed on a single day or spread over several days. ESAC has coordinated three European point prevalence surveys in 2006, 2008, and 2009; full reports are available on the ESAC website. The European Centre for Disease Control is co-ordinating a point prevalence survey in all European countries from 2011–2012.

The point prevalence method can be adapted for regular measurement of quality indicators in a sample of patients (Fig. 19.3).

The antimicrobial management team

Antimicrobial management teams are multidisciplinary and acknowledge the need for a combination of expertise and roles. However, in most hospitals the role of antimicrobial management teams is to develop and audit guidelines about antibiotic use (Table 20.1). There is a shortage of adequately trained specialist physicians or pharmacists, which means that their clinical role is limited to the management of complex infections or high-risk groups of patients (e.g. Intensive Care). Current initiatives promoting prudent antimicrobial prescribing and management have generally failed to include nurses, which subsequently limits the extent to which these strategies can improve patient outcomes. For antimicrobial stewardship programmes to be successful, a sustained and seamless level of monitoring and decision making in relation to antimicrobial therapy is needed. General, ward-based pharmacists already have an important role in antibiotic stewardship in many hospitals. However, the role of nurses is less clearly defined. As nurses have the most consistent presence as patient carers, they are in an ideal position to contribute to antibiotic stewardship (Table 20.6).

Evidence from primary care and secondary care shows that measurement and feedback of information about antibiotic prescribing does change practice (Table 19.2, Fig. 19.3 and Fig. 19.4) Ideally measures should be collected by clinical teams as part of their daily work, which means that they must be simple, reliable, and sustainable (Table 20.5). Point prevalence surveys can be a sustainable method for driving change at the national level. In Scotland progress has been achieved by clinical teams in acute admissions units with two of the key principles of effective prescribing: prescribing in accordance with local policies and documentation in clinical notes (Fig. 19.3). Data collection applies the principles of measurement (Table 20.6) because data are collected by clinical teams on 20 patients per month. Data are shared between teams by posting on a secure website.

Measurement of practice is the foundation for change but the model for improvement also requires tests of change (Box 19.1). More information is required about how to influence prescribing behaviour, which means that qualitative data are required in addition to quantitative data (Table 20.6). Most healthcare professionals have little or no training in qualitative research. Nonetheless, use of *Plan Do Study Act* cycles is a practical method for testing change by clinical teams (Box 19.1).

Table 20.6 Critical gaps in antibiotic stewardship

Gap	Comments
Performance measures	*Establish clinically meaningful outcome measures*
	◆ National prescribing surveillance that includes clinical indication (point prevalence surveys) and develops meaningful benchmarking outcomes
	◆ Establish clear links between process of care (prescribing) indicators and clinical or resistance outcomes
	Include balancing measures of unintended consequences
	◆ Efforts to reduce unnecessary antibiotic prescribing must be balanced by measures of effective treatment of infection
	◆ Promotion of aminoglycosides to reduce risk of *C. difficile* infection must be balanced by measures of nephrotoxicity
	Apply the principles of measurement
	◆ Seek usefulness, not perfection, in the measurement
	◆ Use a balanced set of process, outcome, and cost measures
	◆ Keep measurement simple; think big but start small
	◆ Use qualitative and quantitative data
	◆ Write down clear, operational definitions of the measures
	◆ Measure small, representative samples
	◆ Build measurement into daily work
Influencing prescribing behaviour	*Support junior doctors*
	◆ Most antibiotic prescriptions are written by junior doctors but they may not have made the prescribing decision
	◆ Clinical teams develop prescribing norms and etiquette
	◆ Doctor avoid altering other prescribers' decisions
	◆ Doctors avoid making prescribing decisions outside their own clinical team
	◆ More evidence is required about behaviour change strategies, including decision support systems
	◆ The goal should be to make prudent prescribing the default and routine practice
Multidisciplinary engagement	*Sustainable, local antimicrobial management teams*
	◆ AMTs have primarily involved combinations of specialists who can only review selected patients
	◆ Local champions (doctors and nurses) should be trained to support antibiotic stewardship activities through multidisciplinary ward rounds and team meetings
	Develop the role of nurses in antibiotic stewardship
	◆ Early recognition of sepsis
	◆ Route of administration and appropriate IV to oral switch
	◆ Duration of treatment
	◆ Therapeutic drug monitoring

Conclusions

There is a growing consensus about the structures that need to be in place for an organization to implement antibiotic stewardship (Table 20.1) and the key principles that define prudent antibiotic use (Table 20.2). However, it is also clear that none of this will necessarily change prescribing behaviour. Successful antibiotic stewardship requires social competence in addition to technical (antibiotic specific) competence. There are important gaps in performance measures, understanding of prescribing behaviour,and multidisciplinary engagement (Table 20.6). Antibiotic stewardship needs to be an integral, essential component of infection control, clinical quality improvement and patient safety with appropriate financial and legal support.

Key points

- ◆ The twin goals of antibiotic stewardship are first, to ensure effective, timely treatment of infection and second, to minimize collateral damage from unnecessary use.

- ◆ Doctors are responsible for most antimicrobial prescriptions and most doctors prescribe antimicrobials regularly. Consequently understanding of infection and antibiotic prescribing are a mandatory part of training.

- ◆ There is also a need to develop 'antibiotic officers', physicians trained in antibiotic stewardship who will support change within clinical teams.

- ◆ Non-medical prescribing is increasingly common. This is most likely to impact on antibiotic prescribing in primary care. The limited evidence available has focused on unnecessary antibiotic prescribing for respiratory tract infections and has conflicting results. More evidence is required to support the potential benefits to patients from non-medical prescribing.

- ◆ There is increasing consensus about the components of antibiotic stewardship and the role of the antibiotic management team at the organizational level. The next step is for clinical teams to implement sustainable measures of their antibiotic stewardship and use small tests of change to achieve improvement.

Further reading

Antibiotic stewardship

Allerberger F, Gareis R, Jindrak V et al. (2009), 'Antibiotic stewardship implementation in the EU: the way forward', *Expert Review of Anti–infective Therapy,* **7**: 1175–83.

Charani E, Cooke J, Holmes A (2010), 'Antibiotic stewardship programmes—what's missing?', *Journal of Antimicrobial Chemotherapy,* **65**: 2275–7.

Cooke J, Alexander K, Charani E et al. (2010), 'Antimicrobial stewardship: an evidence-based, antimicrobial self-assessment toolkit (ASAT) for acute hospitals', *Journal of Antimicrobial Chemotherapy,* **65**: 2669–73.

Edwards R, Drumright LN, Kiernan M et al. (2011), 'Covering more territory to fight resistance: considering nurses' role in antimicrobial stewardship', *Journal of Infection Prevention,* **12**: 6–10.

Lewis PJ, Tully MP (2009), 'Uncomfortable prescribing decisions in hospitals: the impact of teamwork', *Journal of the Royal Society of Medicine,* **102**: 481–8.

Nelson EC, Splaine ME, Batalden PB et al. (1998), 'Building measurement and data collection into medical practice', *Annals of Internal Medicine,* **128**: 460–6.

Tonna, AP, Stewart, D, West, B, Gould, I, McCaig, D (2008) 'Antimicrobial optimisation in secondary care: the pharmacist as part of a multidisciplinary antimicrobial programme - a literature review', *International Journal of Antimicrobial Agents* **31**(6): 511–517.

Measurement of antimicrobial use

Ansari F, Molana H, Goossens H et al. 2010), 'Development of standardized methods for analysis of changes in antibacterial use in hospitals from 18 European countries: the European Surveillance of Antimicrobial Consumption (ESAC) longitudinal survey, 2000–06', *Journal of Antimicrobial Chemotherapy*, **65**: 2685–91.

Ansari F, Erntell M, Goossens H et al. (2009), 'The European surveillance of antimicrobial consumption (ESAC) point-prevalence survey of antibacterial use in 20 European hospitals in 2006', *Clinical Infectious Diseases*, **49**: 1496–504.

European Surveillance of Antimicrobial Consumption (ESAC). Available at: http://app.esac.ua.ac.be/public/.

Polk RE, Fox C, Mahoney A et al. (2007), 'Measurement of adult antibacterial drug use in 130 US hospitals: comparison of defined daily dose and days of therapy', *Clinical Infectious Diseases*, **44**: 664–70.

Non-medical prescribing

Cooper R, Guillaume L, Avery T et al. (2008), 'Nonmedical prescribing in the United Kingdom: developments and stakeholder interests', *Journal of Ambulatory Care Management*, **31**: 244–52.

Non-medical prescribing in the UK: http://www.dh.gov.uk/en/Healthcare/Medicinespharmacyandindustry/Prescriptions/TheNon-MedicalPrescribingProgramme/index.htm.

National Prescribing Centre. Patient Group Directions. (2009), Available at: http://www.elmmb.nhs.uk/EasySiteWeb/getresource.axd?AssetID=1901&type=full&servicetype=Attachment (1st May 2011, date last accessed). Further information on patient group directions is available at www.pgd.nhs.uk/.

Tonna AP, Stewart DC, West B et al. (2010), 'Exploring pharmacists' perceptions of the feasibility and value of pharmacist prescribing of antimicrobials in secondary care in Scotland', *International Journal of Pharmacy Practice*, **18**: 312–9.

Van Ruth LM, Mistiaen P, Francke AL (2008), 'Effects of nurse prescribing of medication: a systematic review', *The Internet Journal of Healthcare Administration*, **5** Available at: http://www.ispub.com/ostia/index.php?xmlFilePath=journals/ijhca/vol5n2/nurse.xml (1st May 2011, date last accessed).

Nurse-prescribing of antibiotics

Butler CC, Rees M, Kinnersley P et al. (2001), 'A case study of nurse management of upper respiratory tract infections in general practice', *Journal of Advanced Nursing*, **33**: 328–33.

Cox C, Jones M (2000), 'An evaluation of the management of patients with sore throats by practice nurses and GPs', *British Journal of General Practice*, **50**: 872–6.

Ladd E (2005), 'The use of antibiotics for viral upper respiratory tract infections: an analysis of nurse practitioner and physician prescribing practices in ambulatory care, 1997–2001', *Journal of the American Academy of Nurse Practitioners*, **17**: 416–24.

Roumie CL, Halasa NB, Edwards KM et al. (2005), 'Differences in antibiotic prescribing among physicians, residents, and nonphysician clinicians', *American Journal of Medicine*, **118**: 641–8.

Part 4

Therapeutic use of antimicrobial agents

Chapter 21

Respiratory tract infections

Respiratory infections are caused by viruses, or bacteria, or both. If the illness is entirely viral in origin, an antibiotic will not help. If there is a bacterial component, antibiotic treatment will sometimes help, and may be vital. It is often difficult to recognize when bacteria may be involved in respiratory infection as secondary bacterial infection may complicate viral respiratory infections. However, the key question in the decision about treatment with antimicrobials is: do the benefits to the patient outweigh the risks? It is not necessary to prescribe antimicrobials for all bacterial respiratory infections.

When considering the role of antimicrobial chemotherapy it is important to reflect on the epidemiology of infection in the twentieth century. In the USA mortality fell by 50% from 1900–1917, then rose again in 1918, because of the influenza pandemic, then declined progressively throughout the first half of the century, before the arrival of antimicrobial chemotherapy or vaccines. The introduction of antimicrobial chemotherapy did accelerate the decline in mortality from some respiratory infections (e.g. otitis media, pneumonia, and tuberculosis) but had no impact on others (e.g. bronchitis). Two conclusions can be drawn from this information. First, it is clear why there is so much concern about the possibility of an influenza pandemic given the massive impact on mortality of the 1918 pandemic. Second, antimicrobial chemotherapy has not had the dramatic effect on mortality from infections that is popularly attributed to it. The major impact in the first half of the twentieth century came from improvements in public health, which is why death from all infections still increases with increasing socio-economic deprivation in the twenty-first century. Antimicrobial chemotherapy is just one component of an overall strategy to prevent and treat infections.

Upper respiratory tract infection

Antibiotic treatment of upper respiratory infection

Before discussing specific upper respiratory infection it is important to emphasise that antibiotic treatment makes very little difference to clinical outcome. The evidence to support this statement comes from randomized controlled trials and several systematic reviews in the Cochrane Library. In the UK a large observational study of 3.36 million episodes of respiratory tract infection showed that over 2000 people with upper respiratory tract infection would need to be treated with an antibiotic to prevent one hospitalization with complications (Fig. 21.1)

Sore throat

This is one of the commonest acute problems seen in general medical practice, with an incidence of 100 cases per 1000 inhabitants per year, although only a minority of these will present to a doctor. It is commoner in females than men. Symptoms include: sore throat with anorexia, lethargy, and systemic illness. On examination there may be inflamed tonsils or pharynx, a purulent exudate on tonsils, fever, and anterior cervical lymphadenopathy.

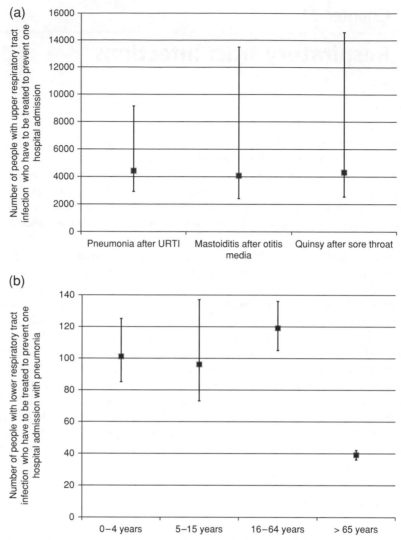

Fig. 21.1 The number of people who need to be treated with an antibiotic to prevent one hospital admission from a complication in an observational study of 3.36 million episodes of respiratory tract infection. The risk or hospitalization was adjusted for age, sex, and social deprivation. The bars are 95% confidence intervals, (a) Number of people with upper respiratory tract infection who need to be treated with an antibiotic to prevent hospitalization with specified complications, (b) Number of people with lower respiratory tract infection who need to be treated with an antibiotic to prevent hospitalization with pneumonia. Drawn from data in Table 4 of Petersen, I, Johnson, AM, Islam, A, Duckworth, G, Livermore, DM, Hayward, AC (2007) Protective effect of antibiotics against serious complications of common respiratory tract infections: retrospective cohort study with the UK General Practice Research Database. *BMJ* **335**(7627): 982–988.

Sore throat may be part of the early symptom complex of many upper respiratory viral infections, in which case cough is a common additional feature. Occasionally, it may be a presenting symptom of acute epiglottitis or other serious upper airway disease.

There is no evidence that bacterial sore throats are more severe or long-lasting than viral ones. The most commonly identified organism is *Streptococcus pyogenes*, the group A β-haemolytic streptococcus. Most other cases are caused by adenoviruses. There is no reliable way to distinguish between bacterial and viral causes based on symptoms and signs.

The gold standard for diagnosis of streptococcal infection in the throat includes a positive anti-streptolysin O (ASO) titre in addition to culture of *Str. pyogenes* from the throat. There is a high asymptomatic carrier rate for the organism (up to 40%) and it is common to culture it from sore throats when there is no serological evidence of infection. Moreover a negative culture does not rule out *Str. pyogenes* as a cause of sore throat. Neither culture of throat swabs nor rapid tests based on detection of streptococcal antigen are helpful in most cases.

Most people with sore throat manage the condition successfully without seeing a doctor. Paracetamol is an effective analgesic, with less risk of adverse effects than non-steroidal anti-inflammatory drugs. Aspirin should be avoided in children because of the risk of Reye's syndrome. The immediate benefits from antimicrobial chemotherapy are actually very meagre. Symptoms usually persist for five to seven days with or without antibiotics, which only shorten illness by 24 h. The same control of symptoms can probably be achieved with paracetamol.

Streptococcal sore throat is important because it may lead to serious complications, particularly rheumatic fever, which is still prevalent in many countries. Evidence about the effectiveness of antibiotics for preventing nonsuppurative and suppurative complications comes from studies on military personnel living in overcrowded barracks in the late 1940s and early 1950s. This evidence has little relevance to management of sore throat in modern communities, at least in the developed world, where rheumatic fever is now very uncommon. Similarly experience with the use of antibiotics to prevent cross-infection in sore throat comes mainly from army barracks and other closed institutions. It is very unlikely (and unproven) that trying to eradicate *Str. pyogenes* with routine antibiotic therapy for sore throat will produce any measurable health gain in the general public in Western countries, whereas it is likely that this would increase the prevalence of antimicrobial resistance.

A patient information leaflet may be of value in the management of acute sore throat and may assist in managing future episodes at home without general practitioner involvement. Patients who are sceptical about withholding antibiotics can be given a prescription with the suggestion that they do not use it unless their symptoms persist for more than three days. Only about 30% of patients who are given delayed prescriptions go to the pharmacy to get their antibiotics.

If antibiotics are to be prescribed the drugs of choice are penicillin V or a macrolide, and these should be given for at least 10 days to eradicate the organism and prevent recurrence. Glandular fever commonly causes symptoms and signs that are indistinguishable from streptococcal throat infection (including a very impressive purulent exudate on the tonsils). Ampicillin, amoxicillin, and co-amoxiclav should not be used, as they will cause a rash if the sore throat is the herald of glandular fever. Tetracyclines are also inappropriate because of the high incidence of resistance among streptococci.

Other infections that may present with sore throat

Croup

Noisy difficult breathing, hoarseness, and stridor are common signs of croup, a distressing condition that is usually viral in origin. Treatment is supportive; the condition is usually self-limiting and resolves in two to four days if uncomplicated, but severe cases may require endotracheal intubation or tracheostomy. Acute epiglottitis is a much less common, but much more dangerous, cause of croup caused by infection with *Haemophilus influenzae* type b; it can occur in adults as well as in children. There is systemic illness as well as local respiratory difficulty, and the swollen oedematous epiglottis can cause complete airways obstruction with dramatic suddenness. It is this complication that makes acute epiglottitis such a life-threatening condition. Treatment is as much concerned with maintaining the airways as with controlling the infection.

If breathing difficulty is present in a patient with croup, urgent referral to hospital is mandatory and attempts to examine the throat should be avoided.

Diphtheria

Although rare in countries with effective vaccination policies, diphtheria is still prevalent in many parts of the world. Diagnosis is made on clinical grounds, notably the presence of a characteristic membranous exudate on the tonsils and pharynx. Treatment with antitoxin should be given immediately without waiting for laboratory confirmation. Antibiotics have no part to play in treating the infection, but penicillin or erythromycin is effective in eradicating the infection to prevent spread.

Thrush

Oral thrush, infection of the mucous membrane with the yeast *Candida albicans*, is predominantly a neonatal infection. Candida is a common vaginal commensal, especially in pregnancy, and the infant acquires infection during passage through the birth canal. It presents in the first few days of life as white curdy patches on cheeks, lips, palate, and tongue. Treatment is with local nystatin.

In adults, oral thrush may follow treatment with antibacterials or corticosteroids. However, it may be indicative of serious underlying disease, such as diabetes or immunodeficiency (Chapter 31). In all these conditions one of the oral polyene or azole derivatives may be used to control the candida.

Acute otitis media

Three-quarters of cases of acute otitis media occur in children; one in four children will have an episode during their first 10 years of life. Acute otitis media should be distinguished from otitis media with effusion, commonly referred to as glue ear; as many as 80% of children suffer this infection at least once before the age of four.

Acute otitis media is an inflammation of the middle ear of rapid onset presenting with local symptoms (earache, rubbing, or tugging of the affected ear) and systemic signs (fever, irritability, disturbed sleeping). It is often preceded by other upper respiratory symptoms such as cough or rhinorrhoea. On examination a middle ear effusion may be present but in addition the drum looks opaque and may be bulging.

The condition is caused predominantly by *H. influenzae* and *Streptococcus pneumoniae*. Staphylococci, *Str. pyogenes*, and α-haemolytic streptococci are less often involved. However, acute otitis media should not be treated routinely with antibiotics. As with sore throat, antibiotics only have a small impact on the duration of acute symptoms, which can be controlled equally effectively with paracetamol. If an antibiotic is to be prescribed a five day course is sufficient; the antibiotic of choice is amoxicillin; erythromycin and co-amoxiclav are logical alternatives and may be necessary if β-lactamase-producing *H. influenzae* is involved. Decongestants, antihistamines, and mucolytics are not effective. As with sore throat, patient information leaflets and delayed antibiotic prescriptions are effective strategies for reducing the unnecessary use of antibiotics.

Glue ear is an inflammation of the middle ear with accumulation of fluid in the middle ear but without symptoms or signs of acute inflammation. It is often asymptomatic and earache is uncommon. On examination a middle ear effusion is present but with a normal-looking ear drum. Antibiotics should not be given.

Acute sinusitis

Acute sinusitis presents with pain originating in the maxillary, frontal, ethmoid, or sphenoid sinuses, with the maxillary sinus being by far the commonest. Onset of facial pain is often preceded by non-specific symptoms of upper respiratory inflammation and there may be systemic signs of inflammation. The bacterial causes of acute sinusitis are the same as acute otitis media. If X-ray or culture confirms the clinical diagnosis then antibiotics can substantially reduce the duration of symptoms. However, neither of these investigations is routinely available in primary care. Culture of the sinuses requires percutaneous sinus puncture and aspiration, which is not a procedure that most general practitioners are trained to do (or that many patients would consent to). Unfortunately antibiotic treatment of patients with symptoms suggestive of sinusitis but without confirmation by X-ray or culture is no more effective than symptomatic relief.

As with acute otitis media antibiotics for acute sinusitis should be reserved for the more severe cases. Penicillin V or amoxicillin are as effective as newer antibiotics. The recommended duration of treatment is 10 days in the absence of evidence that shorter courses are as effective.

Antibiotic treatment of lower respiratory tract infections

Acute cough is the most common symptom of lower respiratory infection, whether as a new symptom or as an exacerbation of chronic symptoms. Cough is not a universal feature: some patients with pneumonia present with pleuritic chest pain or with symptoms of systemic inflammatory response (fever, malaise, headache, or myalgia) without cough. The most important diagnosis to make is pneumonia because it can be life threatening and its outcome can be improved with antimicrobial chemotherapy. However, it is not possible to distinguish reliably between pneumonia and other causes of lower respiratory tract infection from clinical history and signs. Consequently, in primary care management must be based on an assessment of severity of illness and need for referral to hospital.

In comparison with upper respiratory tract infection, the evidence for benefits and risks of antibiotic treatment of lower respiratory tract infection is more complex. In a large observational study the number of people who needed to be treated with antibiotics to prevent one hospitalization with pneumonia was about 100 for those aged <65 and 40 for those aged >65 (Fig. 21.1b). However, a cluster randomized trial in general practice showed that two strategies (training in consultation skills or near patient testing for C-reactive protein) resulted in 50% reduction in prescribing of antibiotics for lower respiratory tract infection without any measurable change in time to recovery (Fig. 21.2). This evidence shows that doctors in primary care can reliably identify patients with lower respiratory tract infection and low risk of complications. Nonetheless the risk of complications from pneumonia means that interventions to reduce prescribing need to be supported by balancing measures that will detect unintended increase in complications.

Epidemiology

The incidence of lower respiratory tract infection in the UK is between 40 and 90 cases per 1000 population per year, being commoner in the very young and old and in the winter months. In the UK there is about a fourfold higher incidence in the most deprived communities in comparison with the most affluent communities.

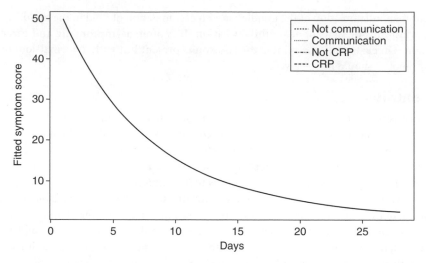

Antibiotic prescribing at index consultation	Usual care (n=120)	CRP test (n=110)	Communication skills training (n=84)	CRP test and communication skills training (n=117)
% of patients	67%	39%	33%	23%
95% CI*	54% to 80%	26% to 53%	20% to 47%	12% to 35%

*Calculated and inflated for clustering by using standard deviation inflated by variance inflation factor.

Fig. 21.2 Corrected symptom scores for treatment groups in a cluster randomised clinical trial of the effect of point of care testing for C-reactive protein and training in communication skills on antibiotic use in lower respiratory tract infections in general practice. The symptom scores corrected by a four level autoregressive moving averages model to account for practice, general practitioner, patient, and repeated measurements over time. The four lines in this figure are indistinguishable meaning that treatment groups had identical clinical recovery despite fewer antibiotics prescribed in intervention groups (see Table 21.1). 'No test' and 'No training' represent usual care in the two control arms of the trial. Reproduced from British Medical Journal, Cals, JW, Butler, CC, Hopstaken, RM, Hood, K, Dinant, GJ (2009), *BMJ* **338:** b1374, with permission from BMJ Publishing Group Ltd.

Mortality is highest in the elderly. The 30-day mortality associated with lower respiratory tract infection in people over 65 years old is 10%. However, many of these elderly people die 'with' rather than 'of' the infection. Bronchopneumonia is often recorded as the immediate cause of death in people with chronic, life-threatening diseases. Mortality from 'pneumonia' has actually increased in developed countries since the introduction of antibiotics, but more people are living longer and most of this mortality is from bronchopneumonia.

Most people with lower respiratory infections manage their own symptoms without seeking medical attention. Of one million people with lower respiratory tract infection only 300 000 will see a primary care physician. Of these one in four (70 000) will be treated with antibiotics, although only about one in 10 (7000 people) will have a diagnosis of pneumonia. From the original 300 000 people who presented to a primary care physician only about 200 (0.7%) will be admitted to hospital with pneumonia.

Management in primary care

The key to management of lower respiratory tract infection in primary care is to distinguish between patients who have severe infection that should be referred to hospital and the majority (99%) who can be managed safely at home. There are four questions to address:

◆ Has the patient been previously well or is there underlying chronic respiratory or other disease?

◆ Has there been the development or deterioration in either dyspnoea or sputum purulence?

◆ Are there any new localizing physical signs in the chest to suggest pneumonia?

◆ Are any features of severity present (Box 21.1)?

The answers to these questions distinguish between four broad populations of people with lower respiratory tract infection. These will be discussed starting with the most severe (but least common).

Patients with features indicating severe infection

Referral to hospital should be considered in patients who exhibit one or more of the features of severity (Box 21.1), especially if they are over the age of 50. This applies whether or not the patient has additional physical signs indicating pneumonia because the absence of these signs is not a reliable method for excluding pneumonia. The final decision should be based on clinical judgment that includes social factors. Even a relatively well patient who lives in poor social circumstances or in an isolated rural area with no home support may require referral to hospital. Conversely patients who are 65 years old and have signs of pneumonia can be managed safely at home if they have sufficient social support.

Suspected community-acquired pneumonia without features of severity

These patients have new focal signs in the chest (crackles or altered breath sounds), but are not severely ill. In the absence of chest X-ray (not available in many primary care settings) pneumonia can be diagnosed from symptoms of an acute lower respiratory infection (cough or dyspnoea or pleuritic chest pain) with at least one systemic symptom of infection (fever or tachycardia) and new focal signs on chest examination. However, only 50% of those with all of these features will actually have an abnormal chest X-ray.

Below the age of 45 very few patients with pneumonia also have chronic obstructive pulmonary disease. Between the ages of 45 and 64 the proportion is up to 10% and rises to 20% between the

---

Box 21.1 Features of severity of lower respiratory tract infection that can be easily assessed in primary care (items in bold are most important)

◆ **Raised respiratory rate (>30/min)**

◆ **Low blood pressure (<90 mm Hg systolic and or <60 mm Hg diastolic)**

◆ **Confusion of recent onset**

◆ Age >50 years

◆ Coexisting disease present (e.g. severe chronic obstructive pulmonary disease, cardiac failure, cerebrovascular, neoplastic, renal or liver disease)

◆ Very high or very low temperature (<35 °C or >40 °C) Tachycardia (>125/min)

ages of 75 and 84. Pneumonia in these patients is more likely to be associated with severity criteria (Box 21.1).

A wide variety of organisms can cause pneumonia, including viruses. The commonest bacterial cause is *Str. pneumoniae*, which accounts for about 70 to 80% of cases in which a bacterial pathogen is identified. Atypical bacteria (*Mycoplasma pneumoniae, Chlamydophila (Chlamydia) pneumoniae, Chlamydophila psittaci, Legionella pneumophila*, and *Coxiella burnetii*) collectively account for 10 to 20% of cases and the remainder are caused by *H. influenzae* or *Staphylococcus aureus*. The latter is particularly associated with secondary bacterial infection following influenza.

With current technology neither sputum culture nor blood tests such as C-reactive protein or white cell count provide sufficient added value to the diagnosis to justify routine use. Sputum culture may be recommended in areas with a high prevalence of penicillin-resistant pneumococci.

Pneumonia is a life-threatening illness. None the less, patients with no features of severity (Box 21.1) can be managed safely at home with oral amoxicillin, a macrolide, or a tetracycline. There is no need to give combination therapy. A macrolide or tetracycline may be preferred if there are clinical features suggesting infection with one of the atypical bacteria (e.g. prominent upper respiratory symptoms, headache, or symptom duration for >1 week) particularly in younger patients or during an epidemic year for *M. pneumoniae*.

Patients with underlying chronic respiratory disease

These patients often have no new signs in the chest other than dyspnoea and sputum purulence. In the absence of signs of severity (Box 21.1) or of pneumonia the diagnosis is an acute exacerbation of the underlying condition. The likely bacterial pathogens are *H. influenzae, Str. pneumoniae*, and *Moraxella catarrhalis*. The development of green (purulent) sputum is a good indicator of a high bacterial load in the sputum. However, even in these patients antibacterial treatment has only a slight impact on the course of an acute exacerbation, shortening an illness of five to seven days by no more than one day. Antibacterial treatment does not benefit patients with acute exacerbations of chronic obstructive pulmonary disease who do not have purulent sputum. The prevalence of resistance to aminopenicillins in *H. influenzae* is 10 to 30% and is much higher in *Mor. catarrhalis*. Despite this the clinical effectiveness of amoxicillin is just as good as co-amoxiclav or fluoroquinolones, probably because of the modest benefit from any antibacterial treatment. For the same reason routine sputum culture is not recommended and should be reserved for patients with symptoms that persist despite treatment with amoxicillin. A macrolide or tetracycline is appropriate for patients who are allergic to penicillin, or who have not responded to amoxicillin treatment. Fluoroquinolones should not be used empirically in the management of exacerbations of respiratory disease in primary care.

Non-pneumonic lower respiratory infection (acute bronchitis)

Most patients with no signs in the chest, who have been previously well and do not have other features of severity, have non-pneumonic infections, most of which are caused by viruses. A few cases are caused by *M. pneumoniae, Bordetella pertussis, C. pneumoniae, Str. pneumoniae*, or *H. influenzae*. Patients will have an illness lasting several days with or without antibiotics, which should not be prescribed unless patients have signs in the chest or features of severity (Box 21.1). Sputum purulence alone is not an indication for antibiotics in a previously well patient with no chest signs. As with sore throat and acute otitis media, patient information leaflets and delayed prescriptions are effective strategies for reducing unnecessary antibiotic treatment.

Pertussis (whooping cough)

Antibiotics are notoriously ineffective in controlling the distressing cough of pertussis; neverthe-less, erythromycin has been shown to eradicate the organism from the respiratory tract and can also be used for the protection of susceptible close contacts. Vaccination is the only reliable way of preventing and controlling this early childhood infectious disease.

Cystic fibrosis

The susceptibility of patients with cystic fibrosis to pulmonary infection is well recognized and is often the cause of early death. Most lung infections in patients with cystic fibrosis are managed in the community, usually by outreach teams from secondary care. One of the striking features of chest infections in cystic fibrosis is that relatively few pathogens are involved. Early in the disease the organisms implicated are frequently *Staph. aureus* or *H. influenzae*, or both. As patients progress through adolescence to adulthood, these pathogens are replaced by *Pseudomonas aeruginosa*. Major problems arise when *Ps. aeruginosa* is replaced by *Stenotrophomonas maltophilia* or *Burkholderia cepacia*; these organisms are often resistant to many antibiotics and treatment should be guided by laboratory findings. The selection of antibiotics in patients with cystic fibrosis should be determined by the specialist services that manage the patient.

Management in hospital

Community-acquired pneumonia

In hospital the clinical diagnosis can be confirmed with a chest X-ray, although it should be recognized that sensitivity is not 100%. The gold standard for diagnosis of bacterial pneumonia is culture of bacteria from lung tissues or a needle aspirate from the lung but these tests are too dangerous to use in routine clinical practice. The point is that some patients with pneumonia can have a normal chest X-ray at presentation, so if the clinical features strongly suggest pneumonia it is reasonable to treat and repeat the chest X-ray after 24–48 h.

The severity criteria for community-acquired pneumonia are based on assessments of confusion, urea concentration, respiratory rate, and blood pressure for those 65 years of age and older (CURB-65 score; Table 21.1). It is similar to but importantly different from the classification of severity of sepsis (Chapter 26). The CURB-65 score is specifically designed to be used in patients who present to hospital in order to identify low-risk patients who do not need to be admitted to hospital, whereas the classification of sepsis is intended to be used for any patient with infection (community- or hospital-acquired) to identify patients who are deteriorating and require more intensive therapy. The CURB-65 score identifies low-risk patients more accurately than the sepsis severity score. There are more complex pneumonia-specific scores (for example the pneumonia severity index used in North America) but these are no more accurate than CURB-65. In addition

Table 21.1 The CURB-65 severity score for patients presenting to hospital with community acquired pneumonia and the mortality range measured in two prospective cohort studies. CURB-65: score one point for each of: Confusion; urea >7 mmol/l; respiratory rate ≥30/min; low systolic (<90 mm Hg) or diastolic (≤60 mm Hg) blood pressure); age ≥65 years

Risk	CURB-65 score	30–day mortality
Low risk	0–1	0–1%
Intermediate	2	8–9%
High risk	>2	22–23%
All patients	Not applicable	9–10%

Data from Lim WS, van der Eerden MM, Laing R, Boersma WG, Karalus N, Town GI, Lewis SA, Macfarlane JT. Defining community acquired pneumonia severity on presentation to hospital: an international derivation and validation study. *Thorax* 2003; **58**: 377–382.

to considering severity of pneumonia, recent surveys about hospital antibiotic policies show increasing concern about risk of infection with *C. difficile*. Pneumonia occurs commonly in older patients who are at high risk of infection with *C. difficile*. Consequently some hospitals are recommending narrower spectrum therapy for high-risk and low-risk pneumonia than is recommended in national guidelines.

Between 30 and 50% of patients who present to hospital with community-acquired pneumonia are found to be in the CURB-65 low-risk group. However, about half of these patients have other reasons for admission. Some will have co-morbidities that require inpatient management. In particular, patients with chronic obstructive pulmonary disease and pneumonia could be in respiratory failure and yet have a CURB-65 score of 0 (if they have a respiratory rate <30/min, which is likely if they have Type 2 respiratory failure). In addition to medical reasons for admission some patients will have poor social circumstances or insufficient support to be managed at home.

The management of patients admitted to hospital should be determined by their CURB-65 score. Low-risk patients who are admitted for other reasons can be managed in the same way as low-risk patients in the community, with either amoxicillin, a macrolide, or a tetracycline. Some guidelines do recommend that all patients admitted to hospital with pneumonia should receive antibiotics for pneumonia caused by atypical bacteria but several clinical trials shows that treatment with an aminopenicillin alone is just as effective for patients with low or intermediate risk pneumonia.

At the other end of the scale, patients at high risk should be treated with intravenous antibiotics that are effective against the full range of pathogens that may cause community-acquired pneumonia. Possible regimens include benzyl penicillin or co-amoxiclav a macrolide, or a fluoroquinolone with good activity against *Str. pneumoniae* (e.g. levofloxacin) for patients with penicillin allergy. The choice between benzylpenicillin versus co-amoxiclav for severe pneumonia is determined by hospital specific risk of *C. difficile* infection. The patient must receive the antibiotic(s) immediately and certainly within four hours of admission as later administration is associated with increased mortality from severe sepsis. If patients are admitted through an Accident and Emergency Department they must receive their first dose of antibiotics there before transfer to the ward. If they are admitted direct to a ward the first dose must be clearly written for immediate administration, not left until the next drug round. In addition to intravenous antibiotics patients with severe pneumonia must have their oxygen requirements assessed by pulse oximetry or blood gas measurement within four hours of admission and receive high flow oxygen (5 litres per minute) if they are hypoxic. Adequate fluid replacement is also essential. Patients should be referred to a high dependency or intensive care unit if their vital signs do not improve rapidly. When young patients die from community-acquired pneumonia it is usually because of failure to recognize the need for intensive care.

The management of patients at intermediate risk falls between these two extremes and is a matter for clinical judgment. If in doubt it would be wise to treat as severe pneumonia while waiting for senior review.

Hospital-acquired pneumonia

Pneumonia is the leading cause of mortality resulting from infection acquired in hospital. The incidence of hospital-acquired pneumonia in intensive care units ranges from 10 to 65%, with case fatalities of 13 to 55%. It is often associated with mechanical ventilation. The risk of hospital-acquired pneumonia can be substantially reduced by using non-invasive methods for respiratory support instead of ventilation and by having clear care protocols for protecting host defences against respiratory infection during mechanical ventilation. Chemoprophylaxis plays a role through the use of selective decontamination of the digestive tract (see Chapters 18 and 31), which reduces the numbers of Gram-negative bacilli and hence the risk of infection.

The micro-organisms causing pneumonia within five days of admission are quite different from those seen in disease with a later onset. The bacteria responsible for early onset pneumonia are *Str. pneumoniae, H. influenzae, Staph. aureus*, and only rarely enteric Gram-negative bacilli. In contrast late onset infection is almost always caused by Gram-negative bacteria, mainly entero-bacteria but also *Ps. aeruginosa* and *Acinetobacter spp.* Meticillin-resistant *Staph. aureus* (MRSA) is becoming increasingly common in some units. Since tracheal aspirates are poor indicators of the cause of ventilator-associated pneumonia, bronchoalveolar lavage is recommended to con-firm the diagnosis.

Empirical treatment for early onset pneumonia in patients who have not received antibiotics should be with co-amoxiclav or cefuroxime. Treatment of patients who have already received antibiotics or have late onset disease should be with a broad-spectrum cephalosporin such as cefotaxime, a fluoroquinolone, or piperacillin plus tazobactam. Combination therapy is no more effective than monotherapy. Subsequent treatment should be directed by the results of broncho-alveolar lavage.

Other respiratory tract infections

Pneumonia developing in association with neutropenia following treatment with cytotoxic drugs, or in patients with immunosuppression, including those suffering from AIDS, may be due to *Pneumocystis carinii*, other fungi, or viruses. Appropriate treatment is discussed in Chapters 31 and 32. The treatment of tuberculosis is considered in Chapter 30; influenza and other respiratory viral infections are dealt with in Chapter 32.

Key points

- Respiratory tract infections are the commonest indication for antibiotic treatment in primary care and in hospitals.

- Most respiratory infections in primary care are caused by viruses and will not benefit from antibiotic treatment. However, the key question in the decision about treatment with antimicrobials is: do the benefits to the patient outweigh the risks? It is not necessary to prescribe antimicrobials for all bacterial respiratory infections.

- Upper respiratory tract infections, sore throat, and otitis media do not benefit from antibiotic treatment even when caused by bacteria unless there is clinical evidence of complications.

- Bronchitis in adults aged <65 does not benefit from antibiotic treatment. However, in older adults it is more difficult to distinguish between bronchitis and pneumonia.

- Severity of suspected pneumonia should be assessed with the CURB65 score in primary care and the CURB65 score in hospitals.

- Patients with severe pneumonia should be treated with intravenous antibiotics that are effective against the full range of pathogens that may cause community-acquired pneumonia. The choice of antibiotic is influenced by the risk of *C. difficile* infection in the hospital.

Further reading

All respiratory infections

Health Protection Agency 'Management of infection guidance for primary care for consultation & local adaptation', Available at: http://www.hpa.org.uk/servlet/Satellite?c=Page&cid=1197637041219&pagename= HPAweb%2FPage%2FHPAwebAutoListName (26th February 2011, date last accessed).

Scottish Intercollegiate Guidelines Network (Available at: www.sign.ac.uk).

Guideline 117: management of sore throat and indications for tonsillectomy
Guideline 66: diagnosis and management of childhood otitis media in primary care
Guideline 59: community management of lower respiratory tract infection in adults

Pneumonia

Barker, B, Macfarlane, J, Lim, WS, Douglas, G (2009), 'Local guidelines for management of adult community acquired pneumonia: a survey of UK hospitals', *Thorax*, **64** (2): 181.

British Thoracic Society (2002), 'Guidelines for the management of community acquired pneumonia in childhood. Thorax', **57** Suppl 1: i1–i24. Available at: http://thorax.bmjjournals.com/cgi/content/full/57/90001/i1.

Dryden, M, Hand, K, Davey, P (2009), 'Antibiotics for community-acquired pneumonia', *Journal of Antimicrobial Chemotherapy*, **64**(6): 1123–25.

Lim, WS, Baudouin, SV, George, RC, Hill, AT, Jamieson, C, Le Jeune, I, Macfarlane, JT, Read, RC, Roberts, HJ, Levy, ML, Wani, M, Woodhead, MA(2009), 'BTS guidelines for the management of community acquired pneumonia in adults: update 2009', *Thorax* ,**64** Suppl 3: iii1–55.

Chapter 22

Topical use of antimicrobial agents

The concept of applying drugs directly to clinical lesions is appealing: problems of absorption and pharmacokinetics do not apply and agents too toxic for systemic use may be safely applied to skin or mucous membranes. The major drawback is that, even in the most superficial skin lesion, there may be areas inaccessible to a topical approach. Furthermore, collections of pus may prevent the agent reaching the infecting organisms and for this reason the management of any abscess includes drainage of pus.

Although skin, the largest and most accessible organ of the body, is the most obvious target for topical antimicrobial agents, other sites are available for this approach to therapy: the mucous membranes of the mouth and vagina, and the external surfaces of eyes and ears. Direct application of antibiotics into normally sterile sites, such as joints, peritoneal cavity, spinal fluid, or the urinary bladder, or instillation into surgical wounds prior to suture, may also be considered as a form of topical therapy, but will not be specifically dealt with in this chapter. Application of topical agents to mucous membranes or damaged skin may lead to considerable systemic absorption and the possibility of systemic toxicity should be borne in mind.

The chief reasons for using topical antimicrobial agents are:

◆ to achieve high drug concentrations at the site of infection;

◆ to treat trivial infections where use of a systemic drug is unjustified;

◆ to prevent infection in a susceptible site (e.g. burns);

◆ to enable the use of agents that are too toxic for systemic use;

◆ cost: topical agents are generally cheaper than systemic drugs.

Antiseptics

Disinfectant is a general term for chemicals that can destroy vegetative micro-organisms; those disinfectants that are sufficiently non-injurious to skin and exposed tissues to be used topically are called antiseptics. In order to achieve adequate antimicrobial activity, high concentrations of antiseptics are required and this serves to distinguish them from antibiotics in Waksman's original sense of 'substances produced by micro-organisms antagonistic to the growth or life of others in high dilution'. In many cases, true antibiotics are used topically in high concentration and might thus be classed as antiseptics. In fact, antiseptics and antibiotics are often used in exactly the same situations in dermatological practice and there has been some difference of opinion as to which class of agent to use in, for example, the treatment of infected ulcers or wounds. Antiseptics are usually cheaper and have the advantage that bacterial resistance rarely develops. Preparations commonly employed include chlorhexidine, cetrimide, iodophors (non-irritant iodine complexes), triclosan, and solutions liberating hypochlorite, such as Eusol or Dakin's solution.

Some concern has been expressed about the effect on tissue viability of many chemicals applied directly. There is some evidence *in vitro* of a direct toxic effect on epidermal cells and white blood cells of many antiseptics at concentrations well below those used topically.

Methods of application

Drugs that are dissolved in aqueous solutions (lotions) have the disadvantage of running off the skin and cooling it by evaporation. This method of delivering antimicrobial agents to the site of infection is inefficient and not often used, except as ear or eye drops. For use in eye infections, frequent application on to the cornea and conjunctiva is necessary, because the drug is only in contact for a short time and much of the active component runs down the cheek as an expensive tear! The value of aqueous preparations resides mainly in their irrigant and cleansing action and much of the therapeutic success may be due to these properties.

It is usual to apply drugs to the skin in a fat base, as either an oil and water cream, or a largely lipid ointment. Drug solubility affects the achievable concentration in each component, and availability at the lesion depends on diffusion from the applicant and absorption from the skin. Antibiotics that are lipid soluble and freely diffusible, for example fusidic acid, are at an advantage in this respect.

Sticky ointments may remain in contact with the infected site for a considerable time and application may be needed only once daily, but this obviously depends on the frequency of washing or removal of dressings.

Some of the commonly used topical preparations are listed in Table 22.1. Many of the formulations designed for topical use contain combinations of antimicrobial agents. Mixtures are intended to cover a wide antibacterial spectrum and to be compatible.

Choice

The results of laboratory tests may be helpful if adequate specimens are sent to the laboratory, but swabbing chronic ulcers or other skin wounds is not helpful (Chapter 29). Frequently, colonizing microbes are isolated from the surface of deep lesions leaving the true underlying pathogen undetected. The clinician must be careful not to use a battery of antimicrobials to treat harmless commensals colonizing an unoccupied niche. The golden rule is 'treat the patient, not the wound'.

Conventional antimicrobial sensitivity testing is often irrelevant because susceptibility of organisms to antiseptics can usually be assumed. Moreover, laboratory criteria of susceptibility to antibiotics usually apply to systemic use, not the high concentrations achievable by topical application. Nevertheless, complete resistance in laboratory tests is a contra-indication to use of a particular agent. Regular monitoring of hospital patients with large skin lesions, such as ulcers and burns, is useful to determine the nature and prevalence of resistant organisms, as well as the extent of cross-infection.

Choice, if not based on microbiological evidence, must include agents active against all likely pathogens. Topical antiseptics and hydroxyquinolines are to be preferred to antibiotics on microbiological grounds of avoidance of resistance, but many users prefer antibiotics because it is claimed that a quicker response is generally obtained. Tetracyclines are often recommended by clinicians, but not by microbiologists, who point to the prevalence of tetracycline resistance and the readiness with which such prevalence increases under selective pressure. Combinations of antibiotics, such as bacitracin and neomycin, or bacitracin, neomycin, and polymyxin are often used, and a corticosteroid is sometimes added for good measure. These antibiotics are not usually used for systemic therapy, so possible problems of compromising the activity of systemically useful agents by encouraging the emergence of resistance are minimized (see below). Nevertheless, it should be remembered that the topical use of neomycin might generate strains of bacteria cross-resistant to other aminoglycosides such as gentamicin.

One antibiotic, mupirocin (pseudomonic acid), has been marketed solely for topical use. The spectrum of activity of this agent is virtually restricted to Gram-positive cocci. Mupirocin is unsuitable for systemic use since it is quickly metabolized in the body. It has a unique mode of action (on protein synthesis) and cross-resistance is not a problem.

Table 22.1 Commonly used topical antimicrobial agents for skin infections. The numerous topical antiseptics available are omitted

Infection	Agent	Application	Comments
Bacterial	Chloramphenicol[a]	Ointment	Very broad spectrum
	Clindamycin[a]	Ointment	Used for acne
	Erythromycin[a]	Ointment	Used for acne
	Fusidic acid[a]	Ointment	Only active against *Staph. aureus* and *Str. pyogenes*
	Gentamicin[a]	Cream/ointment	Ototoxic and nephrotoxic if used over large areas of broken skin
	Metronidazole[a]	Gel	Used in rosacea and acne
	Mupirocin	Ointment	Macrogol-based ointment or nasal cream. Only active against gram positive cocci and mainly used for eradication of MRSA carriage
	Neomycin	Cream/ointment/powder	Often combined with gramicidin or bacitracin and/or polymyxin B. Ototoxic and nephrotoxic if used over large areas of broken skin
	Polymyxins[a]	Ointment/powder	Nephrotoxic and neurotoxic if used over large areas of broken skin
	Silver sulfadiazine (sulphonamide)	Cream	May cause sensitization
	Tetracycline[a]	Ointment/cream/drops	Broad-spectrum; resistance common
Fungal	Imidazoles (clotrimazole, etc.)	Cream/powder	For dermatophyte or yeast skin infections but ineffective against nail infections
	Nystatin (and other polyenes)	Cream	For dermatophyte or yeast skin infections but ineffective against nail infections
	Tioconazole and amorolfine	Nail lacquer/cream	For limited dermatophyte nail infections
Viral	Aciclovir[a] and penciclovir[a]	Ointment/cream	Antiviral agents; for use on herpes lesions
	Idoxuridine	Ointment/drops	

[a] Compounds that are also used systemically.

In practice, one of the most important limitations to choice is the availability of a particular drug as a topical product. Manufacturers are well aware that it makes little commercial sense to market a relatively cheap topical formulation if it is going to encourage resistance that diminishes the usefulness of more expensive parenteral forms of the drug. Here, at least, the interests of industry and the consumer coincide.

Bacterial skin infections

Trivial skin sepsis, often due to staphylococci, is common, but usually self-limiting in healthy individuals. In general, mild infections of the skin respond to local measures involving cleansing of the crusted areas and application of topical agents, such as fusidic acid or mupirocin, to the raw surfaces. More severe staphylococcal and streptococcal skin lesions may require systemic therapy (Chapter 29).

Table 22.2 Commonly used topical antimicrobial agents for other sites. The numerous topical antiseptics available are omitted

Site	Agent	Application	Comments
Ear, bacterial	Chloramphenicol[a]	Ear drops	For otitis externa
	Aminoglycosides (framycetin, gentamicin[a] and neomycin)	Ear drops	For otitis externa, should not be used in otitis media because of risk of ototoxicity with a perforated ear drum
	Polymyxins[a]	Ear drops	For otitis externa, should not be used in otitis media because of risk of ototoxicity with a perforated ear drum
	Fluoroquinolones (ciprofloxacin and ofloxacin)[a]	Ear drops	For otitis externa and otitis media. Not licensed in the UK
Ear, fungal	Clotrimazole	Ear drops	For fungal otitis externa
Eye, bacterial	Aminoglycosides (framycetin, gentamicin[a], and neomycin)	Eye and ear drops	
	Chloramphenicol[a]	Eye drops or ointment	Drug of choice for superficial eye infections
	Fusidic acid[a]	Eye drops	For staphylococcal infections only
	Polymyxins[a]	Eye drops or ointment	
	Fluoroquinolones (ciprofloxacin and ofloxacin)[a]	Eye drops	
Eye, viral	Aciclovir[a]	Eye ointment	For local treatment of superficial Herpes simplex (dendritic ulcer)
	Ganciclovir[a]	Eye drops	For treatment of herpes keratitis
Mouth, fungal	Amphotericin[a]	Lozenges or suspension	For mild oral candida (thrush), not absorbed
	Miconazole	Oral gel	For mild oral candida (thrush). Enough oral absorption to cause drug interactions, check before use
	Nystatin	Pastilles or suspension	For mild oral candida (thrush), not absorbed
Vaginal, fungal	Imidazoles (e.g. clotrimazole, econazole)	Creams, ointments and pessaries	Vaginal candidiasis (thrush)
	Nystatin		

[a] Compounds that are also used systemically.

Nasal carriage

In recurrent sepsis with *Staph. aureus* it may be necessary to attempt to eradicate the organism from the body. This is also desirable in patients and staff colonized with antibiotic-resistant strains, particularly meticillin-resistant *Staph. aureus* (MRSA), which can cause serious cross-infection problems. The external surface of the skin can be washed in antiseptics, but nasal carriage of staphylococci is often resistant to this treatment. For this purpose, nasal creams should be applied at least twice a day for 5 days. Chlorhexidine/neomycin cream (Naseptin) has been widely used, but does not appear to be as effective as mupirocin in the eradication of nasal carriage of MRSA. The normal dermatological preparation of mupirocin, which is in a macrogol (polyethylene glycol) excipient, is unsuitable for nasal application and a paraffin-based ointment should be used for this purpose.

Acne

The role of bacteria in the pathogenesis of acne vulgaris is still under debate, although commensal diphtheroids, such as *Propionibacterium acnes*, are thought to play some part. Systemic antibiotics, including tetracycline and erythromycin, do improve severe intractable cases and success has also been claimed for topical antimicrobial agents, in particular for clindamycin. Treatment with any of these agents needs to be prolonged and is an adjunct to other measures aimed at improving the condition.

Burns

The treatment of burns is an enormous specialized topic that cannot be covered adequately in this chapter. However, topical agents do have definite value in the prevention of infection in patients with burns so it is appropriate that their use should be mentioned.

Initially, a thermal burn renders the skin sterile, but bacterial colonization is inevitable, even with scrupulous aseptic technique. Indeed, infection, usually with *Str. pyogenes, Staph. aureus*, or *Pseudomonas aeruginosa*, is an important determinant in the outcome of extensive burns, since it is a major cause of delay in skin healing and of death.

Prophylaxis with topical antibiotics and antiseptics has been shown significantly to reduce colonization and sepsis. Mafenide, a sulphonamide derivative, was widely used, but has been largely replaced in the UK by silver sulfadiazine or chlorhexidine. None of these agents will reliably prevent infection by multiresistant Gram-negative rods, especially *Ps. aeruginosa* (an organism that has replaced *Str. pyogenes* as the major scourge of burns units), or fungi. Aggressive surgical approaches of early wound closure by skin grafting after debridement has reduced the requirement for topical applications to burned surfaces.

In cases in which infection becomes established, systemic drugs will often have to be employed, the choice being dictated by laboratory tests. However, since the penetration of antibiotics to surface lesions with a poor blood supply may be inadequate, topical dressings are additionally required.

Urinary and respiratory infections are commonly encountered in the burned patient and may result in bacteraemia with sepsis, which has a poor prognosis. These infections require, of course, systemic therapy, but choice may be limited by bacterial resistance since many burns units are notorious for the prevalence of highly resistant strains, especially of *Ps. aeruginosa*.

Skin ulcers

Ulceration of the skin of the leg or the area overlying the sacrum may arise from a variety of pathological states and colonization is usually a sequela, not an initiating event. Disorders of the circulation, including obliterative arterial disease, small-vessel damage consequent on diabetes mellitus, and varicose veins are the most common underlying conditions; correction of the underlying cause is essential to the healing of any ulcer. Continuous pressure is another common factor in the formation of a break in the skin, particularly in the bed-ridden. Such pressure sores (bed sores) are difficult to prevent without scrupulous nursing care. This problem has led to the development of special air beds and cushions to minimize local vascular occlusion to the skin overlying bony areas such as the sacrum.

The presence of colonization in a skin ulcer may be detected by odour and appearance of pus, which in the case of pseudomonas infection may be characteristically green. However, colonization is not an indication for antibacterial treatment, which should be reserved for patients with spreading cellulitis or systemic inflammatory response (Chapter 29). Swab reports showing the presence of potential pathogens do not prove infection since colonization of a large raw skin area is inevitable. *Staph. aureus*, environmental and gut bacteria are the organisms most commonly found in these sites. *Ps. aeruginosa* is frequently found in long-standing ulcers because of its intrinsic resistance to many antibiotics and chemical agents used as antiseptics.

Some chemical antiseptics are cytotoxic and impair wound healing, consequently older remedies such as honey, sugar, and vinegar may be as effective as modern antiseptics. Topical antibiotics should be avoided. Many weeks of regular dressing combined with bed rest may be required to heal large ulcers; admission to hospital often speeds up the process. Skin grafting is frequently used for the most recalcitrant cases.

Superficial fungal infections

Confirmation of the diagnosis of superficial fungal infections such as ringworm and tinea pedis of the skin, or thrush of the mouth or vagina, depends on laboratory investigation of appropriate specimens from the affected area (nail, hair, skin scrapings, swabs of lesions of mucous membranes). Microscopy alone will be sufficient to establish a fungal cause in most cases, but culture is necessary to identify the aetiological agent. Susceptibility testing presents technical difficulties, but dermatophytes may usually be assumed to be susceptible to appropriate agents (see Table 4.1). *Candida albicans* may acquire resistance to some drugs, but this is of great importance only in invasive candidiasis.

The limiting factor in treating dermatophyte infections is penetration of the agent. For superficial skin infections old-fashioned remedies, such as benzoic acid-containing ointments (e.g. Whitfield's ointment) are perfectly effective, but for hair and nail infections, agents that penetrate into keratinized tissue are needed. Oral griseofulvin and terbinafine are suited to this purpose, since they are absorbed from the gastrointestinal tract and are preferentially concentrated in keratin. Because of the slow turnover of nail and hair, treatment for several months may be required; indeed, fungal infections of toenails may not completely clear even after a year's treatment with griseofulvin, despite susceptibility of the infecting fungus. In such cases terbinafine (see Chapter 7) may be successful. Topical treatment with amorolfine or tioconazole, which are formulated to penetrate nails, are less effective than terbinafine.

Thrush responds in most cases to an appropriate antifungal agent, applied topically (e.g. nystatin or an imidazole), but precipitating factors, such as diabetes or antibiotic therapy, must also be corrected if they are present. If there is clinical evidence for invasive infection, as, for example, *Candida* oesophagitis, appropriate systemic drugs, such as amphotericin, 5-fluorocytosine, fluconazole, ketoconazole, or itraconazole must be added.

Disadvantages of topical therapy

Topical therapy is not without its hazards. Although the direct toxic effects of drugs given systemically are reduced, exposed tissues and mucous membranes offer a fairly efficient site for drug absorption. For example, aminoglycoside ototoxicity has been reported following local application of neomycin, especially in the newborn. A more frequently observed effect is sensitization to the agent so that subsequent use of the drug, either topically or parenterally, produces a hypersensitivity reaction. Penicillin, in particular, is prone to sensitize the host and because of possible anaphylactic reactions it is not advisable to use any β-lactam antibiotic on the skin. A further hazard of topical therapy is that local irritation may lead to a delay in wound healing, even though the actual infection is controlled.

Superinfection with resistant bacteria or with fungi is a common consequence of using any topical antibiotic for a prolonged period. Widespread use of one particular agent will lead to a larger reservoir of resistant organisms and the possibility of cross-infection. This is particularly likely to occur in burns units and dermatology wards, where there are many patients with large open skin lesions. Prevention of infection and cross-infection by aseptic methods is desirable, but often difficult in practice.

Of equal concern is the development of bacterial resistance during therapy. It has been shown that topical neomycin can select resistant *Staphylococcus epidermidis* strains, which can transfer resistance to *Staph. aureus* on the skin. The emergence of gentamicin-resistant *Ps. aeruginosa* and coliforms has been associated with topical use of that aminoglycoside, particularly on leg ulcers. In some instances the resistance is plasmid mediated. In this manner, topical agents select multiresistant organisms, which may subsequently cause systemic infection in the patient or, by cross-infection, others.

Tetracycline eye drops select for tetracycline-resistant bacteria in the mouth flora when used for mass population treatment of trachoma. The explanation is likely to be that medications administered to the eye can readily reach the nasopharynx via the naso-lachrymal duct. Selection of resistant bacteria is the most powerful argument against the indiscriminate use of topical antibiotics, and since antiseptics lack this disadvantage they are to be preferred wherever possible.

Key points

♦ Although skin, the largest and most accessible organ of the body, is the most obvious target for topical antimicrobial agents, other sites are available for this approach to therapy: the mucous membranes of the mouth and vagina, and the external surfaces of eyes and ears.

♦ The major drawback to topical treatment of skin infections is that, even in the most superficial skin lesion, there may be areas inaccessible to a topical approach. Furthermore, collections of pus may prevent the agent reaching the infecting organisms and for this reason the management of any abscess includes drainage of pus.

♦ Application of topical agents to mucous membranes or damaged skin may lead to considerable systemic absorption and the possibility of systemic toxicity should be borne in mind.

♦ Superinfection with resistant bacteria or with fungi and selection of resistant strains during treatment are both common consequence of using any topical antibiotic for a prolonged period.

♦ Widespread use of one particular agent will lead to a larger reservoir of resistant organisms and the possibility of cross-infection. This is particularly likely to occur in burns units and dermatology wards, where there are many patients with large open skin lesions.

Chapter 23

Urinary infections

Urinary tract infection is the second most common clinical indication for empirical antimicrobial treatment in primary and secondary care; respiratory tract infections are the commonest clinical indication in both settings. Urine samples constitute the largest single category of specimens examined in most medical microbiology laboratories. Healthcare practitioners regularly have to make decisions about prescription of antibiotics for urinary tract infection. Criteria for the diagnosis of urinary tract infection vary depending on the patient and the context. Because it is such a common problem it is an excellent opportunity for students to understand how to interpret microbiology results in the context of clinical symptoms and signs.

Bacteriuria

Normal urine is sterile, so bacteriuria (the presence of bacteria in a urine sample) is abnormal. In domiciliary practice four bacterial species account for 95% of isolates, whereas in hospital there is a wider range of pathogens.

The clinical significance of bacteriuria depends on how the sample was obtained, how it was transported to the laboratory, and the clinical history. Before considering the clinical significance of bacteriuria in the context of specific problems it is important to understand what the microbiology laboratory means by the term 'significant bacteriuria'.

Diagnostic methods

Urine sampling and testing

The laboratory confirmation of bacteriuria is made by quantitative culture of an uncontaminated urine specimen. The most reliable methods for obtaining a urine sample without contamination by skin or perineal flora are by suprapubic aspiration of the bladder with a syringe and needle or by urethral catheterization. Neither of these is practical or acceptable in clinical practice so urine samples are collected during micturition. The practice of cleansing the perineum and taking the specimen in the middle of micturition minimizes the risk of contamination by the perineal flora. However, it is critical that cultures of urine are done as quickly as possible, otherwise a few contaminating bacteria from skin and perineal flora will multiply in a few hours at room temperature and give false positive results. Refrigeration and rapid processing in the laboratory can reduce this problem. Alternatively, culture of urine as soon as it is passed can circumvent the possibility of contaminants growing in the urine during transit. This is achieved by using dip-inoculum methods, which consist of agar attached to slides or spoons that are dipped in the urine, drained, and transported in a stoppered bottle to the laboratory where any bacterial colonies are counted after overnight incubation at 37°C. A rough quantification is possible by this method or by other simple methods of direct plating of a fixed volume of urine on appropriate culture media. Simple identification of the resulting significant isolates is made and antimicrobial susceptibility tests performed as described in Chapter 12.

Criteria of infection

When more than 10^5 organisms/ml (10^8/l) of a single bacterial species are cultured from a freshly voided midstream specimen of urine, the term 'significant' bacteriuria is used because it is highly unlikely that such a large number of bacteria could be the result of contamination of the sample. In other words the laboratory finding of 'significant' bacteriuria means that it is very likely that the bacteria were present in the urine in the body, before micturition.

The symptoms of urinary tract infection can be associated with lower counts of bacteria: 10^3 organisms/ml in men and 10^2 organisms/ml in women. However, most clinical laboratories cannot detect such low levels of bacteria with routine methods, so in practice the threshold for significant bacteriuria remains at 10^5 organisms/ml.

Although normal urine is sterile a few healthy people have bacteriuria without any symptoms. Most information comes from women, in whom the prevalence of bacteriuria increases with age (Fig. 23.1). The prevalence at any given age is related to sexual activity: 5% of married women aged 24–44 are likely to have asymptomatic bacteriuria compared with <1% of nuns of the same age.

There is less information about men. As with women the prevalence of bacteriuria in men increases with age but it is always lower than in women of the same age. In the elderly the prevalence in men and women increases with deterioration of health and reaches 100% in anybody who has an indwelling urinary catheter present for >4 weeks (Table 23.2).

The important point to remember is that bacteriuria is not a disease, it is a laboratory finding (see Key points at end of chapter).

Urine dipstick testing

Urine dipsticks use reagents to detect the presence of chemicals in the urine. The presence of nitrites in urine is associated with bacteriuria because nitrites are products of bacterial metabolism;

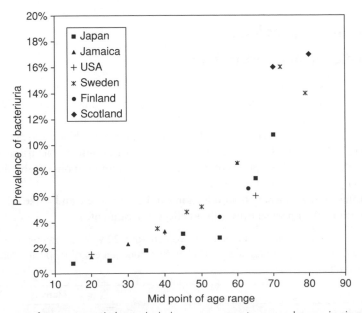

Fig. 23.1 Presence of asymptomatic bacteriuria in non-pregnant women by age in six countries. From S2.1.2 in Supplementary Materials supporting SIGN Guideline 88 (Management of suspected bacterial urinary tract infection in adults).

Table 23.1 Prevalence of resistance to antibiotics in urinary isolates from women aged <65 presenting to community health centres in 17 countries. Data from Table 5 of Kahlmeter, G (2003) An international survey of the antimicrobial susceptibility of pathogens from uncomplicated urinary tract infections: the ECO.SENS Project. *Journal of Antimicrobial Chemotherapy* **51**(1): 69–76

Pathogen	n	Ampicillin	Co-amoxiclav	Trimethoprim	Ciprofloxacin	Nitrofurantoin
E. coli	2478	30%	3%	15%	2%	1%
P. mirabilis	192	16%	1%	25%	2%	100%
Klebsiella spp.	97	83%	4%	12%	1%	100%
Other Enterobacteriaceae	122	46%	21%	9%	1%	40%
S. saprophyticus	116	2%	2%	0	0	0

however, nitrites can be found in sterile urine as well. The presence of leucocyte esterase is associated with the presence of white blood cells in the urine, which may in turn be associated with urinary tract infection. However, any cause of inflammation of the urinary tract will result in white cells in the urine. Other substances (blood or protein) can be present in the urine of patients with symptomatic urinary tract infection, but they are even less specific to the diagnosis than nitrites or leucocyte esterase.

Rigorous analysis of the value of urine dipstick testing has been largely disappointing (see Key points at end of this chapter). In fact the only patient group in which dipstick testing appears to be helpful is adults with a single symptom (dysuria or frequency). In patients with very clear symptoms of infection the likelihood of bacteriuria is so high that dipstick testing contributes nothing to management. In contrast dipsticks result in too many false negative results to be used for screening of asymptomatic bacteriuria in pregnancy because of the dire consequences of a false negative result.

Common clinical problems

Symptomatic urinary tract infection

Lower urinary tract infection

Infection of the tissues of the bladder or urethra causes increased frequency of micturition with severe burning pain on passing urine (dysuria). The walls of the bladder and urethra have a relatively poor blood supply so bacteria are not able to penetrate into the blood and people with lower urinary tract infection do not have a systemic inflammatory response. In fact if a patient presents with dysuria, frequency, and symptoms of systemic inflammatory response, it should be assumed that they have upper urinary tract infection.

The symptoms of lower urinary tract infection can be very severe and make it impossible for patients to continue their normal lives without effective treatment.

Table 23.2 Prevalence of bacteriuria in men and women aged 70 years or greater. From data in Supplementary Materials supporting SIGN Guideline 88 (Management of suspected bacterial urinary tract infection in adults)

Category	Men	Women
Healthy, ambulatory	7%	17%
Institutionalized	37%	57%
Indwelling urinary catheter for >4 weeks	100%	100%

Cystitis means inflammation of the bladder and is sometimes used as a pseudonym for lower urinary tract infection, although strictly the term should be bacterial cystitis to distinguish from other causes of cystitis (e.g. chemical cystitis or interstitial cystitis).

Upper urinary tract infection

Infection of the kidney causes loin pain and flank tenderness but these are likely to be accompanied by symptoms of lower urinary tract infection as well. The kidney has an excellent blood supply so, in contrast to lower urinary tract infection, patients with upper urinary tract infection commonly have a systemic inflammatory response and may develop bacteraemia with severe sepsis or even septic shock.

Pyelonephritis means inflammation of the kidney and collecting system and is sometimes used as a pseudonym for upper urinary tract infection.

Uncomplicated urinary tract infection

This means lower urinary tract infection in non-pregnant women with no underlying anatomical abnormalities that predispose to recurrent urinary tract infection. The adjective 'uncomplicated' is being used in two different ways:

1. The likelihood that the infection can be resolved successfully with a short (three day) course of antibiotics. This is why lower urinary tract infection in men is classified as complicated, because it is likely to be associated with prostatitis, in which case it is likely to relapse unless antibiotics are continued for two weeks.

2. The likelihood that there will be no clinical complications from the infection. This is why all upper urinary tract infections and also symptoms of lower urinary tract infections in pregnant women are classed as complicated, because both problems are associated with immediate risk to the patient from sepsis or severe sepsis.

Antibiotic treatment

Symptomatic infection

Patients with symptomatic infection of the lower or upper urinary tract benefit from antibiotic treatment. Symptoms would resolve without antibiotic treatment in about 50% of people with lower urinary tract infection but they resolve much faster with antibiotic treatment. Patients with symptoms of upper urinary tract infection require urgent effective antibiotic treatment to minimize the risk of bacteraemia.

In general practice about half the women presenting with frequency and dysuria have sterile urine cultures. This condition is sometimes referred to as the 'urethral syndrome' or symptomatic abacteriuria—a common, but largely unexplained condition. Some cases may be due to sexually transmitted organisms, such as chlamydia, and some may represent the early stages of urinary infection. Counselling is more important than antimicrobial therapy, but persistent symptoms need further investigation.

Asymptomatic bacteriuria

There are only two groups of patients in whom asymptomatic bacteriuria should be treated with antibiotics:

1. In very young children whose kidneys are still growing there is evidence that asymptomatic bacteriuria is associated with scarring of the kidney and predisposes to hypertension or chronic renal impairment. Young children who have had symptomatic urinary tract infection are therefore followed up after treatment to ensure that they do not have continuing bacteriuria.

2. In pregnancy asymptomatic bacteriuria is associated with increased risk of pyelonephritis later in pregnancy and with pre-term delivery. Moreover there is good evidence that antibiotic treatment of asymptomatic bacteriuria reduces the risk of both these outcomes. Consequently all pregnant women should be screened in the first trimester of pregnancy and women with bacteriuria should be treated.

Asymptomatic bacteriuria should not be treated with antibiotics in any other people. Placebo controlled trials have failed to show convincing benefit in patients with diabetes, in institutionalized elderly men or women, or in those with long-term indwelling catheters, whereas the same trials did show increased risk of adverse events in the treated patients, including colonization with antibiotic-resistant bacteria.

Choice of agent

Lower urinary tract infection

In lower urinary tract infection seen in general practice, over 90% of patients become asymptomatic after a few days' appropriate antibiotic therapy and remain free from bacteriuria for several weeks or more. Most current practice guidelines recommend empirical treatment with a 'best guess' antibiotic selected based on knowledge of likely pathogens and local resistance patterns. In domiciliary practice *Escherichia coli* predominates, accounting for at least 80% of isolates and most will be fully sensitive to trimethoprim or nitrofurantoin (Fig. 23.2). However, ampicillin-resistant organisms are now sufficiently common for this drug to be abandoned in favour of trimethoprim or one of the other oral agents. The use of co-trimoxazole is not recommended in the treatment of urinary infection, since the sulphonamide component plays an insignificant role and trimethoprim alone is less toxic. Two agents, nitrofurantoin and nalidixic acid, achieve adequate concentrations only in urine and are exclusively used in lower urinary tract infection. Nitrofurantoin has the distinct advantage of being unrelated to other antibiotics. In contrast

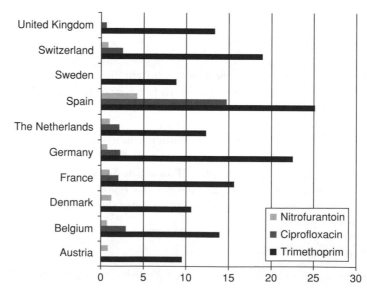

Fig 23.2 Prevalence of resistance to antibiotics in urinary isolates of *Esch. coli* from women aged <65 presenting to community health centres in 10 countries. Drawn from data in Table 5 of Kahlmeter, G (2003) An international survey of the antimicrobial susceptibility of pathogens from uncomplicated urinary tract infections: the ECO.SENS Project. *Journal of Antimicrobial Chemotherapy* **51**(1): 69–76.

nalidixic acid is a quinolone and is likely to select for bacteria that are resistant to fluoroquinolones such as ciprofloxacin. For that reason nitrofurantoin is usually recommended as the preferred alternative to trimethoprim for lower urinary tract infection.

For bacteria that are resistant to nitrofurantoin and trimethoprim or for patients who cannot tolerate these drugs, there is a range of alternative oral agents, including oral cephalosporins, co-amoxiclav, fluoroquinolones, and pivmecillinam. The reason that these drugs are not used first line is that they are no more effective than nitrofurantoin or trimethoprim and should be reserved for patients in whom these first-line agents are ineffective or contraindicated.

The prevalence of resistance in *Esch. coli* is variable between countries (Fig. 23.2). In 2003 the prevalence of trimethoprim resistance in *Esch. coli* isolated from urine was 8.8% in Sweden but 25.1% in Spain. Ciprofloxacin resistance in *Esch. coli* isolates from urine was uncommon in most European countries in 2003 but was 14.7% in Spain. The prevalence of multiresistant *Esch. coli* with extended spectrum β-lactamases (ESBL) has been increasing in all European countries over the past ten years and even in primary care patients may present with infections caused by bacteria that are resistant to all available oral antibiotics. Fosfomycin is an antibiotic that was discovered over 35 years ago but until recently was only used in a few European countries. An oral formulation is available and fosfomycin may provide the only option for oral treatment of some urinary tract infections in primary care. Fosfomycin can be obtained on a named patient basis in countries where it is not licensed for use.

Upper urinary tract infection

Upper urinary tract infection can be accompanied by bacteraemia, making it a life-threatening infection. However, infection should respond to effective antibiotic treatment in 90% of patients.

Nitrofurantoin is not an effective treatment for upper urinary tract infection because it does not achieve effective concentrations in the blood. Resistance to trimethoprim is too common to recommend this drug for empirical treatment of a life-threatening infection. Consequently, empirical treatment should be with a broad-spectrum antibiotic such as co-amoxiclav or ciprofloxacin.

Because of the potentially serious consequences of upper urinary tract infections it is recommended that urine cultures should be obtained before starting antibiotic treatment in all patients. This is because community-acquired infection can be caused by pathogens that are resistant to either co-amoxiclav, ciprofloxacin or any of the other oral antibiotics used in general practice and this is not an acceptable risk with a life-threatening infection.

Therapeutic regimens

In the special circumstances of urinary infection, unlike those in other parts of the body, the drugs used are often preferentially excreted into the urine and may attain very high concentrations there, sometimes for long periods. Moreover, in the treatment of lower urinary tract infection (in contrast to pyelonephritis or infections complicating urinary tract abnormalities) antibacterial drugs are generally needed only to tip the balance in favour of normal clearance mechanisms. Several studies have shown that much-curtailed regimens, lasting one to three days, are as successful as prolonged therapy in curing acute urinary infections. Indeed, longer courses are wasteful of resources especially since many patients, wiser than their doctors, abandon treatment once the symptoms abate.

Short-course treatment has an additional potential benefit in serving to identify those few patients (the ones who fail short-course therapy) who are likely to require more extensive urological investigation. Most current guidelines recommend three days' treatment with trimethoprim for uncomplicated lower urinary tract infection but there is less certainty about nitrofurantoin.

UK guidelines recommend three days' therapy but guidelines in other countries recommend treatment for five or seven days.

Management of common clinical problems

Acute symptomatic infections in children

Diagnosis of symptomatic urinary tract infection is rarely straightforward, especially in younger children. They may present with generalized symptoms (fever, vomiting, general malaise) rather than with symptoms in the urinary tract. Consequently, clinically, suspicion should be confirmed by urine culture. If it is difficult to obtain a high-quality clean catch midstream specimen of urine then diagnosis may have to rely on obtaining urine by catheterization or suprapubic needle aspirate. In a child with a low clinical suspicion of urinary tract infection in whom these tests are considered unnecessarily invasive urine dipstick testing can be used, followed by culture of urine only if the dipstick results suggest bacteriuria. However, false negative dipstick tests do occur.

Acute symptomatic infections in adult women

Clinical diagnosis of lower urinary tract infection is reliable in young adult women who have dysuria and frequency but no history of vaginal discharge. Neither dipstick tests nor urine culture are necessary to confirm the diagnosis and empiric antibiotic treatment (three days of trimethoprim or nitrofurantoin) should be given on the basis of these symptoms alone. If the symptoms are less clear-cut (e.g. the patient has frequency or dysuria but not both) then urine dipstick testing should be done. If this is positive then three days of trimethoprim or nitrofurantoin should be given, but if it is negative bacteriuria should be confirmed with culture before treatment is given.

If the woman has symptoms of upper tract infection (loin pain or systemic inflammatory response) then a urine culture should be taken before empiric treatment is started in order to identify resistant bacteria. Empiric treatment should be with co-amoxiclav, pivmecillinam, or a fluoroquinolone for seven days.

Urinary tract infection is difficult to diagnose in older women because it is more likely to present with vague, generalized symptoms. Moreover the prevalence of asymptomatic bacteriuria increases steadily with age and with increasing co-morbidity. Over 50% of institutionalized elderly women have asymptomatic bacteriuria all of the time. The decision to give antibiotic treatment should be based on clinical diagnosis of infection, supported by acute local or systemic symptoms of inflammation. Smelly urine just means that the patient has bacteriuria, which is not unusual and does not require antibiotic treatment.

Recurrent symptomatic infections in women

Recurrent urinary tract infection in healthy non-pregnant women is defined as three or more episodes during a 12 month period. Antibiotics can be used to reduce the frequency of recurrent infection in two ways. A single dose of either trimethoprim or nitrofurantoin taken at night reduces the risk of symptomatic infection to about one-fifth of the risk with no treatment. However, the risk of recurrent urinary infection returns to pretreatment levels as soon as treatment is stopped. An alternative, equally effective strategy for women with infection associated with sexual intercourse is to take a single postcoital dose of antibiotic. Prophylactic antibiotics for recurrent infection have side effects (oral or vaginal candidiasis and gastrointestinal symptoms) but infection by bacteria resistant to the prophylactic antibiotic does not appear to be a significant risk.

In postmenopausal women, oestrogen replacement is not consistently effective in preventing recurrent urinary tract infection and is less effective than antibiotic prophylaxis.

Cranberry products (juice and capsules or tablets containing concentrated extracts) are effective for preventing recurrent infection in young women after antibiotic treatment of an acute attack. The effectiveness of prophylaxis with antibiotics or cranberry products against recurrent urinary tract infections decreases with age. Cranberry products are nearly as effective as trimethoprim in preventing urinary tract infection and have significantly fewer adverse effects.

Acute symptomatic infections in men

Uncomplicated lower urinary tract infection does not occur in men. Urinary tract infections in men are generally viewed as complicated because they result from an anatomic or functional anomaly or instrumentation of the genito-urinary tract. Consequently, urine cultures should be obtained before antibiotic treatment is started. It is impossible to distinguish reliably between urinary tract infection and prostatitis, consequently two weeks' empirical treatment with a fluoroquinolone is recommended.

Catheterized patients

Between 2 and 7% of patients with indwelling urethral catheters acquire bacteriuria each day, even with the application of best practice for insertion and care of the catheter. All patients with a long-term indwelling catheter are bacteriuric, often with two or more organisms. The presence of a short- or long-term indwelling catheter is associated with a greater incidence of fever of urinary tract origin. Fever without any localizing signs is a common occurrence in catheterized patients and urinary tract infection accounts for about a third of these episodes.

In catheterized patients the common occurrence of fever, the consistent presence of bacteriuria, and the variable presence of a broad range of other associated clinical manifestations (new onset confusion, renal angle tenderness or suprapubic pain, chills, rigors, etc.) makes the diagnosis of symptomatic urinary tract infection difficult.

The presence of one of the following symptoms is an indication for empiric antibiotic treatment:

- new costovertebral tenderness;
- rigors;
- new onset confusion;
- fever greater than 37.8°C or 1.5°C above baseline on two occasions during 12 h.

Urine culture should be used to test the susceptibility of the bacteria that are inevitably present in the urine. Antibiotic treatment should never be given simply because of change in the smell or appearance of the urine in patients with indwelling urinary catheters.

Key points

- Bacteriuria is not a disease, it is a laboratory finding.
- Tests for bacteriuria do not establish the diagnosis of urinary tract infection, which should be based on symptoms and signs.
- Bacteriuria alone is rarely an indication for treatment.
- Bacteriuria can only be an absolute indication for antibiotic treatment when there is convincing evidence that eradication of bacteriuria results in meaningful health gain at acceptable risk.
- Treatment of asymptomatic bacteriuria is indicated only in children and pregnant women.
- The main value of urine culture is to identify the bacteria responsible for an infection and their sensitivity to antibiotics.
- Urine dipstick tests have a very limited role in the diagnosis of urinary tract infection. They are not sufficiently accurate to be used for screening of asymptomatic bacteriuria in pregnancy and are only helpful in the management of patients who do not have clear symptoms of lower urinary tract infection.

Further reading

Albert X, Huertas I, Pereiró I, Sanfélix J, Gosalbes V, Perrota C (2004), 'Antibiotics for preventing recurrent urinary tract infection in non-pregnant women', *The Cochrane Database of Systematic Reviews*, Issue 3. Art. No.: CD001209. DOI: 10.1002/14651858.CD001209.pub2.

Cincinnati Children's Hospital Medical Center (2005), 'Evidence based clinical practice guideline for medical management of first time acute urinary tract infection in children 12 years of age or less. Cincinnati (OH): Cincinnati Children's Hospital Medical Center'. Available at: http://www.guideline. gov/summary/summary.aspx?doc_id=7272&nbr=004334&string=uti+AND+children.

European Antimicrobial Resistance Surveillance Network (EARS-NET). Annual reports are available open access from the European Centre for Disease Control: http://www.ecdc.europa.eu/en/activities/ surveillance/EARS-Net/Pages/index.aspx.

Loeb, M, Brazil, K, Lohfeld, L, McGeer, A, Simor, A, Stevenson, K, Zoutman, D, Smith, S, Liu, X, Walter, SD (2005), 'Effect of a multifaceted intervention on number of antimicrobial prescriptions for suspected urinary tract infections in residents of nursing homes: cluster randomised controlled trial', *British Medical Journal*, **331**(7518): 669.

Scottish Intercollegiate Guidelines Network (2006), 'Management of suspected bacterial urinary tract infection in adults. SIGN, Edinburgh', Available at: http://www.sign.ac.uk/pdf/sign88.pdf.

Turner, D, Little, P, Raftery, J, Turner, S, Smith, H, Rumsby, K, Mullee, M (2010), 'Cost effectiveness of management strategies for urinary tract infections: results from randomised controlled trial', *British Medical Journal*, **340**: c346.

Chapter 24

Sexually transmitted infections

Sexually transmitted infections (Table 24.1) formerly referred to as venereal diseases, are common (Fig. 24.1) but remain under-diagnosed because of the reluctance of some to seek medical help when genital symptoms develop. Some, such as syphilis and human immunodeficiency virus (HIV) infection (see Chapter 33), are potentially serious and have life-threatening complications; others, such as trichomonal vaginal discharge, are merely a nuisance. The stigmatization of sexually transmitted infections has been reduced in many societies particularly following the rapid emergence of HIV infection in the last two decades of the twentieth century. Realization that prevention of transmission of pathogens, notably by practising safe sex, is of paramount importance has eroded taboos that have existed for centuries. The explosive increase in sexually transmitted diseases worldwide makes it important for all doctors to have knowledge of their treatment. While genito-urinary medicine clinics specialize in their diagnosis, management, and follow up, community-based doctors deal with an increasingly large proportion of cases.

Laboratory diagnosis

Direct microscopic examination is of utmost importance in genito-urinary medicine as it confirms many clinical diagnoses, and for this reason many clinics have some laboratory function on site. In most cases a sufficiently accurate microbiological diagnosis can be made to enable specific chemotherapy to be given. Microscopy of a genital discharge can give accurate, rapid confirmation of a clinical diagnosis in many cases. Typical Gram-negative intracellular diplococci in a Gram-stained film of a urethral discharge are strongly supportive of the diagnosis of acute gonorrhoea in a man. Conversely, in a patient with dysuria and discharge, large numbers of neutrophils (pus cells), but no diplococci, in 'threads' of urethral discharge that are present in an early stream urine sample suggest chlamydial (formerly referred to as 'non-specific') urethritis. The examination of exudate from a syphilitic chancre must be done by dark ground microscopy within a few minutes of collecting the specimen; the presence of motile spirochaetes confirms the diagnosis; it is not possible to cultivate these organisms in artificial media. The unstained 'wet' film of vaginal secretions can be used to diagnose trichomoniasis, by virtue of seeing the motile *Trichomonas vaginalis* protozoa, and may also reveal *Candida* or bacteria-studded epithelial cells ('clue' cells) suggestive of bacterial vaginosis.

For several reasons culture and other methods detection of the presence of sexually transmitted pathogens should also be attempted. Multiple infections may be present simultaneously and it is routine practice therefore to screen patients with symptoms or signs of genital infection for the common causes. The antimicrobial susceptibility of pathogens can give important case-specific and epidemiological information (see Gonorrhoea, below). Culture of cervical swabs and from extra-genital sites in both sexes is necessary because examination of Gram-stained smears is unreliable. Few genital pathogens can be cultivated easily. The most commonly sought, *Neisseria gonorrhoeae*, is a fastidious organism requiring special media and growth conditions. Selective media containing antibiotics to inhibit commensal bacteria are used. Isolation of *Chlamydia trachomatis* requires cell culture as this is an obligate intracellular pathogen. The laborious steps required to culture and then visualize *C. trachomatis* led to the development of enzyme immunoassays to detect antigenic

Table 24.1 Common genital tract infections and their treatment

Condition	Pathogen	Antimicrobial agent
Urethral discharges		
Gonorrhoea	*Neisseria gonorrhoeae*	Cefixime, ceftriaxone
Non-specific urethritis	*Chlamydia, Ureaplasma* or *Mycoplasma* spp.	Tetracyclines (azithromycin)
Vaginal discharges		
Thrush	*Candida albicans*	Nystatin (clotrimazole)
Trichomoniasis	*Trichomonas vaginalis*	Metronidazole
Non-specific vaginosis	*Gardnerella vaginalis* and *Mobiluncus* spp.	Metronidazole
Genital sores		
Syphilis	*Treponema pallidum*	Penicillin (doxycycline)
Chancroid	*Haemophilus ducreyi*	Erythromycin (tetracyclines)
Lymphogranuloma venereum	LGV (chlamydia)	Tetracyclines (erythromycin)
Herpes	Herpes simplex virus	Aciclovir
Warts	Human papillomaviruses	Local podophyllin (cryotheraphy)

Compounds in brackets are examples of alternative drugs.

chlamydial particles. Both of these detection methods have been displaced in favour of more rapid and sensitive DNA amplification methods. These improved detection methods can be applied to urine samples, so diagnosis is not reliant on invasive sampling, for example involving a swab inserted into the urethra; such approaches make it more likely that a patient will (re)seek medical help.

Genital tract infections and their treatment

Some patients with sexually transmitted infections either default treatment or do not remain abstinent until the antimicrobial treatment course has been completed, risking disease transmission

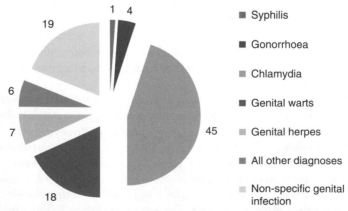

Fig. 24.1 Relatives proportions (%) of new diagnoses of sexually transmitted infection made in UK genitourinary medicine clinics and community settings in 2010. Reproduced with permission of the Health Protection Authority.

and/or re-infection. It is therefore important to render as many patients as possible non-infectious after a single visit to the clinic. Short-course or ideally single dose treatment, where therapy compliance is directly observed, is therefore increasingly preferred. Concomitant treatment of the sexual partner(s) is essential to prevent re-infection, and the value of contact tracing has been shown, particularly in the control of spread of antibiotic-resistant strains of *N. gonorrhoeae*.

Gonorrhoea

Acute gonococcal urethritis occurs two to 10 days after contact and in men is nearly always obvious, presenting as a visible thick yellow discharge accompanied by dysuria. Asymptomatic cases represent less than 5% of male infections, but about 50% of female infections. Prompt treatment with appropriate antibiotics will cure patients with no residual effects: it is hard to imagine that gonorrhoea was once treated by weeks of local irrigation and many sufferers were left with urethral strictures. Nowadays, the major problems of the disease are seen in women, especially with disseminated gonococcaemia. It is one of the main causes of infertility in the world.

N. gonorrhoeae was originally sensitive to many antimicrobial agents. However, the emergence of resistance has led to changes in the recommended treatment options. Penicillin replaced sulphonamides as the drug of choice once it became available in the later stages of the Second World War. In the late 1950s *in vitro* testing showed that some strains of *N. gonorrhoeae* were becoming less sensitive to penicillin. Increasing the dose of penicillin to keep ahead of bacterial resistance worked successfully until the emergence of high-level, plasmid-mediated resistance in the 1970s.

In acute disease, in areas in which resistance is uncommon or when susceptibility is already known, a single dose of a penicillin giving high tissue concentrations for 12 h is sufficient. Intramuscular injections of procaine penicillin were often used for this purpose, but these have been largely replaced by single oral doses of amoxicillin together with probenecid to delay renal excretion. In the 1980s and 1990s widespread penicillin, resistance led to a switch in empirical therapy to a fluoroquinolone, such as a single dose (250–500 mg) of ciprofloxacin. As happened with penicillin, disseminated resistance to fluoroquinolones occurred, leading to many clinics having again to alter empirical therapy for gonorrhoea in the late 1990s and early part of the this century (Fig. 24.2). β-lactamase-producing strains of *N. gonorrhoeae* still respond to intramuscular treatment with cephalosporins such as ceftriaxone, or to oral therapy with cefixime. If there is known hypersensitivity to penicillin, cephalosporins may be used, but if the reaction was previously severe the danger of cross-allergy is too great and a non-β-lactam alternative (e.g. ciprofloxacin, azithromycin, or spectinomycin) can be employed. Data on the prevalence of antibiotic resistance in *N. gonorrhoeae* (Table 24.2) show that the great majority of isolates remain susceptible to ceftriaxone and cefixime, but occasional strains are now being seen with increased MICs to these agents and, more worryingly, treatment failures have been reported. UK data for 2009 show that 1.2% of gonococcal isolates demonstrated decreased susceptibility to cefixime (MIC≥0.25 mg/l), and 0.3% to ceftriaxone (MIC≥0.125 mg/l). Using a slightly lower cut off of MIC≥0.125 mg/l, 10.6% of isolates showed decreased susceptibility to cefixime. Isolates with decreased susceptibility to cefixime and ceftriaxone were predominantly found among men who have sex with men of white ethnicity, who reported having frequent new partners. Notably, all isolates with decreased susceptibility to cefixime and ceftriaxone were also found to be ciprofloxacin (MIC≥1 mg/l) and tetracycline (MIC≥2 mg/l) resistant.

Such observations are likely to lead in the near future to the use of alternative agents (such as i.m. ceftriaxone plus p.o. azithromycin) for the empirical treatment of gonococcal infection. Azithromycin-resistant strains remain uncommon, but reduced susceptibility has been documented, and there is increasing use of this antibiotic for the treatment of chlamydial infection detected via screening programmes. Unfortunately, such intensive antibiotic prescribing may well compromise the utility of azithromycin in the future.

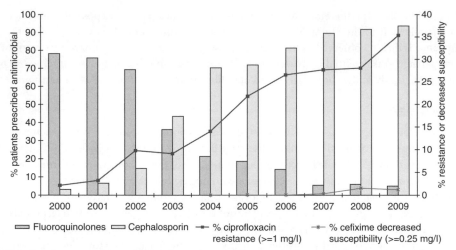

Fig. 24.2 Relative prescribing of cephalosporins and fluoroquinolones for the treatment of gonorrhoea in genitourinary medicine clinics in England and Wales, and prevalence of resistance to ciprofloxacin, 2000–2009. Reproduced with permission of the Health Protection Authority.

Antibiotic treatment usually results in a rapid and complete cure in acute gonorrhoea. Occasional complications such as epididymitis, arthritis, and pelvic infection in women require admission to hospital and prolonged antibiotics. Non-genital gonococcal infection also requires more than a single dose of penicillin to achieve cure (see below).

Non-gonococcal urethritis or cervicitis

After penicillin became available for the treatment of gonorrhoea it was evident that some treated individuals still had symptoms of urethritis or cervicitis or both. The terms non-specific or non-gonococcal urethritis were used to refer to such cases or when gonococci could not be demonstrated despite symptoms. It is now clear that most of these infections are caused by *C. trachomatis*. Indeed, numbers of *C. trachomatis* sexually transmitted infections now far exceed cases of gonorrhoea in most developed countries. Of great concern, *C. trachomatis* is a major cause of pelvic

Table 24.2 Prevalence of resistance in *N. gonorrhoeae* isolates from laboratories in England and Wales, 2003 and 2009

Antimicrobial agent (breakpoint concentration)	Prevalence of resistance (%)	
	2003	**2009**
Penicillin (≥1 mg/l or β-lactamase positive)	10	22
Tetracycline (≥2 mg/l)	38	53
Ciprofloxacin (≥1 mg/l)	9	35
Azithromycin (≥1 mg/l)	0.9	1.3
Spectinomycin (≥128 mg/l)	0	0
Ceftriaxone (≥0.125 mg/l)	0	0.3
Cefixime (≥0.25 mg/l)	0	1.2

Data from gonococcal antimicrobial resistance surveillance programme (GRASP). Available at: http://www.hpa.org.uk/Topics/InfectiousDiseases/InfectionsAZ/Gonorrhoea/AntimicrobialResistance/.

inflammatory disease in women (see below), which can lead to infertility. Some cases of non-gonococcal urethritis are probably due to ureaplasmas or mycoplasmas, but as these cell wall deficient bacteria may be found in some healthy individuals, diagnosis of infection is difficult and not routinely practised. *T. vaginalis*, herpesvirus, urinary tract infection, and local causes such as trauma also account for some cases of urethritis/cervicitis.

The now widespread availability of nucleic acid tests for *C. trachomatis* infection means that cumbersome invasive sampling, and internal examination in females, is no longer mandatory. Furthermore, screening of urine samples from young sexually active people, particularly those frequently changing sexual partners, is increasingly used to detect subclinical chlamydia infection.

Tetracyclines, especially doxycycline, given for at least seven days are effective. Failure of therapy occurs and may reflect poor compliance or re-infection. A single dose of azithromycin is as effective as one to two weeks of tetracycline therapy and clearly overcomes compliance problems. It is considerably more expensive than tetracyclines, but improved overall compliance and efficacy has led to increasing preference for this treatment option. Erythromycin can also be used for one to two weeks, but the relatively poor gastrointestinal side effect profile does not encourage compliance. Genuine relapses of infection are possibly due to latent phase chlamydial infection. Antimicrobial resistance is thought to be rare, but as routine culture and susceptibility testing of *C. trachomatis* is not practised limited data are available. Chlamydiae are eukaryotic cells, and although these bacteria lack a peptidoglycan cell wall, ampicillin and penicillin still achieve some cellular penetration. In pregnancy, erythromycin is the preferred treatment option for *C. trachomatis* infection, but amoxicillin or clindamycin can be used if it is not tolerated. Azithromycin has not been approved for use in pregnancy.

Pelvic inflammatory disease

In women, upper genital tract infection with sexually transmitted pathogens, anaerobes, streptococci or Gram-negative bacilli commonly results in pelvic inflammatory disease, which gives rise to serious complications of tubal blockage or dysfunction. The condition is difficult to diagnose because of the variety of symptoms, its often chronic nature, and difficulty in obtaining microbiological confirmation of the presence of pathogens in the peritoneal cavity. The disease is becoming more common, primarily because of the increases in sexually transmitted infections: it develops in 10 to 40% of women with inadequately treated chlamydial or gonococcal cervicitis. Pelvic inflammatory disease increases the chance of ectopic pregnancy sevenfold, as a result of tubal damage. Also, the risk of subsequent infertility increases with each episode. Chronic disease, a condition with considerable morbidity, commonly occurs, typified by chronic lower abdominal or pelvic pain.

Unless there is a known cause combination antimicrobial therapy is usually prescribed to cover the many different pathogens. In severe cases intravenous therapy with a cephalosporin such as cefotaxime or ceftriaxone, combined with a tetracycline with or without metronidazole is used. Oral therapy can comprise a fluoroquinolone, such as levofloxacin, moxifloxacin, or gatifloxacin with or without metronidazole. Therapy duration is usually two weeks.

Throughout the world chlamydiae cause substantial morbidity in terms of pelvic infection and infertility as well as the blinding eye disease, trachoma. Trachoma is treated using 1% tetracycline eye ointment (applied twice daily for six weeks), oral erythromycin, or if affordable with single-dose azithromycin.

Neonatal gonococcal or chlamydial infection

Ophthalmia neonatorum occurs within the first month, and usually a few days after birth, in babies born to infected mothers. Gonococci in the female genital tract are implanted in the conjunctivae during delivery and the neonate develops a purulent discharge from one or both eyes. There may be considerable cellulitis and if untreated the infection may lead to destruction of the cornea. Treatment should be prompt, with parenteral penicillin if the strain is sensitive and frequent local instillations of saline. Silver nitrate drops placed in the eyes immediately after birth may prevent the condition, but this has no activity against chlamydiae (see below). This therapy (Credé's method) is still used in areas where the danger of infection is high but carries a risk of inducing a chemical conjunctivitis especially if the concentration of silver nitrate is too high. Topical povidone iodine (Betadine) is an inexpensive alternative used to prevent eye infection in developing countries, and has the advantage of broader antimicrobial activity than silver nitrate.

Neonatal conjunctivitis due to chlamydiae is a less severe form of ophthalmia neonatorum than gonococcal infection. It may be so mild as to be unsuspected clinically and, like all the conditions due to chlamydiae, it is underdiagnosed. In spite of its mild, self-limiting course it can cause permanent eye damage and, whenever suspected, chlamydial conjunctivitis should be treated. Erythromycin or tetracycline eye ointment can be used, but as local treatment can be difficult to apply adequately, many clinicians also advise giving erythromycin orally to prevent the development of chlamydial pneumonia. Erythromycin is used to treat infants because systemic tetracycline stains teeth and bones. Therapy needs to be for at least two weeks as with all complicated chlamydial infections. It is self-evident that the parents should be examined and treated as for non-specific urethritis (see above).

Syphilis

Syphilis may manifest as a primary illness, typified by the painless ulcer (chancre), or in more chronic forms (secondary or tertiary syphilis) that can affect nearly every organ. The old student adage 'know syphilis and you will know medicine' reflects the many ways in which syphilis can present and how it can mimic many other conditions. The progression of the infection varies greatly; even in untreated cases, latent periods of many years frequently occur. A diagnosis of syphilis used to be viewed with dread, in a similar way to identifying HIV infection, at least prior to the discovery of effective and non-toxic antimicrobial options.

Heavy metals, in particular mercury, were used for many centuries to treat syphilis. The development early in the twentieth century of arsenicals such as Salvarsan heralded the start of modern chemotherapy. Penicillin has been the mainstay of therapy since 1943 when the drug was first used to treat the disease. *Treponema pallidum* is exquisitely sensitive to penicillin: as little as 0.002 mg/l is bactericidal. There is no evidence of resistance to penicillin, but occasional treatment failures do occur. The aim of treatment is to maintain tissue levels of penicillin above 0.03 mg/l to ensure treponemal killing. Early syphilis is treated with intramuscular procaine penicillin usually given with probenecid for two weeks. In countries where it is still available, benzathine penicillin is used. Doxycycline, azithromycin, or ceftriaxone are alternatives in patients hypersensitive to penicillin. Erythromycin is associated with treatment failure and should not be used. Many antimicrobial agents may only suppress the disease, which can reappear in its later manifestations. This danger exists in treating a patient with non-syphilitic sexually transmitted infections who may also be incubating syphilis. For this reason serological tests for syphilis should be done on all high-risk patients.

In tertiary syphilis treatment for several weeks is necessary. Slow-release penicillins do not achieve adequate cerebrospinal fluid concentrations and frequent high doses of benzylpenicillin are recommended in the treatment of neurosyphilis. Similarly, high doses and longer duration of penicillin administration are recommended in patients co-infected with HIV, in whom a higher incidence of treatment failure has been noted. This presumably reflects the importance of the natural T-cell response in combating syphilis infection.

A common hazard of syphilis therapy is the Jarisch–Herxheimer reaction observed within a few hours of treatment with penicillin (or arsenicals). This is a hypersensitivity reaction due to spiro-chaetal endotoxin and is not related to penicillin allergy. The Herxheimer response is of little significance in primary cases, but may occasionally be fatal in some tertiary or late cases.

Genital herpes simplex virus

Herpes simplex virus types 1 and 2 generally cause infection 'above and below the belt' respec-tively, although sexual practices obscure this association. Genital infection is characterized by vesicles, usually on the penis or labia, similar to 'cold sores' found around the mouth. Proctitis is common in men who have sex with men. The painful vesicles burst to form superficial erosions, which can be secondarily infected. Women may carry the virus in the cervix and this may be a source of infection to the newborn, which may occasionally be fatal. Topical aciclovir can be used, or oral therapy for severe attacks or to reduce the frequency of symptoms.

Vaginal discharge

The normal bacteria flora of the adult vagina before the menopause consists of numerous lacto-bacilli, diphtheroids, and anaerobes. These maintain a local pH of 4–5, which is inhibitory to coliforms. However, yeasts can flourish in such relatively acidic conditions.

Candidiasis

Candida albicans, the commonest pathogenic yeast, may be found in up to a quarter of healthy women of child-bearing age and frequently the delicate balance between the resident flora and intruding *Candida* is disturbed to produce clinical 'thrush'. Oral antibiotics, in particular tetracy-clines, are prone to produce this side effect, which is also more common in pregnancy. Men, espe-cially if uncircumcised, may occasionally have clinical balanitis caused by *Candida* and healthy individuals frequently carry the organism. Sexual transmission is probable in these circumstances, but thrush can occur without intimate contact. Local applications of nystatin or one of the imida-zoles such as clotrimazole are sufficient, but prolonged and repeated courses are required. Persistent infections are sometimes treated with oral fluconazole, along with therapy for the partner.

Trichomonal infection

T. vaginalis is a flagellate protozoon commonly found throughout the world. It favours a more alkaline pH than *Candida* and causes a foul-smelling yellow vaginal discharge often noticed because of staining of clothes and itching. It has been found in a high proportion of asymptomatic women in antenatal clinics, but may cause symptoms subsequently, especially after menstruation. In some patients the organism invades the anterior urethra and symptoms of dysuria and frequency may lead the clinician to make a tentative diagnosis of urinary tract infection. Some patients labelled as having 'urethral syndrome' may be suffering from trichomoniasis. The organism is sometimes car-ried transiently and asymptomatically by men, but a low-grade non-specific urethritis may occur.

Trichomonal infection is treated with a single oral high dose (2 g) of metronidazole or tinida-zole. Longer courses of therapy are not more effective. Treatment of partners is required to reduce the risk of recurrence. Metronidazole used to be avoided during pregnancy because of a possible, albeit unproven, teratogenic effect. However, a possible association between trichomoniasis and premature rupture of membranes means that its use can be justified in this setting.

Bacterial vaginosis

This is a term employed for a symptomatic discharge for which no obvious cause can be found. As with non-specific urethritis there are likely to be many possible aetiological agents, not all microbial.

Bacterial vaginosis is now known to be associated with an increased risk of premature delivery, and with pelvic inflammatory disease in women undergoing termination of pregnancy. There is evidence that a proportion of these cases are associated with a pleomorphic, Gram-variable rod, *Gardnerella* (formerly *Haemophilus*) *vaginalis*, although the bacterium can be found in normal healthy individuals. Oral metronidazole given for seven days is the treatment of choice for bacterial vaginosis, even though *G. vaginalis* is relatively resistant to this agent; its role may be to inhibit associated anaerobic, curved bacteria called *Mobiluncus*. Topical metronidazole or clindamycin can also be used. In treatment-resistant cases intravaginal boric acid has been successful. In recurrent infection of women, male partners are sometimes treated.

Warts

Genital (condylomata acuminata) and common skin warts are caused by human papillomavirus (HPV). Importantly, certain types of virus (e.g. types 16 and 18) are carcinogenic and can cause cervical, vulval, penile, or anal cancer in some infected individuals. The treatment of genital warts occupies a good part of the work of genito-urinary medicine clinics and is often unrewarding. A long course of chemical applications such as podophyllin, trichloracetic acid, or salicylic acid, or burning the lesions with diathermy or liquid nitrogen, is often required; in some patients the warts disappear spontaneously. Imiquimod cream may be helpful by inducing the production of interferon-α and other cytokines. Genital warts in immunocompromised patients, including HIV-infected individuals, are relatively refractory to treatment; combinations of the above options are often required.

Two vaccines are now available, one covering HPV types 16 and 18, and the other additionally confers protection against types 6 and 11, which cause 90% of genital warts. Mass population vaccination campaigns targeting girls aged 12-13 years have now been employed with these vaccines, and there is already evidence that a reduction in the incidence of associated cancers is occurring. Public health decisions about which vaccine to use and whether only to vaccinate girls will continue to be scrutinized to determine the most efficacious approach.

Chancroid (soft sore)

Chancroid is caused by *Haemophilus ducreyi* but is rarely seen in the UK. In tropical and subtropical countries epidemics occur and the infection enhances the spread of HIV. The genital lesions are painful and often multiple with large associated inguinal glands, which may suppurate to form a 'bubo'. Erythromycin for seven days or single-dose azithromycin is usually effective. Ceftriaxone can also be used but may be less efficacious in HIV-infected individuals. Tetracyclines and co-trimoxazole work in most cases unless bacterial resistance is common. Short courses (three days) of co-amoxiclav or fluoroquinolones have also been used successfully.

Lymphogranuloma venereum

This is also a predominantly tropical condition, caused by specific serovars of *Chlamydia trachomatis*. It starts as a small ulcer, which may be unnoticed until inguinal glands enlarge and become matted together. Associated inflammation may give the appearance of elephantiasis as a late complication and breakdown of abscesses may give rectovaginal fistulae. Tetracyclines, sulphonamides, or erythromycin may be used but, as with other chlamydial infection, two to three weeks of therapy is required.

Key points

◆ Directly observed, stat, oral treatment is preferable for sexually transmitted infections.

◆ The recommended treatment of gonorrhoea has changed from penicillin to ciprofloxacin and now to cefixime (or ceftriaxone plus azithromycin) because of resistance emergence.

◆ Azithromycin is increasingly used to treat *C. trachomatis* infection, but occasional reports of resistance are starting to appear.

◆ Two HPV vaccines are available, one covering the oncogenic types (16 and 18) and the other additionally confers protection against types 6 and 11, which cause 90% of genital warts.

Further reading

Centers for Disease Control and Prevention. *Sexually transmitted diseases.* Available at: http://www.cdc.gov/STD/.

World Health Organization. *Sexually transmitted infections.* Available at: http://www.who.int/topics/sexually_transmitted_infections/en/.

Health Protection Agency. *Sexually transmitted infections.* Available at: http://www.hpa.org.uk/Topics/InfectiousDiseases/InfectionsAZ/STIs/.

Chapter 25

Gastrointestinal infections

Gastrointestinal disease caused by bacteria, viruses, protozoa, and helminths are among the commonest infections suffered by mankind. Worldwide it has been estimated that on any one day 200 million people are suffering from acute infective gastroenteritis. Over two million children in Asia, Africa, and Latin America die each year of gastrointestinal infection. The very young, elderly, and malnourished are particularly at risk from the electrolyte and fluid losses that complicate severe diarrhoea or vomiting. Restoration of fluids and electrolytes is the mainstay of treatment; oral rehydration therapy has had a significant impact in reducing mortality in developing countries. Even in countries with well-developed healthcare systems the true numbers of cases of infective gastroenteritis are certainly greater than those diagnosed in symptomatic patients, and greater still than those detected by testing faecal samples. Fig. 25.1 shows that for every one case of intestinal infection identified by laboratory testing, many more people have symptoms of this infection. This under-reporting of cases of gastroenteritis means that the full socio-economic impact of these infections, for example lost work days, is unknown but certainly considerable.

Transmission and acquisition

Gastrointestinal pathogens are transmitted directly from person to person or indirectly through faecal contamination of the environment, food, or water supply. Viral gastroenteritis, which is highly infectious and affects all ages, is often transmitted by aerosols from vomit. Some pathogens, most notably salmonellae, are common to human beings and animals. The high frequency of gastroenteritis in developing countries reflects the scarcity of clean water supplies or safe sewage disposal, the close proximity of human beings living with animals, and the extent of poverty and malnutrition.

Travel-associated diarrhoea often affects residents of industrial countries travelling to developing countries. The onset is usually within five to 15 days of arrival and generally follows ingestion of salads, raw vegetables, and untreated water (or ice). Enterotoxigenic *Escherichia coli* is the most common cause.

There are major differences in the numbers of micro-organisms needed to cause gastroenteritis. For example, the infective dose of shigella is about 10–100 bacteria, whereas ingestion of 10^5–10^8 bacteria are required to cause salmonella or *Escherichia coli* gastroenteritis. This partly explains the ease of spread and epidemic nature of some types of gastroenteritis (e.g. *Shigella sonnei* dysentery in young children).

Viral gastroenteritis is also highly infectious, affects all ages, and has become much more common in recent years in the UK and Europe. The term 'winter vomiting disease' is sometimes used but this name is misleading because cases are increasingly seen throughout the year. Most importantly, viral gastroenteritis spreads rapidly, typically among people in close contact, such as children in nurseries, patients and healthcare workers in hospitals, and holidaymakers on cruise ships. Such outbreaks can severely affect normal activity—in a hospital it can force wards closures and cancellations of operations. In viral gastroenteritis not only is the diarrhoea infectious, but

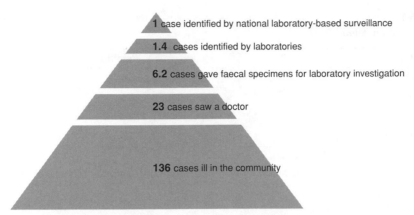

1 case identified by national laboratory-based surveillance

1.4 cases identified by laboratories

6.2 cases gave faecal specimens for laboratory investigation

23 cases saw a doctor

136 cases ill in the community

Fig. 25.1 Under ascertainment of gastroenteritis in England. From Handysides S (1999), 'Underascertainment of infectious intestinal disease', *Communicable Disease and Public Health* **2**: 78–79, with permission of the Health Protection Authority.

crucially, vomiting creates a 'cloud' of virus that can contaminate surfaces or possibly be inhaled by others.

Food may be contaminated by various gut pathogens, or their toxins at source, in the abattoir, subsequent to marketing, or during preparation. When illness occurs as a sudden outbreak that can be traced to a common foodstuff, the term food poisoning is used. Non-microbial food poisoning occasionally results from the ingestion of chemicals, fungi, and other toxins such as scombrotoxin and ciguatoxin.

Clinical manifestations

The incubation period of gastrointestinal infections varies according to the ingested dose, the site of infection in the gut, and the pathogenic mechanism of diarrhoea. The shortest incubation periods are seen with *Staphylococcus aureus* food poisoning where a preformed toxin produces symptoms within half an hour to eight hours of ingestion. Longer incubation periods are associated with salmonellosis and shigellosis, in which microbial replication within the bowel may take a day or so before symptoms occur. Symptoms of nausea and vomiting are more frequently associated with small-bowel infection. Large-bowel involvement is often associated with tenderness over the colon. In dysentery, diarrhoea is accompanied by a profuse, bloody exudate. Regardless of the major site of action, colicky pain is the commonest symptom associated with gastrointestinal infection. The severity of illness is essentially dictated by the degree of fluid loss. Losses of less than 3% body weight are usually undetectable. As fluid and electrolyte loss increase then mental impairment occurs. Once fluid loss exceeds 10% body weight, oliguria, cyanosis, and cardiovascular collapse develop and may be fatal unless rapidly corrected. Systemic symptoms of fever, headache, and rigors are seen in shigellosis and salmonellosis where the intestinal mucosa is involved. Bacteraemia may complicate a severe attack of gastrointestinal salmonellosis and occasionally result in metastatic infection such as septic arthritis.

General management

Fluid replacement

The management of acute gastroenteritis is largely dictated by the severity of the illness. Most attacks are self-limiting and adequate oral fluid replacement is usually possible. Admission to

Table 25.1 Formula for oral rehydration glucose-salts solution recommended by the World Health Organization (updated 2003)

Substance	Weight (g)
Sodium chloride	2.6
Potassium chloride	1.5
Sodium citrate	2.9
Glucose (anhydrous)	13.5

To be dissolved in 1 litre of clean drinking water.

Data from World Health Organization at: http://www.who.int/child-adolescent-health/New_Publications/CHILD_HEALTH/WHO_FCH_CAH_06.1.pdf.

hospital may be required if vomiting persists or clinical dehydration develops from severe or protracted diarrhoea. Other indications include extremes of age, fever, abdominal pain, and other significant pre-existing disease. In most instances, oral fluid replacement is successful. In infants oral treatment with a glucose–electrolyte solution is usually given; milk feeding is temporarily stopped as lactose deficiency frequently complicates gastroenteritis in early childhood. Gut bacteria break down unhydrolysed lactose remaining in the bowel to lactic and acetic acid, which produce diarrhoea through the effects of an osmotic load. Older children and adults can usually replace fluid losses by drinking water, fruit juices, or soft drinks. Few patients require intravenous fluid and electrolyte replacement. However, under such circumstances normal saline and bicarbonate are usually rapidly effective in the severely dehydrated.

The glucose-salts solution recommended for oral rehydration by the World Health Organization (WHO) and the United Nations Children's Fund (UNICEF) is shown in Table 25.1. Over-the-counter preparations available in the UK generally contain less sodium chloride and more glucose. They may be useful in moderate attacks of diarrhoea, but are not as effective as the WHO formulation in severe dehydration. Glucose facilitates the absorption of sodium (and hence water) on a 1:1 molar basis in the small intestine; sodium and potassium are needed to replace the body losses of these essential ions during diarrhoea (and vomiting); and citrate corrects the acidosis that occurs as a result of diarrhoea and dehydration.

Use of antibiotics in gastrointestinal infections

Since most episodes of acute gastroenteritis are self-limiting, antibiotics are not generally indicated. Furthermore, the use of antibiotics carries the risk of directly irritating an inflamed bowel mucosa, or of inducing diarrhoea due to *Clostridium difficile* infection (see below). In addition, their use may encourage transferable drug resistance (see Chapter 10).

There are some specific circumstances where antibiotics are appropriate for gastrointestinal infections and associated with clear benefits. Table 25.2 summarizes the chief indications for antimicrobial therapy.

Gut sedatives and adsorbents

Various agents are frequently prescribed for the symptomatic control of gastrointestinal symptoms, yet there is little definite evidence for their efficacy. They act by slowing gastrointestinal motility or fluid adsorption. Diphenoxylate with atropine, loperamide, and codeine slow

Table 25.2 Major gastrointestinal infections and appropriate antimicrobial therapy

Organism	Site of infection	Disease produced	Antimicrobial therapy	Comments
Bacillus cereus	Small bowel	Food poisoning	None	Reheated rice often incriminated
Campylobacter jejuni (coli)	Small bowel	Enteritis	Erythromycin,[c] ciprofloxacin[c]	Antibiotics in severe cases only
Clostridium botulinum	Central nervous system	Botulism (neural paralysis)	Penicillin	Antitoxin more important than antibiotics
Clostridium difficile	Large bowel	Antibiotic associated diarrhoea; pseu-domembranous colitis	Metronidazole; vancomycin	Antibiotic-associated; stop offending antibiotic(s) if possible
Clostridium perfringens	Small bowel	Food poisoning	None	Due to toxin production
Entamoeba histolytica	Large bowel[b]	Amoebic dysentery	Metronidazole	See Chapter 35
Escherichia coli	Small/large bowel	Traveller's diarrhoea	(Ciprofloxacin)[c]	Mostly self-limiting
Esch. coli serotype O157[a]	Small/large bowel; kidneys	Haemolytic uraemic syndrome	None	Antibiotics contraindicated
Giardia lamblia	Small bowel	Giardiasis	Metronidazole	See Chapter 35
Norovirus	Small bowel[b]	'Winter vomiting disease'	None	Outbreaks occur
Rotavirus	Small bowel[b]	Diarrhoea	None	Outbreaks occur
Salmonella enterica serotypes Typhi and Paratyphi	Extra-intestinal	Enteric fever	Ciprofloxacin, chloramphenicol or co-trimoxazole	Antibiotic treatment mandatory; resistance occurs
Other salmonellae	Small bowel[b]	Diarrhoea	None	Ciprofloxacin in systemic infection
Shigella sonnei	Large bowel[b]	Sonnei dysentery	None	Usually self-limiting
Other shigellae	Large bowel[b]	Bacillary dysentery	Ciprofloxacin; co-trimoxazole	Antibiotics in severe cases only
Staphylococcus aureus	Small bowel	Food poisoning (vomiting)	None	Due to enterotoxin
Vibrio cholera	Small bowel	Cholera	Doxycycline; ciprofloxacin	Fluid replacement essential
Yersinia enterocolitica	Small bowel	Mesenteric adenitis/ileitis	Ciprofloxacin, co-trimoxazole	Antibiotics in severe cases only

[a]Other serotypes are sometimes involved.

[b]Mucosal invasion.

[c]Routine use not recommended.

gastrointestinal motility, and may have an additional mild analgesic effect. Adsorbants include kaolin, chalk, aluminium hydroxide, and cellulose, which tend to increase the stool bulk. Their use should not minimize the importance of adequate fluid and electrolyte replacement. This is especially important in infancy and early childhood where bowel sedatives may induce an ileus and mask fluid loss. Moreover, excessive dosing with diphenoxylate may induce respiratory depression in the young child. Bowel sedatives should also be used cautiously in those with fever or bloody diarrhoea since it is possible to potentiate toxin mediated or invasive bacterial disease.

Specific infections

Virus infections

Viral infections of the bowel commonly cause sporadic and epidemic disease in the community and in healthcare institutions. Numerically the most important are infections with norovirus (including 'Norwalk' virus) and rotavirus, which often causes diarrhoea in infants and young children. Several other viruses, including enteric adenoviruses, caliciviruses, and astroviruses may also be involved. The infections are usually self-limiting and there is currently no effective antiviral therapy. Severe infections respond to fluid replacement therapy. Rotavirus vaccines are becoming available, and should prove especially beneficial in reducing mortality in children in developing countries.

Cholera

Cholera is prevalent throughout the Indian subcontinent and South-east Asia from where it has spread to many parts of Africa and central and South America. *Vibrio cholerae* multiplies and survives, possibly for years, in the environment, and as such does not require a human host to maintain its life cycle. *V. cholerae* is present in large numbers in the stools of infected patients, and is spread primarily by faecal contamination of water supplies.

The onset of cholera is sudden with the development of profuse, pale, watery diarrhoea, which may reach several litres a day; the classical rice-water stools that are isotonic with plasma. The patient rapidly becomes dehydrated and, unless fluid and electrolytes are replaced, becomes apathetic and confused with subsequent hypotension and death. Mortality is highest in old, very young, or malnourished people.

Cholera is one of the few gastrointestinal infections for which there is little argument concerning the merits of antibiotic treatment as an adjunct to fluid and electrolyte replacement therapy. The duration of diarrhoea is decreased and the volume of stool is reduced by almost half by the use of an oral tetracycline such as doxycycline, prescribed as a single dose of 300 mg in adults. Resistance to tetracyclines is, unfortunately, increasing. Alternatives include co-trimoxazole, azithromycin, or ciprofloxacin (although fluoroquinolone resistant strains have emerged in India). The vibrio is eliminated from the bowel and toxin production ceases rapidly. The carrier state does not occur but transmission from dead bodies has been reported.

Campylobacter infection

Campylobacter jejuni (or occasionally *Campylobacter coli*) is among the commonest causes of sporadic acute gastrointestinal infection throughout the world. The organism produces infection in all age groups, but most frequently in young adults and pre-school children. Epidemics have occurred involving several thousand people following the ingestion of contaminated milk or water supplies. Campylobacters cause infection in domestic and farm animals, poultry and wild birds, and hence there are many opportunities for spread to humans. Importantly, campylobacter infection is occasionally complicated by the development of Guillain–Barré syndrome or reactive arthritis.

Campylobacter gastroenteritis generally lasts for a few days, but may occasionally be more protracted with marked abdominal symptoms of colicky pain and tenderness as well as profuse diarrhoea. Acute appendicitis may be mimicked. Attacks are self-limiting and managed mainly by increasing the oral fluid intake. Although campylobacter infection is common, fatalities are rare. Excretion ceases soon after clinical recovery. Antibiotic therapy is not beneficial in most cases. Cases with severe or prolonged symptoms may benefit from oral therapy with erythromycin or a fluoroquinolone such as ciprofloxacin. However, the prevalence of resistance to these agents has increased, probably related to their use in animal husbandry.

Helicobacter infection

Helicobacter pylori is an important cause of chronic gastritis and gastroduodenal ulceration. It is also likely to be responsible for some cases of gastric carcinoma. Treatment of *H. pylori* infection usually involves seven days' therapy with two antibiotics (various combinations of clarithromycin, metronidazole and amoxicillin are often used) together with a proton pump inhibitor such as omeprazole. Treatment fails in approximately 10% of patients. There is evidence for increasing antibiotic resistance among *H. pylori* strains, particularly in individuals who have previously received metronidazole. Resistance to metronidazole occurs in approximately 50% of infected individuals in many European countries with levels of up to 90% in developing countries. Resistance to clarithromycin is currently below 10% in many European countries, but rates may be increasing. Pre-treatment resistance to clarithromycin can reduce the effectiveness of therapy by about 50%. Resistance to amoxicillin or tetracycline is presently uncommon.

Salmonellosis

Intestinal salmonellosis

Gastrointestinal salmonellosis is second only to campylobacter as a bacterial cause of community acquired gastrointestinal infection; several thousand cases are reported annually in the UK. There are more than 2400 different serotypes of *Salmonella enterica*, although relatively few regularly cause human disease. Some common serotypes are Typhimurium, Enteritidis, Hadar, and Virchow. Frozen poultry and eggs are a common source of infection, which is easily transmitted among battery hens and during the evisceration of carcasses. Measures to control infection in chickens have markedly reduced the incidence of salmonella infection in the UK.

Illness is commonly associated with systemic features of fever and malaise, in addition to the gastrointestinal symptoms. Bloodstream invasion may occur following mucosal penetration. Bloodstream infection complicating salmonella gastroenteritis is more likely in the very young and the elderly, and in those with underlying diseases such as alcoholism, cirrhosis, and AIDS. Achlorhydria from pernicious anaemia, atrophic gastritis, gastrectomy, or therapy with H_2-receptor antagonists or proton pump inhibitor enhances the risk of salmonellosis by eliminating the protection afforded by the normal gastric acid so that the number of bacteria needed to be ingested to cause infection is reduced.

Treatment of acute gastrointestinal salmonellosis is essentially directed at the replacement of any lost fluid or electrolytes, either by mouth or intravenously. Antibiotics are usually unnecessary unless there is secondary bloodstream invasion, since they do not reduce the duration of illness. Antibiotic treatment may also be associated with increased incidence of carriage of salmonellae. For severe or invasive infections fluoroquinolones are useful, although resistance is becoming more common. Co-trimoxazole or a cephalosporin, such as ceftriaxone, provide alternative choices. The emergence of multiresistant strains, some with transferable genes, compromises treatment choices in some parts of the world. Local epidemiological surveillance data can help guide empirical therapy.

Enteric (typhoid and paratyphoid) fever

Enteric fever is caused by *Salmonella enterica* serotypes Typhi or Paratyphi A, B, or C. This is primarily a septicaemic illness acquired by ingestion of the bacterium followed by mucosal invasion. The pathogen gains access to the lymphatics and blood from where it infects the liver and other parts of the reticuloendothelial system. The bowel is also involved since the lymphoid tissue in Peyer's patches is inflamed and often ulcerates. Notably, constipation is more common than diarrhoea. Perforation and peritonitis are not uncommon in untreated cases. Enteric fever is potentially fatal and, unlike gastrointestinal salmonellosis, should always be treated with antibiotics. The bacteria are often located intracellularly and drugs active *in vitro* may not evoke a satisfactory clinical response.

The antibiotic of choice for enteric fever is ciprofloxacin, which produces the most rapid resolution of fever and best cure rates. Treatment must be continued for two weeks and, even so, relapse may occur. Relapses should be treated for a further two weeks. Resistance to fluoroquinolones has emerged. Alternative agents with variable activity include chloramphenicol, co-trimoxazole, and high-dose amoxicillin. For multiresistant strains cephalosporins such as ceftriaxone or cefixime (which can be given orally) have proved useful. Because of the threat of multiresistant strains, the susceptibility of clinical isolates should be tested in the laboratory whenever possible. In severe infection steroids given in the first 48 h may be beneficial.

Although typhoid vaccines are available they are not recommended for international travel unless there is a high risk of exposure.

Salmonella carriage

Salmonellae may be excreted in faeces for several weeks after clinical recovery. If this continues for more than three months it is likely that the patient will become a persistent carrier. Chronic carriage is uncommon (<5%) but more frequent in infants and in people with biliary disease (including bile stones) or schistosomal bladder infection. The chronic carrier is normally harmless to the individual, but may be a threat to the household and the community if lapses in personal hygiene cause contamination of food or water supplies. Importantly, humans are the only natural host for *Salmonella* Typhi and so it is important to identify and treat carriers as a public health control measure. Chronic excretion precludes employment as a food handler. Ciprofloxacin is the preferred treatment for carriers; alternatively, prolonged high-dosage ampicillin may be curative.

Shigellosis

Shigellosis in its most severe form is characterized by profuse diarrhoea with blood and pus (i.e. classic bacillary dysentery). Infection is more common in underdeveloped countries where sanitation and levels of hygiene are low. In developed countries shigellosis (usually caused by *Sh. sonnei*) occurs particularly among young children in nurseries and schools, and also in long-stay institutions such as prisons and psychiatric hospitals. The spectrum of illness ranges from mild diarrhoea to a fulminating attack of dysentery. The more severe forms of disease are associated with *Shigella dysenteriae*, whereas milder symptoms are caused by *Sh. Sonnei, Shigella flexneri,* and *Shigella boydii* tend to produce disease of intermediate severity. *Shigella* spp. are among the most virulent gastrointestinal pathogens, requiring only few bacteria to produce disease. The bacteria multiply in the small bowel with subsequent invasion of the mucosa of the terminal ileum and colon. The intense inflammatory response produces a hyperaemic bowel which readily bleeds, although bloodstream invasion is uncommon. Some strains, notably *Sh. dysenteriae*, produce an enterotoxin (Shiga toxin) that stimulates fluid secretion in the small bowel, so that watery diarrhoea may precede frank dysentery. Occasionally, haemolytic uraemic syndrome (see below) occurs.

Treatment of shigellosis is dependent on the severity of the diarrhoea and blood loss. Mild attacks, including most *Sh. sonnei* cases, may be managed by oral rehydration with glucose-salts solution. More severe cases may require admission to hospital and intravenous fluids. In severe shigellosis there is a definite place for antibiotic therapy. In addition treatment is sometimes used to shorten symptoms and bacterial excretion, particularly in outbreaks. Three days of treatment with oral ciprofloxacin, co-trimoxazole, ampicillin, or tetracycline have been widely used. However, resistance to each of these agents occurs, and laboratory testing of susceptibility is important.

Escherichia coli

Distinct types of *Esch. coli* cause a wide spectrum of gastrointestinal infection.

- *Enterotoxigenic Esch. coli* cause most cases of traveller's diarrhoea. The toxins have many similarities to cholera toxin and the pathophysiology of the illness is similar, though fatalities are uncommon.

- *Enteropathogenic Esch. coli* is now largely confined to developing countries where it remains a leading cause of severe diarrhoea in the very young.

- *Entero-invasive Esch. coli* can produce severe invasive (dysentery-like) infection of the bowel, but are fortunately uncommon.

- *Enterohaemorrhagic Esch. coli* (principally *Esch. coli* O157) produce a shiga-like toxin. In addition to haemorrhagic colitis these strains can cause renal impairment and haemolysis (haemolytic uraemic syndrome); this develops in approximately 5% of affected children during outbreaks.

- *Entero-aggregative Esch. coli* show characteristic patterns of adherence to epithelial cells.

Antimicrobial therapy is usually unnecessary in the treatment of gastrointestinal infections with *Esch. coli*. Indeed, in haemolytic uraemic syndrome antibiotic administration is contraindicated because of the chance of exacerbating symptoms, presumably because of antibiotic-mediated bacterial cell lysis and toxin release.

The use of antibiotics to prevent traveller's diarrhoea is not recommended because of the possibility of encouraging the emergence of multiresistant strains, the risk of side effects, and the generally mild nature of the infection. If diarrhoea develops fluoroquinolones can alleviate symptoms within 24 h. If the importance of the trip warrants the use of prophylaxis, fluoroquinolones, tetracyclines, or co-trimoxazole appear to be effective.

Yersiniosis

Infection with *Yersinia enterocolitica* may produce mesenteric adenitis, terminal ileitis, and acute diarrhoea. Erythema nodosum and a reactive arthritis may complicate such infections. The illness is usually self-limiting and, unless complicated by extra-gastrointestinal symptoms, is infrequently suspected. Ciprofloxacin, co-trimoxazole, or tetracycline are effective in severe cases.

Intestinal parasites

Some protozoa and helminths may cause symptoms ranging from mild diarrhoea to severe dysentery. These are considered in Chapters 8 and 35.

Antibiotic-associated diarrhoea and *C. difficile* infection

The use of antimicrobial agents is sometimes complicated by diarrhoea. This is most often due to a direct effect on gut motility or the bowel mucosa. However, about 20% of cases are caused by toxin producing strains of *Clostridium difficile*. *C. difficile* may have a competitive advantage over the normal gut flora following antibiotic exposure, notably in the elderly. Less commonly, *Clostridium perfringens, Staph. aureus* and *Klebsiella oxytoca* may also cause antibiotic-associated diarrhoea/colitis. Colitis and occasionally pseudomembranous colitis can complicate *C. difficile* infection. Colonic perforation is the major cause of death and severe cases may require surgical intervention (colectomy). Some *C. difficile* strains are associated with epidemic infection, especially in hospitals, and strains with increased virulence have spread rapidly in North America and Europe. Such strains cause more severe disease and decrease the chances of survival, especially in the elderly.

All antibiotics may induce *C. difficile* infection and toxin production, but clindamycin, and broad-spectrum β-lactam antibiotics (especially amoxicillin, ampicillin, and cephalosporins) are most commonly incriminated. Fluoroquinolones have also been implicated, but these studies have commonly not controlled for exposure to *C. difficile* and have been performed during outbreaks. *C. difficile* infection should be suspected in any patient with diarrhoea in hospital (Fig. 25.2). However, *C. difficile* infection is increasingly being seen in the community and should be suspected in any patient who has recently been in hospital or received antibiotics (Fig. 25.2). Rarely *C. difficile* infection is community acquired and only 30–50% of these cases have received antibiotics within the previous three months. This condition is, ironically, treated with antibiotics after stopping the causative agent. Oral metronidazole or vancomycin are usually effective; metronidazole is recommended for non-severe cases and vancomycin is reserved for severe cases (Figure 25.1). In general, if non-*C. difficile* treatment antibiotics are continued response is less likely.

Between 15–30% of patients may have recurrent symptoms. Recent studies have shown that oral fidaxomicin (approved for use in USA in 2011 and likely in Europe from 2012) halves the risk of recurrent *C. difficile* infection compared with patients treated with oral vancomycin. Oral rifaximin, given after a course of oral vancomycin, may also reduce recurrent infection. These options are expensive and targeted use in those patients most likely to benefit will be key to cost-effective prescribing. Management of a second episode is the same as for the initial episode (Fig. 25.2). Thereafter vancomycin is used, initially in standard dose and then sometimes in a tapering regimen (Fig. 25.3). The rationale for this is that *C. difficile* forms spores that are resistant to treatment and interruption of therapy allows the spores to become (antibiotic-susceptible) mature bacteria. Thereafter, there are several options that have been tested in case series but not in randomized controlled trials (Fig. 25.3).

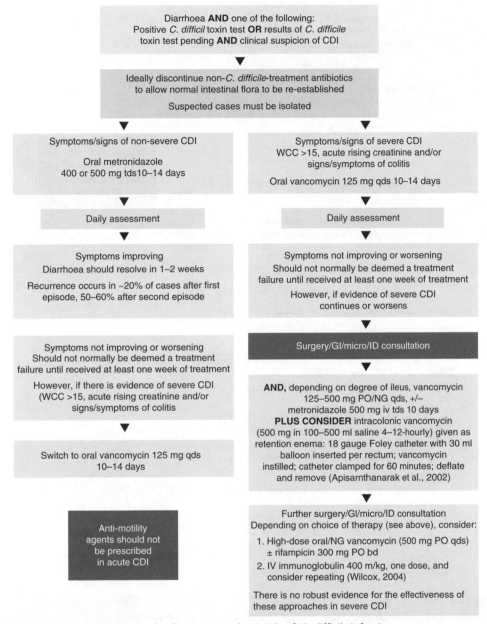

Fig. 25.2 Treatment algorithm for first or second episode of *C. difficile* infection.
Redrawn from '*Clostridium difficile* infection: How to deal with the problem', http://www.dh.gov.uk/prod_consum_dh/groups/dh_digitalassets/documents/digitalasset/dh_093218.pdf.
Reference cited in Figure 25.2:
Apisarnthanarak A, Razavi B and Mundy LM (2002), 'Adjunctive intracolonic vancomycin for severe *Clostridium difficile* colitis: case series and review of the literature', *Clinical Infectious Diseases* **35**: 690–96.

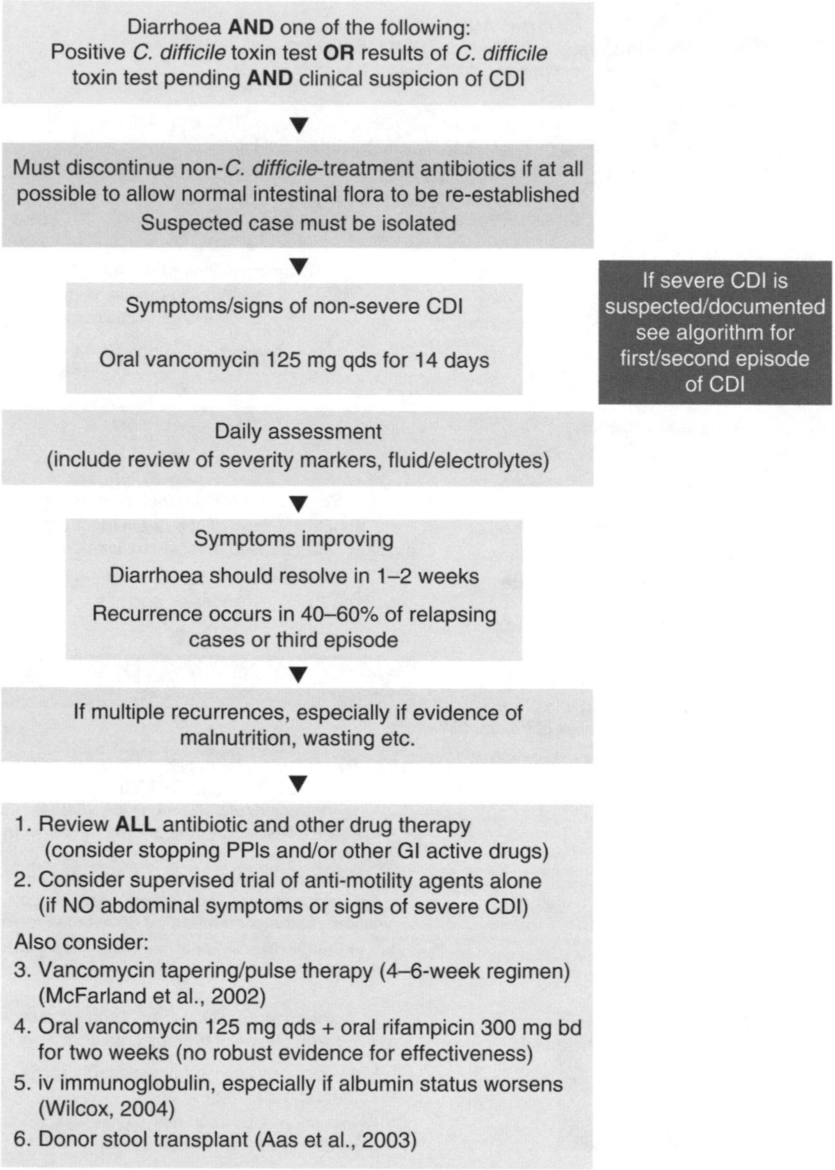

Diarrhoea **AND** one of the following:
Positive *C. difficile* toxin test **OR** results of *C. difficile* toxin test pending **AND** clinical suspicion of CDI

Must discontinue non-*C. difficile*-treatment antibiotics if at all possible to allow normal intestinal flora to be re-established
Suspected case must be isolated

Symptoms/signs of non-severe CDI

Oral vancomycin 125 mg qds for 14 days

If severe CDI is suspected/documented see algorithm for first/second episode of CDI

Daily assessment
(include review of severity markers, fluid/electrolytes)

Symptoms improving

Diarrhoea should resolve in 1–2 weeks

Recurrence occurs in 40–60% of relapsing cases or third episode

If multiple recurrences, especially if evidence of malnutrition, wasting etc.

▼

1. Review **ALL** antibiotic and other drug therapy (consider stopping PPIs and/or other GI active drugs)
2. Consider supervised trial of anti-motility agents alone (if NO abdominal symptoms or signs of severe CDI)

Also consider:
3. Vancomycin tapering/pulse therapy (4–6-week regimen) (McFarland et al., 2002)
4. Oral vancomycin 125 mg qds + oral rifampicin 300 mg bd for two weeks (no robust evidence for effectiveness)
5. iv immunoglobulin, especially if albumin status worsens (Wilcox, 2004)
6. Donor stool transplant (Aas et al., 2003)

Fig. 25.3 Treatment algorithm for recurrent *C difficile* infection (third or subsequent episode) Redrawn from '*Clostridium difficile* infection: How to deal with the problem', http://www.dh.gov.uk/prod_consum_dh/groups/dh_digitalassets/documents/digitalasset/dh_093218.pdf.
References cited in Figure 25.3:
Aas J, Gessert CE and Bakken S (2003), 'Recurrent *Clostridium difficile* colitis: case series involving 18 patients treated with donor stool administered via a nasogastric tube', *Clinical Infectious Diseases* **36**: 580–5.
McFarland LV, Elmer GW and Surawicz CM (2002), 'Breaking the cycle: treatment strategies for 163 cases of recurrent *Clostridium difficile* disease', *American Journal of Gastroenterology* **97**: 1769–75.
Wilcox MH (2004), 'Descriptive study of intravenous immunoglobulin for the treatment of recurrent *Clostridium difficile* diarrhoea', *Journal of Antimicrobial Chemotherapy* **53**: 882–4.

Key points

- On any one day 200 million people are suffering from acute infective gastroenteritis.

- The very young, elderly, and malnourished are particularly at risk from the electrolyte and fluid losses that complicate severe diarrhoea or vomiting.

- Restoration of fluids and electrolytes is the mainstay of treatment; oral rehydration therapy has had a significant impact in reducing mortality in developing countries.

- Gastrointestinal pathogens are transmitted directly from person to person or indirectly through faecal contamination of the environment, food, or water supply.

- Since most episodes of acute gastroenteritis are self-limiting, antibiotics are not generally indicated. Furthermore, the use of antibiotics carries the risk of directly irritating an inflamed bowel mucosa, or of inducing diarrhoea due to *Clostridium difficile* infection.

- About 20% of cases of antibiotic associated diarrhoea are caused by toxin producing strains of *Clostridium difficile.*

- All antibiotics may induce *C. difficile* infection and toxin production, but clindamycin, and broad-spectrum β-lactam antibiotics (especially amoxicillin, ampicillin, and cephalosporins) are most commonly incriminated.

- *C. difficile* infection should be suspected in any patient with diarrhoea in hospital, in any patient who has recently been in hospital or any patient who has recently received antibiotics in the community.

- Oral metronidazole or vancomycin are usually effective but recurrence is common.

Further reading

A wide variety of information about specific gastrointestinal pathogens is available from the UK Health Protection Agency at: http://www.hpa.org.uk/infections/topics_az/list.htm.

Health Protection Agency & Department of Health 'Clostridium difficile infection: How to deal with the problem', available at: http://www.dh.gov.uk/prod_consum_dh/groups/dh_digitalassets/documents/digitalasset/dh_093218.pdf.

World Health Organization information about oral rehydration with glucose-salts solution is available at: http://www.who.int/childadolescenthealth/New_Publications/CHILD_HEALTH/WHO_FCH_CAH_06.1.pdf.

Chapter 26

Serious bloodstream infections

The blood is normally sterile in health. However, in disease, micro-organisms invade the bloodstream as either part of the disease process (e.g. malaria), or in the case of blood-borne viruses (e.g. HIV, hepatitis B and C) as a result of the intimate association between an infected target tissue and the blood. In the case of bacterial infections, the blood may be infected as a consequence of a primary endovascular infection (e.g. infective endocarditis) or more commonly as a result of infection affecting a major organ or other body tissues.

Bacteraemia

Bacteraemia simply refers to the presence of viable bacteria in the blood. The patient may be completely asymptomatic or present with fever, rigors, tachycardia, shock, and multi-organ failure, sometimes leading to death. When bacteraemia is associated with clinical signs and symptoms it was often referred to as 'septicaemia'; however, this term is imprecise and should no longer be used. Bacteraemia is a laboratory finding. The clinical features of systemic response to infection should be described using objectively defined criteria that define and distinguish between sepsis, severe sepsis and septic shock (Chapter 13). The sepsis syndrome is a consequence of the release of cytokines (inflammatory mediators such as tumour necrosis factor, interleukin-1, and interleukin-6) stimulated by microbial products (structural component of organisms, such as lipopolysaccharide, teichoic acid, or exotoxins). The sepsis syndrome can be associated with any infection and is not restricted to patients with bacteraemia. It may also be triggered by non-infective causes.

Assessment of sepsis and the systemic inflammatory response

Sepsis is defined as the combination of symptoms or signs of a localized primary site of infection plus a systemic inflammatory response. The presence of systemic inflammatory response is often the first sign that infection is spreading from the primary site and that the patient may be bacteraemic (see Chapter 13). The systemic inflammatory response syndrome (SIRS) is defined as in Table 26.1.

Severe sepsis is defined as sepsis plus evidence of organ dysfunction, hypoperfusion, or hypotension. Evidence of perfusion abnormalities affecting the vital organs (brain, heart, kidneys, lungs) includes acute confusion, hypotension, oliguria, and hypoxia or lactic acidosis.

Septic shock is defined as sepsis with hypotension that persists despite adequate fluid resuscitation, along with the presence of perfusion abnormalities. The more severe the host response to trigger of sepsis, the higher the mortality (see Chapter 13).

The distinction between sepsis, sepsis syndrome, and septic shock, including refractory shock, is clinically useful and of prognostic importance. The judicious use of fluid replacement, vasopressor and inotropic drugs, mechanical ventilation and dialysis support in response to target organ failure can be life-saving. It is essential that there be a prompt assessment of the likely source and nature of the triggering infection. Relevant microbiological samples should be collected, including blood cultures.

Table 26.1 Features and criteria that establish systemic inflammatory response syndrome—defined by the presence of two or more of the following indicators

Temperature	>38°C or <36°C
Heart rate	>90 beats/min
Respiratory rate	>20 breaths/min or alveolar pressure of carbon dioxide $(PaCO_2)$ <4.3 kPa
Peripheral white blood cell count (WBC)	>12 × 10⁹/L or <4 × 10⁹/L

Any traumatic procedure that facilitates entry of organisms from an infected cutaneous lesion or bacteria-laden mucosal surface may cause bacteraemia (Table 26.2). In addition, invasive infections such as pneumococcal pneumonia, meningitis, or osteomyelitis may be associated with bacteraemia.

In the last 50 years, changes have taken place in the type of organism most frequently encountered. In the pre-antibiotic era *Streptococcus pyogenes* and *Str. pneumoniae* accounted for most positive blood cultures and fatalities, but by 1960 *Staphylococcus aureus* had become dominant. Today, staphylococci and pneumococci are still important, but are outnumbered by Gram-negative bacilli as causes of sepsis and death (Table 26.3). Anaerobes such as *Bacteroides fragilis* are also encountered more frequently, perhaps because of improved anaerobic techniques.

The increase in bacteraemic infections due to Gram-negative bacilli follows the success of antibiotics in controlling many Gram-positive infections, but advances in medical and surgical expertise have also played an important part: Gram-negative sepsis is a complication of severe urinary tract infections. It is also common in patients undergoing intra-abdominal surgery or aggressive immunosuppressive therapy and invasive procedures, and in those whose normal defences are already compromised by underlying disease. These infections are mostly hospital acquired, and because of the widespread use of antibiotics the infecting organisms are often multiresistant.

Vascular catheters are widely used in medical management and have resulted in an increase in bacteraemia caused by Gram-positive cocci, notably *Staph. aureus* and *Staph. epidermidis*. Polymicrobial bacteraemia and recurrent bacteraemia have also become more common in recent years.

Bacteraemia may be transient (lasting for several minutes) intermittent, or continuous (lasting for several hours to days). The danger of transient bacteraemia depends on the host and the organism. Thus, transient bacteraemia due to viridans streptococci after dental extraction is of no

Table 26.2 Procedures that may produce transient bacteraemia

Predominant organism	Procedure
Viridans streptococci	Dental extraction
	Periodontal surgery
	Surgery or instrumentation of the upper respiratory tract
Enterococci	Surgery or instrumentation of:
	urinary tract
	gastrointestinal tract
	biliary tract
	Obstetric or gynaecological surgery
Staphylococcus aureus	Manipulation or drainage of a septic focus

Table 26.3 Distribution of micro-organisms in blood cultures at Nottingham University Hospitals (2006–2010)

Gram-negative	Percent	Gram-positive	Percent
Escherichia coli	27.9	Staphylococcus aureus MSSA	11.8
Klebsiella spp.	7.6	Staphylococcus aureus MRSA	3.1
Proteus spp.	2.7	Streptococcus pneumoniae	4.7
Salmonella spp.	0.6	Coagulase negative staphylococci	11.2
Other Enterobacteriaceae	8.6	Haemolytic streptococci (group A, B, C, and G)	4.4
Pseudomonas spp.	5.4	Other streptococci	5.4
Haemophilus influenzae	0.7	Enterococci	7.3
Neisseria meningitidis	0.5	Others	1.5
Others	1.6	Anaerobes	1.9
Anaerobes	3.3	Candida spp	2.5
Total*	58.9	Total*	53.8

*totals include 12.7% polymicrobial

MSSA=meticillin-sensitive Staph. aureus

MRSA = meticillin-resistant Staph. aureus

Data supplied by Ros Montgomery, HSBMS, Nottingham University Hospitals

consequence in an otherwise healthy individual, but in those patients with abnormal heart valves it may produce endocarditis (see below). *Staph. aureus* may localize in the metaphyses of long bones in children or the vertebrae in adults and lead to osteomyelitis. Transient bacteraemia with Gram-negative bacilli following instrumentation of an infected urinary tract may produce rigor and fever.

Continuous bacteraemia is the hallmark of intravascular infection and also occurs in infections in patients with neutropenia, overwhelming sepsis, acute haematogenous osteomyelitis, and infections with intracellular organisms such as *Salmonella enterica* serotype Typhi.

Most other bacteraemias are intermittent and are characteristic of abscesses and certain types of chronic infection such as meningococcal or gonococcal sepsis.

Laboratory investigation and antibiotic therapy

There are no specific clinical findings that are diagnostic of bacteraemia or fungaemia or, for that matter, that differentiate between Gram-negative and Gram-positive sepsis. Hence the importance of blood cultures so that the pathogen is identified and specific therapy instituted as soon as possible. Mortality in patients with shock is over 50%. If death is to be prevented and shock avoided, the clinician must react promptly to the early signs of sepsis with appropriate 'best-guess' parenteral therapy.

Most episodes of bacteraemia are intermittent, hence the importance of more than one set of blood cultures before starting antibiotics. Ideally, at least two sets should be taken from separate venepunctures at intervals of a few minutes to a few hours (depending on the clinical urgency). Since bacteraemias are usually low-grade, the volume of blood drawn at each venepuncture is important: in adults at least 10 ml should be taken; in infants and young children 1–3ml. Specimens from other likely foci of infection must also be sent to the laboratory; these may include urine, sputum, cerebrospinal fluid, pus, pleural, and joint fluids. A Gram-stained smear of a specimen from the presumed site of infection can provide an early clue on which the choice of best-guess therapy can be based.

Secondary bacteraemia

When bacteraemia is secondary to a primary focus of infection that is readily confirmed or clinically suspected it is often possible to predict the most likely pathogen. The initial selection of antibiotics is guided by the nature of the infection and whether it was acquired in the community or hospital. The most appropriate antibiotic or combination can then be chosen in the light of local knowledge of resistance patterns. The initial antibiotic regimen can be changed later once microbiological information becomes available.

Primary bacteraemia

In some patients there is no clue as to the primary focus of infection or its likely source. Such episodes of 'primary' bacteraemia of unknown source are more common in neonates and immunocompromised patients.

The neonate

The newborn baby is more susceptible to bacterial invasion of the bloodstream. However, the recognition and localization of infection may be difficult because the manifestations are frequently non-specific. However, it is imperative that the diagnosis is made early, specimens collected, and antibiotic treatment started at once.

The initial empirical choice in a neonate with 'early-onset' (<7 days) sepsis is usually a combination of benzylpenicillin and gentamicin, which covers the two most common organisms, *Escherichia coli* and group B haemolytic streptococci (*Str. agalactiae*) as well as other streptococci, many other Gram-negative bacteria and *Listeria monocytogenes*. If, however, there is an obvious staphylococcal skin infection, flucloxacillin should be substituted for benzylpenicillin.

Empirical treatment for 'late-onset' (>7 days) sepsis varies according to the clinical setting. The combination of cefotaxime and gentamicin should be considered in neonates who are ventilated, known to be colonized with enterobacteria, or have had previous exposure to antibiotics. *Staph. epidermidis* is the commonest isolate in patients with infection associated with intravenous catheters and vancomycin is the only reliable agent against these organisms, so that a combination of vancomycin with gentamicin or cefotaxime would be a reasonable choice in neonates in whom catheter-associated sepsis is strongly suspected.

Immunocompromised patients

Bacteraemia is common in immunocompromised patients, especially bone marrow transplant patients and those with haematological malignant disease complicated by profound neutropenia, mucosal ulcerations, as a result of cytotoxic and immunosuppressive drugs. Despite the fact that blood cultures from these patients increasingly yield Gram-positive cocci, it is infection caused by Gram-negative bacilli and, in particular *Pseudomonas aeruginosa*, that are the most life threatening.

Treatment is with a broad-spectrum synergistic combination of antibiotics as initial empirical therapy. Widely used regimens include an aminoglycoside (e.g. gentamicin) together with either an antipseudomonal penicillin (e.g. piperacillin/tazobactam) or an expanded spectrum cephalosporin with antipseudomonal activity (e.g. ceftazidime). If blood cultures are positive modifications to the regimen are made. Vancomycin or teicoplanin may be added to the regimen of those who have vascular catheters *in situ* and where MRSA is suspected.

If fever persists for more than 72 h despite broad-spectrum antibiotics and blood cultures remain negative, the patient should be reassessed and repeat blood cultures obtained. Empirical antifungal therapy with amphotericin should be considered in selected patients who remain febrile and neutropenic for seven days despite broad-spectrum antibiotics.

Normal individuals

Primary bacteraemia in previously healthy individuals is rare. The most common type seen the UK is that due to *Neisseria meningitidis*. In infants, children or young adults it can produce a fulminating sepsis with petechial rash progressing to shock and death, sometimes in a matter of hours. Mortality can be as high as 30%. General practitioners suspecting this condition should give benzylpenicillin immediately before transferring the patient to hospital. Since it is unlikely that subsequent blood or cerebrospinal fluid cultures from these patients would be positive, a throat or pernasal swab should be obtained and a special request made for the isolation of *N. meningitidis*.

Str. pneumoniae occasionally causes bacteraemia in an otherwise healthy, but febrile child. Those aged six months to two years are most at risk. Although such bacteraemias may resolve spontaneously, a few patients remain ill and some develop severe disease, including meningitis. It is important that such patients are treated with antibiotics. Other important causes of primary bacteraemia include *Salmonella enterica* serotypes Typhi and Paratyphi (see p. 266) which complicate overseas travel.

Management of septic shock

Septic shock is characterized by hypotension, decreased systemic vascular resistance, myocardial depression, maldistribution of blood flow, and multi-organ system failure. The management of septic shock and severe sepsis is based on three basic principles:

♦ to stabilize the patient haemodynamically with the administration of intravenous fluids, oxygen, inotropic agents, and vasopressors;

♦ to provide organ support using mechanical ventilation and dialysis as necessary;

♦ to eradicate the source of infection with appropriate antibiotics and drainage or debridement of the septic focus, whenever possible.

Even when managed aggressively in intensive care units, the mortality in those with multi-organ failure stage is depressingly high (about 50%). The pathophysiology of sepsis is extremely complex and characterized by an intense inflammatory response and the release of an array of cytokines and other mediators. A variety of novel approaches has been investigated and targeted both microbial initiators of sepsis as well as components of the inflammatory cascade. Examples include monoclonal antibodies against lipid A of Gram-negative bacteria and against various cytokines, such as interleukin-1 and tumour necrosis factor. To date, none has shown clinical benefit. More recently, recombinant activated Protein C (drotrecogin alfa) has shown some benefit in reducing mortality in selected patients with septic shock and organ dysfunction.

Infective endocarditis

Endocarditis is inflammation of the endocardial surface of the heart. When caused by micro-organisms it is known as 'infective' endocarditis, and may be caused by bacteria including, rickettsiae, chlamydiae, and also fungi. Endocarditis usually affects the heart valves but may involve the adjacent endocardium. The terms acute and subacute endocarditis originated in the pre-antibiotic era when all patients with endocarditis died. Those who died in less than 6 weeks due to infection of normal valves by virulent organisms such as *Staph. aureus, Str. pneumoniae*, or *N. gonorrhoeae* were said to have acute bacterial endocarditis. In contrast, those who suffered a more indolent course due to infection of abnormal valves by organisms of relatively low virulence (e.g. viridans streptococci), died much later and were said to have subacute bacterial endocarditis.

Nowadays, the majority of patients with infective endocarditis are cured provided the diagnosis is made, and treatment with appropriate antibiotics begun sufficiently early. It is also more useful to classify endocarditis according to the infecting organism and the underlying site of infection (e.g. *Staph. aureus* tricuspid endocarditis). In addition, distinguishing native from prosthetic valve infection is also important. These definitions are of relevance in predicting the probable course of the disease and also have therapeutic implications with regard to the antibiotic regimen to be used.

Epidemiology

Infective endocarditis affects about 2000 people per year in England and Wales and has a mortality of 15–30%. With the decline in rheumatic heart disease (in the developed world) and the increase of endocarditis complicating degenerative heart disease, epidemiology of this disease has the following characteristics:

- The mean age of the patient has increased; it is now over 50 years of age for the following reasons:
  - people with congenital heart disease or rheumatic heart disease survive longer because of advances in medical and surgical expertise to correct valve dysfunction;
  - increased life expectancy is associated with a raised incidence of degenerative valve disease. Minor degenerative changes produce valvular lesions that serve as a nidus for infection; even so, almost 30% of elderly patients who develop endocarditis do not have a pre-existing cardiac condition.
  - infectious complications of genitourinary and gastrointestinal disease predispose to bacteraemia in elderly people.
- Acute *Staph. aureus* endocarditis is an important complication of intravenous drug use.
- Mitral valve prolapse with regurgitation predisposes to endocarditis and is now recognized more frequently.
- Prosthetic valve endocarditis has increased in proportion to cardiac valve surgery.
- The 'classic' physical signs of subacute bacterial endocarditis are seen in fewer patients as a result of earlier diagnosis.

Pathogenesis

Infective endocarditis is the consequence of several events (Fig. 26.1):

- haemodynamic or disease-associated damage to the endothelial surface of the valve;
- deposition of platelets and fibrin on the edges of the valve or other damaged endothelial surfaces, initially resulting in the formation of sterile or non-bacterial thrombotic vegetation;
- colonization by micro-organisms transiently circulating in the blood to produce an infected vegetation.

Transient bacteraemia is common. A wide variety of trivial events (e.g. chewing and toothbrushing) can induce bacteraemia with oral streptococci. Some 85% of cases of streptococcal endocarditis cannot be related to any medical or dental procedure. To cause endocarditis, organisms must also be able to survive natural complement-mediated serum bactericidal activity and adhere to thrombotic vegetations. Certain streptococci produce extracellular dextran, which promotes adherence to fibrin–platelet vegetations. These strains cause endocarditis more frequently than non-dextran producing streptococci. However, organisms such as enterococci and *Staph. aureus*

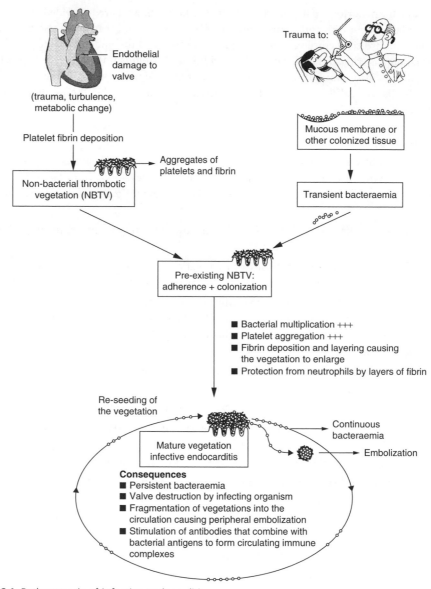

Fig. 26.1 Pathogenesis of infective endocarditis.

that do not produce dextran are also important causes of endocarditis. In these cases host proteins such as fibronectin and fibrinogen may mediate adherence.

Once colonization occurs there is rapid deposition of additional layers of platelets and fibrin over and around the growing colonies, causing the vegetation to enlarge. Within 24–48 h marked proliferation of bacteria occurs, leading to dense populations of organisms (10^9–10^{10} bacteria/g tissue). Micro-organisms deep within the vegetations are often metabolically inactive, whereas the more superficial ones proliferate and are shed continuously into the bloodstream. Fresh vegetations are composed of colonies of micro-organisms in a fibrin–platelet matrix with very few leucocytes.

Aetiological agents

Any organism can cause infective endocarditis, but streptococci and staphylococci account for more than 90% of culture-positive cases. However, the frequency with which various organisms are involved differs not only for the type of valve that is infected (native or prosthetic) but also with the causative event (e.g. dental manipulation, intravenous drug abuse, or a hospital-acquired infection) (Table 26.3).

Native-valve endocarditis

Streptococci Streptococci account for about 65% of all cases of native valve endocarditis. Most common of all are the 'viridans streptococci', which include *Streptococcus mitis, Str. sanguis, Str. mutans*, the *Str. milleri* group, and *Str. salivarius*, which are mouth commensals; most are highly sensitive to penicillin and cause infections primarily on abnormal heart valves. *Str. bovis* is an important cause of endocarditis in elderly people and may be associated with bowel pathology, notably colonic polyps and carcinoma. Recovery of this organism should prompt investigation for colonic disease.

Enterococci are gut streptococci and cause 10% of cases. Haemolytic streptococci of Lancefield groups B and G are occasional causes of endocarditis. Diabetic patients are particularly at risk of group B infections.

Staphylococci Staphylococci account for 25% of cases of native valve endocarditis, but over 90% are due to *Staph. aureus*, which is the leading cause of acute endocarditis. The course is frequently fulminant with widespread metastatic abscesses and death in about 40% of cases. The organism can attack normal or damaged valves and cause rapid destruction of the affected valves. Surgery is often required. *Staph. epidermidis*, in contrast, causes an indolent infection on previously damaged valves.

Other bacteria Other occasional causes are the fastidious, slow-growing Gram-negative bacilli of the 'HACEK' group (*Haemophilus* spp., *Actinobacillus actinomycetemcomitans, Cardiobacterium hominis, Eikenella corrodens*, and *Kingella* spp.).

Gram-negative enteric bacteria rarely cause endocarditis, except in intravenous drug abusers and patients with prosthetic valves. However, salmonellae have an affinity for abnormal cardiac valves and aneurysms of major vessels.

Fungi Fungi are an uncommon cause of native valve endocarditis. Risk factors include major underlying illnesses, prolonged courses of broad-spectrum antibiotics, corticosteroids or cytotoxic agents, and a central venous line *in situ* for a considerable length of time. Fungal endocarditis is more often seen in intravenous drug abusers or after reconstructive cardiovascular surgery. *Candida* and *Aspergillus* species are usually implicated. The course is indolent but grave. Large vegetations frequently embolize, occluding major vessels in the lower extremities. Culture of material obtained at embolectomy may yield the offending organism when blood cultures are negative.

Prosthetic valve endocarditis

Endocarditis complicating prosthetic valve or other devices is divided into 'early' and 'late' onset disease. Early-onset disease usually reflects contamination during the peri-operative period. Despite prophylactic antibiotics, staphylococci account for 50% of all cases; *Staph. epidermidis* is more common than *Staph. aureus*. Early-onset infection is a serious complication and is often associated with valve dehiscence, a fulminant course, and a high mortality. Late-onset prosthetic valve endocarditis occurs after the valve has become endothelialized. The source of infection, as in native valve endocarditis, is seeding of the valves following transient bacteraemia and viridans streptococci again become the commonest organism. Late-onset disease caused by *Staph. epidermidis*, diphtheroids, or other organisms of the early-onset type may just reflect a delayed manifestation of infection acquired in the peri-operative period.

Infective endocarditis and intravenous drug use

The skin is the commonest source of micro-organisms responsible for infective endocarditis in intravenous drug users, although contaminated drug and syringes are other possibilities. *Staph. aureus* is the predominant cause, but other organisms including *Pseudomonas* spp., group A haemolytic streptococci, other streptococci, and fungi are also important. Endocarditis often involves the tricuspid valve, especially when *Staph. aureus* is the causative agent.

Laboratory diagnosis

Blood cultures must be obtained from all patients with fever and heart murmur before contemplating antibiotic therapy, irrespective of the initial diagnosis. Bacteraemia is usually low grade, but continuous, so the timing of blood cultures is not critical. In the absence of previous antimicrobial therapy blood cultures are positive in more than 90% of cases.

At least 10 ml of blood should be withdrawn at each venepuncture and divided equally into two blood culture bottles (one set). Strict attention should be paid to skin preparation and aseptic technique. At least three sets of blood cultures are obtained from three separate venepunctures. *Staph. epidermidis* and diphtheroids are important causes of endocarditis, as well as common blood culture contaminants from the skin, and isolation of the same relatively 'avirulent' organism repeatedly in the absence of an intravascular catheter is highly suggestive of endocarditis.

The interval between each venepuncture depends on the clinical urgency. In acute cases, when antimicrobial therapy should be commenced promptly, three sets from separate venepunctures should be taken at intervals at least 30 min apart before the start of therapy. If there is no urgency, then the three sets can be taken over a 24 hour period. All blood culture bottles must be taken to the laboratory and incubated for up to three weeks to cater for fastidious organisms.

Culture-negative endocarditis

Blood culture may be persistently negative in some patients with suspected endocarditis. Likely explanations are:

 ◆ prior administration of antibiotics (the most common cause);
 ◆ infection with fastidious organisms including those of the HACEK group, *Coxiella burnetii*, *Chlamydia psittaci*, or *Brucella* spp.;
 ◆ infection with *Candida* spp. in which only 50% of blood cultures may be positive;
 ◆ infection of the right side of the heart, which is occasionally accompanied by negative blood cultures;
 ◆ cardiac disease other than infective endocarditis (e.g. left atrial myxoma).

When blood cultures are negative, paired samples of sera (one taken on admission and another 10–14 days later) should be examined for antibodies against other infective causes of endocarditis.

Echocardiography (transthoracic and transoesophageal) is key to the diagnosis, assessment, and management of patients with suspected infective endocarditis, but negative results do not exclude the diagnosis, especially in those with prosthetic valves.

General principles of therapy

The chief aims of management are to sterilize the vegetation and to ensure that relapse will not occur.

Bactericidal antibiotics

In endocarditis, organisms reach extremely high densities within the vegetation and are encased in layers of fibrin, where they are free to divide without interference from phagocytic cells or humoral defences. Hence, bactericidal antibiotics are essential to sterilize the vegetation. The most commonly used bactericidal agents are the penicillins, in particular benzylpenicillin. In penicillin-hypersensitive patients vancomycin or a cephalosporin are suitable alternatives.

Route and duration of therapy

Parenteral high-dose bactericidal therapy is essential to ensure the penetration of relatively avascular vegetations. The duration of therapy is determined by the nature (native or prosthetic valve) and site of the infection and by the susceptibility of the target pathogen. Most patients with endocarditis are cured by four weeks of treatment; some may require treatment for six weeks or more, although a selected group may be cured in only two weeks. Shorter courses are associated with relapse. Oral treatment for the last two weeks of treatment can be considered only after initial parenteral therapy in selected cases of native valve endocarditis where patient compliance with treatment can be assured.

Synergistic combination therapy

Aminoglycosides, though generally bactericidal, have little activity against streptococci and cannot be used alone. However, the combination of gentamicin with penicillin is synergistic and produces a more rapid and complete bactericidal effect than is obtained with penicillin alone. It is therefore common practice to recommend combination therapy in the initial stages of management of infective endocarditis.

Laboratory control of antibiotic therapy

Determination of minimal inhibitory concentration (MIC) and minimal bactericidal concentration

Standard routine sensitivity testing is not recommended in the laboratory management of endocarditis. Instead, the MIC and if considered desirable minimal bactericidal concentration of the antibiotics to be used, for the organism isolated, should be determined. In selective difficult cases, tests for antibiotic synergy may also be required for optimal combination therapy.

Aminoglycoside assays

When aminoglycosides (usually gentamicin) are used to treat endocarditis for their synergistic effects, a serum concentration lower than that normally considered therapeutic for Gram-negative infections is adequate, thus lessening the potential for toxicity. Patients with normal renal function should receive a loading dose appropriate to the age and body weight, followed by a maintenance dose. The serum concentration should be periodically monitored and the dose adjusted accordingly (a pre-dose concentration <1.0 mg/l is adequate).

Specific antimicrobial regimens

Streptococci

Isolates highly sensitive to penicillin (MIC <0.1 mg/l) This includes most viridans streptococci, *Str. bovis*, and other streptococci. Viridans streptococci are highly sensitive to penicillin and a 99% cure rate can be achieved with a—four week regimen of benzylpenicillin alone. Such a regimen is recommended for the treatment of uncomplicated native valve endocarditis in elderly patients, or those with impaired renal function, in whom aminoglycosides are best avoided.

For uncomplicated native valve endocarditis it is common practice in the UK to give two weeks of combination therapy with high-dose benzylpenicillin together with an aminoglycoside and then to consider oral amoxicillin for the last two weeks if patient compliance can be guaranteed. Patients with prosthetic valve endocarditis should be treated for longer to ensure cure; six weeks is recommended.

Isolates relatively resistant to penicillin (MIC 0.1–0.5 mg/l) This category includes some viridans streptococci such as the 'nutritionally variant' streptococci. Viridans streptococci that are relatively resistant to penicillin are increasingly encountered. The relapse rate in endocarditis caused by 'nutritionally variant' streptococci is high, even when two weeks of combination therapy is followed by two further weeks of benzylpenicillin. Endocarditis caused by such strains or other streptococci that are relatively resistant to penicillin is best treated with high-dose benzylpenicillin and gentamicin for four weeks, with appropriate monitoring of serum gentamicin levels.

Isolates resistant to penicillin (MIC >0.5 mg/l) Examples are *Enterococcus faecalis, Ent. faecium*, and other streptococci. Enterococcal endocarditis is the third most common type of endocarditis and is among the most difficult to treat. Mortality is about 20% and relapses are not uncommon. Although penicillin, ampicillin, and vancomycin inhibit the growth of enterococci they are not bactericidal for most strains, and therapy with these agents alone results in a high relapse rate. For a bactericidal effect, it is usually necessary to add an aminoglycoside; this results in marked enhancement of killing. A combination of penicillin or ampicillin with an aminoglycoside is the treatment of choice for enterococcal endocarditis; gentamicin is the preferred aminoglycoside. High-level resistance to gentamicin among enterococci is becoming more common and *in vitro* testing should be a routine procedure in all isolates of enterococci.

Ent. faecium is generally more resistant to β-lactam antibiotics than *Ent. faecalis*; β-lactamase-producing *Ent. faecalis* strains have also been reported. Such patients are best treated with vancomycin and gentamicin. Enterococci are uniformly resistant to all cephalosporins. Patients with enterococcal endocarditis should receive at least four to six weeks of combination therapy.

Staphylococci

Staphylococcus aureus In about one-third of patients with *Staph. aureus* endocarditis there is no evidence of pre-existing valvular heart disease. The infection results in rapid and severe valvular destruction and a mortality of about 40% even with appropriate treatment.

Patients over 50 years of age with *Staph. aureus* endocarditis secondary to infected intravascular devices have the highest mortality rate. Many require surgery to replace the infected valve, because of valvular dysfunction, dehiscence, and myocardial abscesses. In contrast, *Staph. aureus* endocarditis involving the tricuspid valve in intravenous drug abusers is much easier to cure and carries a mortality below 10%.

Since the vast majority of *Staph. aureus* strains produce a β-lactamase that destroys penicillin, the initial choice is a penicillinase-stable penicillin such as flucloxacillin. However, the choice and duration of treatment with a synergistic agent (e.g. gentamicin) remains controversial. While gentamicin is associated with a more rapid clearance of bacteraemia it is no longer recommended because of concerns over toxicity and a lack of clear evidence of benefit. In selected patients, such as an intravenous drug abuser with a right-sided endocarditis, or a patient with uncomplicated native valve endocarditis, who has responded fully to two weeks of combination therapy, oral flucloxacillin may be considered for the remaining two weeks of therapy. The remaining patients should receive high-dose flucloxacillin intravenously for at least four weeks.

If the patient is allergic to penicillin or the *Staph. aureus* is multiresistant, then vancomycin should be used. Rifampicin, a very potent antistaphylococcal agent, should be added in difficult cases but is never used alone, owing to the emergence of resistance. Sodium fusidate provides an alternative to rifampicin. In those intolerant of vancomycin, daptomycin may be substituted.

Staphylococcus epidermidis *Staphylococcus epidermidis* and other coagulase-negative staphylococci rarely infect a native valve, but are a common cause of both early and late onset prosthetic valve endocarditis. It is difficult to cure with antibiotics alone, and surgery is often required, particularly in patients with early-onset endocarditis. Isolates are frequently resistant to flucloxacillin, which must not be used unless the isolate is confirmed to be sensitive. Therapy must therefore be started with vancomycin and rifampicin. If the organism is indeed sensitive to flucloxacillin then flucloxacillin alone is recommended sufficient.

Recommended antibiotic regimens for streptococcal and staphylococcal endocarditis are shown in Tables 26.4 and 26.5 respectively.

Other organisms

Recommended antibiotic regimens for endocarditis caused by Gram-negative bacilli and other organisms are shown in Table 26.6. Culture-negative cases are occasionally caused by *Coxiella burnetii* or *Chlamydia psittaci* and may be detected by serology.

In clinically suspected acute endocarditis, it is prudent to start treatment with a combination of benzylpenicillin, flucloxacillin, and gentamicin and to modify the regimen appropriately once the causative organism has been identified.

Table 26.4 Aetiological agents in infective endocarditis and their approximate frequency

Organism	Predisposing factor			
	Native valve (%)	Prosthetic valve/cardiac surgery		Intravenous drug abuser (%)
		Early-onset (%)	Late-onset (%)	
Streptococci (all)	65	5	35	15
Viridans (α-haemolytic)	35	<5	25	5
Str. bovis	15	<5	<5	<5
Enterococcus faecalis	10	<5	<5	8
Other streptococci	<5	<5	<5	<5
Staphylococci (all)	25	50	30	50
Staph. aureus	23	20	10	50
Staph. epidermidis	2	30	20	<5
Gram-negative aerobic bacilli	<5	20	15	15
Fungi	<5	10	5	5
Miscellaneous bacteria	<5	10	10	10
Culture negative	5–10	5	<5	<5

Table 26.5 Recommended antibiotic treatment regimens for streptococcal endocarditis

Organism	Treatment of choice	Suggested adult dosage/interval/route	Comments
(a) Highly sensitive to penicillin (MIC <0.1 mg/l) Viridans streptococci and *Str. bovis*	Benzylpenicillin (4 weeks) Gentamicin (weeks 1–2)	1.2 g/4 h/i.v.	Native valve endocarditis (NVE): Consider benzylpenicillin alone for 4 weeks for elderly people or those at risk of renal problems Consider change to oral amoxicillin (1 g/6 h) after 2 weeks combination therapy In uncomplicated infections 2 weeks combination therapy may be adequate Prosthetic valve endocarditis (PVE): Gentamicin included for at least 2 weeks, then benzylpenicillin for a further 4 weeks; or oral amoxicillin (1 g/6 h) after 4 weeks benzylpenicillin (ceftriaxone/vancomycin[a])
(b) Relatively resistant to penicillin (MIC 0.1–0.5 mg/l) Nutritionally variant or viridans streptococci	Benzylpenicillin (4 weeks) Gentamicin (4 weeks)	1.2 g/4h/i.v.	The relapse rate is high; combination therapy may be prolonged for 4 weeks
(c) Resistant to penicillin (MIC >0.5 mg/l) Enterococci Viridans streptococci	Ampicillin (4 weeks) Gentamicin (4 weeks)	2 g/4 h/i.v.	Ampicillin more active than benzylpenicillin for enterococci. To avoid relapse, prolong combination therapy for 6 weeks if: (1) PVE; (2) symptoms for >3 months; (3) mitral valve involved; (4) relapse of enterococcal endocarditis (vancomycin or teicoplanin[a])

[a]Alternative drugs if patient is allergic to penicillin.

PVE, prosthetic valve endocarditis.

Table 26.6 Recommended antibiotic treatment regimens for staphylococcal endocarditis

Organism	Treatment of choice	Suggested adult dosage/interval/route	Comments
Meticillin-sensitive	Flucloxacillin (4 weeks) Gentamicin (weeks 1–2)	3 g/6 h/i.v.	In selected patients consider oral flucloxacillin after 2 weeks (see text) In complicated or PVE flucloxacillin may be prolonged for 6 weeks; consider adding rifampicin (300–600 mg b.d. oral)
Meticillin-resistant	Vancomycin Rifampicin or Sodium fusidate (4 weeks)	1 g/12 h/i.v. 300–600 mg/ 12 h/oral 500 mg/8 h/oral	In complicated or PVE treatment is prolonged to 6 weeks. Surgery often required
Vancomycin-resistant	Daptomycin (4 weeks)	6 mg/kg/24h/i.v.	Also appropriate for those intolerant to vancomycin. In complicated or PVE treatment is prolonged to 6 weeks

PVE, prosthetic valve endocarditis.

Table 26.7 Recommended antibiotic treatment regimens for endocarditis other than that caused by streptococci and staphylococci (doses are for adult with normal renal and hepatic function)

Organism	Antibiotic	Suggested dose/interval/ route	Duration (weeks)	Comments
'HACEK' group[a]	Ampicillin + gentamicin	2 g/4h/i.v. Synergistic dose	4	Sensitivity tests difficult to perform or interpret
Enterobacteriaceae	Cefotaxime + gentamicin	2 g/4 h/i.v. Full dose	4–6	Choice depends on sensitivity test results; for salmonellae consider ceftriaxone 2 g/12 h/i.v. preferred; gentamicin in full dose throughout to prevent resistance; mortality high; surgery often required
Ps. aeruginosa	Ceftazidime + gentamicin	3 g/8 h/i.v. Full dose	6	Left-sided endocarditis needs early surgery; right-sided may be treated medically first
Fungi	Amphotericin + flucytosine	1 mg/ kg/24 h/i.v. 37.5 mg/ kg/6 h/oral	6–8	Poor prognosis; early surgical excision plus medical treatment may succeed
Coxiella burnetii	Doxycycline + a quinolone	100 mg/12 h/ oral	Months-years	Rare; surgery often needed
Culture negative				Depends on clinical setting
				NVE: try enterococcal regimen (see Table 26.4) PVE: try *Staph. epidermidis* regimen (see Table 26.5)

[a]See text for meaning of this acronym.
NVE, native valve endocarditis; PVE, prosthetic valve endocarditis.

Surgical management

Emergency valve replacement in patients with infective endocarditis is an important adjunct to medical therapy. In selected patients, it is a life-saving procedure at any stage of the disease. The major indications for surgical intervention include:

◆ refractory heart failure related to structural valvular damage;
◆ myocardial or perivalvular abscess;
◆ untreatable or uncontrolled infection (e.g. infection of a prosthetic valve with fungi or Gram-negative bacilli);
◆ repeated relapses with a difficult organism (e.g. *Ent. faecium*);
◆ multiple embolic episodes.

Prognosis

Infective endocarditis remains a life-threatening infection. The prognosis varies according to the infecting micro-organism, the type of cardiac valve (native versus prosthetic and aortic versus mitral versus tricuspid), the age of the patient, and the presence or absence of complications. Mortality is lowest in viridans streptococcal endocarditis of the native valve and highest in early-onset prosthetic valve endocarditis.

Patients who recover from an episode of infective endocarditis carry a lifelong risk of a further attack. It is important that they maintain high levels of dental hygiene supplemented by regular dental reviews. Antibiotic prophylaxis plays a part in the prevention of endocarditis in selected patients at risk of infective endocarditis (see Chapter 18).

Key points

- Bloodstream infections are usually secondary to infection at another body site.

- The pathogens vary by age, underlying disease, and risk factors such as recent surgery, intra-vascular lines, or bladder catheterization.

- Treatment should be given promptly, usually with intravenous antibiotic and measures to control any complicating sepsis syndrome.

- Infective endocarditis is a serious life-threatening infection of the heart valves (native or prosthetic) and adjacent endocardium.

- Treatment requires high dose, usually parenteral, antibiotic for periods varying from two to six weeks and sometimes longer. Surgical intervention may be required for complicated disease.

Further reading

Dellinger RP, Levy MM, Carlet JM et al. International Surviving Sepsis Campaign Guidelines Committee, American Association of Critical-Care Nurses, American College of Chest Physicians, American College of Emergency Physicians, Canadian Critical Care Society, European Society of Clinical Microbiology and Infectious Diseases, European Society of Intensive Care Medicine, European Respiratory Society, International Sepsis Forum, Japanese Association for Acute Medicine, Japanese Society of Intensive Care Medicine, Society of Critical Care Medicine, Society of Hospital Medicine, Surgical Infection Society, World Federation of Societies of Intensive and Critical Care Medicine (2008) 'Surviving Sepsis Campaign: international guidelines for management of severe sepsis and septic shock'., *Critical Care Medicine*, **36**: 297–327.

Gould FK, Denning DW, Elliott TSJ et al. (2011), 'Guidelines for the antibiotic treatment of endocarditis in adults: report of the Working Party of the British Society for Antimicrobial Chemotherapy', *Journal of Antimicrobial Chemotherapy*, **54**(6): 971–981.

Chapter 27

Bone and joint infections

Septic arthritis

Bacteria can infect joints via the bloodstream (haematogenous septic arthritis) from a distant focus of infection such as a septic skin lesion, otitis media, pneumonia, meningitis, gonorrhoea, or an infection of the urinary tract. However, in adults prosthetic joint infection is now by far the most common presentation. Rarely bacteria may be introduced directly into the synovial space following a penetrating wound or an intra-articular injection. Also, the joint may become infected by direct spread from an adjacent area of osteomyelitis or cellulitis. Once established, septic arthritis can give rise to secondary bacteraemia.

Aetiology

Haematogenous septic arthritis

Staphylococcus aureus accounts for most bacteriologically proven joint infections. Other bacteria are important in specific age groups. *Escherichia coli* and streptococci of Lancefield group B (*Streptococcus agalactiae*) occur in neonates. Pneumococci, *Str. pyogenes*, and coliform bacilli are found in elderly people. *Haemophilus influenzae* of serotype b cause septicaemia and pyogenic arthritis in children under the age of six, but childhood immunization with the *H. influenzae* conjugate vaccine has markedly reduced the incidence of this infection. *Neisseria gonorrhoeae* occasionally causes septic arthritis in young adults. Patients with meningococcal infection may develop septic arthritis during the course of their illness. Other rare causes include *Mycobacterium tuberculosis*, opportunist mycobacteria, *Brucella* spp., fungi, and *Borrelia burgdorferi*, the spirochaete that causes Lyme disease.

Prosthetic joint infection

Acute infections (within one year of the primary operation) are often caused by *Staph. aureus* or *Str. pyogenes*. Infections occurring more than a year after surgery are caused by a much wider range of bacteria, including coagulase negative staphylococci, enterococci, aerobic Gram-negative bacilli, and anaerobic bacteria.

Management

Haematogenous septic arthritis

In 90% of cases a single joint is involved, most commonly the knee, followed by the hip. Typically, the patient is a child with a high temperature and a red, hot, swollen joint with restricted movement. However, septic arthritis is not uncommon in elderly and debilitated people, who may have non-specific symptoms. Patients with rheumatoid arthritis have an increased incidence of septic arthritis and a poorer prognosis, which may in part be attributable to delay in making the clinical diagnosis.

A presumptive diagnosis rests on the immediate examination of the joint fluid, because of the difficulty on clinical grounds in distinguishing other conditions with similar features, such as an exacerbation of rheumatoid arthritis, gout, acute rheumatic fever, or trauma to the joint. Typically, the

Table 27.1 Initial antimicrobial therapy in septic arthritis when bacteria are seen in the Gram-film of the joint aspirate

Description of the Gram-film	Probable organism	Initial choice of antibiotic	Comments
Gram-positive cocci in clusters	Staphylococci	Flucloxacillin	Clindamycin if penicillin-allergic
Gram-positive cocci in chains or pairs	Streptococci	Benzylpenicillin	Clindamycin if penicillin-allergic
Gram-negative coccobacilli	*H. influenzae*	Fluoroquinolone	May change to ampicillin if sensitive
Gram-negative large rods	Coliform bacilli or *Pseudomonas*	Fluoroquinolone	Modify according to culture results
Gram-negative diplococcic	*Neisseria* spp.	Benzylpenicillin	Ciprofloxacin if penicillin allergic or resistant

fluid is cloudy or purulent with a marked excess of neutrophils. The Gram film is of immediate help not only in confirming the diagnosis but also in the choice of the most appropriate antimicrobial therapy (Table 27.1). Despite the microscopic evidence of bacterial infection, culture of synovial fluid may sometimes fail to yield the pathogen, and blood cultures should always be taken at the same time. In suspected gonococcal arthritis, cervical, urethral, rectal, and throat swabs should also be taken for culture before starting antimicrobial therapy.

In young adults who present with acute mono-arthritis but do not have purulent joint fluid a diagnosis of reactive arthritis secondary to sexually transmitted disease should be suspected (Chapter 24).

It is very important that a diagnosis is made rapidly and appropriate therapy started immediately, because permanent damage to the joint may occur and lead to long-term residual abnormalities. Most patients who are treated promptly recover completely. Infection of the hip joint is more difficult to treat since, in addition to antibiotics, open surgical drainage is needed because of the technical difficulty of needle aspiration. The key to success is a combination of antibiotics and drainage. In most cases this is achieved by multidisciplinary management, including input from orthopaedic surgeons, medical microbiologists, and physicians. Surgeons in particular should determine whether drainage of pus should be by repeated needle aspiration or wash-out of the joint in an operating theatre.

The choice of initial antibiotic therapy depends on the age of the patient and the findings in the Gram film. If organisms can be identified with reasonable confidence before culture, the appropriate antibiotic for that particular organism is the automatic choice irrespective of the age (Table 27.1). If bacteria are not seen at this stage, the initial choice is influenced by the age of the patient or the underlying disease. Antibiotics are chosen to cover the most likely bacterial causes of the infection (Table 27.2) and can be modified subsequently if a pathogen is isolated.

Most antimicrobial agents given parenterally achieve therapeutic levels in the infected joint, so the intra-articular injection of antibiotics is not recommended, particularly as it may induce chemical synovitis. A sequential intravenous–oral regimen, carefully monitored at the time of oral therapy, is widely used. In all cases, the initial treatment must be with parenteral antibiotics until the condition of the patient has stabilized (usually seven to ten days) and the joint is reasonably dry. Switch to oral therapy is appropriate once the condition has stabilized as all of the first choice drugs are well absorbed after oral administration. The total duration of treatment is usually between 4 and 8 weeks. Close monitoring is required to ensure not only that signs of joint inflammation

Table 27.2 Initial antimicrobial therapy in septic arthritis when no organisms are seen in the Gram-film of the joint aspirate

Type of patient	Most common organisms	Less common organisms	Initial choice of antibiotic
Neonate (0–2 months)	Staph. aureus Group B streptococci Gram-negative bacilli		Flucloxacillin[b] + gentamicin or cefuroxime/cefotaxime
Infant (2 months–6 years)	Staph. aureus	Str. pyogenes Str. pneumoniae H. influenzae[a]	Flucloxacillin[b] + cefotaxime
Child (7–14 years)	Staph. aureus	MRSA	Flucloxacillin[b]
Adult (>15 years)	Staph. aureus	N. gonorrhoeae, MRSA	Flucloxacillin[b]
Elderly or debilitated	Staph. aureus	Str. pyogenes Str. pneumoniae MRSA Gram-negative bacilli	Flucloxacillin[b] + gentamicin

MRSA, meticillin-resistant Staph. aureus.

[a] Now rare where vaccine has been introduced.

[b] Vancomycin if MRSA likely.

disappear but that inflammatory markers (white blood cell count and C-reactive protein or erythrocyte sedimentation rate) normalize.

Prosthetic joint infection

Most patients with prosthetic joint infection are not systemically unwell. Infection should be suspected in any patient who develops pain or signs of local inflammation in the joint, although it is impossible to distinguish between mechanical loosening of the joint and infection unless there are obvious signs of infection such as purulent discharge from a sinus. Because there is rarely systemic illness it is not necessary to start empirical treatment and the chances of establishing a definitive microbiological diagnosis are greatly enhanced if antibiotics are not given. Serious systemic illness is the only reason for giving empirical antibiotics, as it is extremely unlikely that prosthetic joint infection will resolve with antibiotic therapy alone.

Patients with suspected prosthetic joint infection should be referred urgently to an orthopaedic surgeon who specializes in revision surgery for prosthetic joints and who is likely to work closely with medical microbiologists and infectious diseases physicians. As coagulase-negative staphylococci are frequent causes of prosthetic joint infection and are also common contaminants, interpretation of results is not straightforward. It is of crucial importance that joint tissue specimens are carefully collected to minimize cross contamination, and that all recovered micro-organisms are considered as potential pathogens.

Osteomyelitis

Osteomyelitis is infection of bone and is usually caused by bacteria. Unlike soft tissues, bone is a rigid structure and cannot swell. As infection proceeds and pus forms, there is a marked rise of pressure in the affected part of the bone, which, if unchecked or unrelieved, may impair the blood supply to a wide area and result in areas of infected dead bone. Once this chronic phase of osteomyelitis is established, necrotic bone (sequestrum) must be removed surgically in addition to the use of antibiotics if the infection is to be eradicated.

Pathogenesis and aetiology

Osteomyelitis may be haematogenous (infected through the bloodstream) or non-haematogenous (infected directly through a wound, including a fracture or an overlying chronic ulcer).

Haematogenous osteomyelitis

This type of infection is most commonly caused by staphylococci that reach the site through the bloodstream, usually with no obvious primary focus of infection. Acute haematogenous osteomyelitis is principally a disease of children under 16 years, in whom more than 85% of cases occur. The usual sites are the long bones (femur, tibia, humerus) near the metaphysis, where the blood supply to the bone is most dense. However, when the disease occurs in adults, the vertebrae are commonly affected.

Staph. aureus accounts for about half of all cases and for more than 90% of cases in otherwise normal children. In the elderly with underlying malignancies and other diseases, and in drug addicts, Gram-negative bacilli (coliform bacilli and Ps. aeruginosa) are reported with increasing frequency. Coliforms are particularly likely to cause vertebral osteomyelitis, as it is associated with recurrent urinary tract infection. H. influenzae has become very rare since the introduction of the conjugate vaccine. Other rare causes of haematogenous osteomyelitis include M. tuberculosis, Brucella abortus, and, particularly in parts of the world where sickle-cell anaemia is prevalent, salmonellae.

Non-haematogenous osteomyelitis

When bones are infected by the introduction of organisms through traumatic or post-operative wounds, Staph. aureus is still the commonest cause, but Gram-negative bacteria may also be found. Ps. aeruginosa may occasionally produce osteomyelitis of the metatarsals or calcaneum following a puncture wound of the sole of the foot and Pasteurella multocida infection may follow animal bites. Patients with infected pressure sores over a bone, or those with peripheral vascular disease or diabetes mellitus, may develop osteomyelitis with mixed aerobic and anaerobic organisms (coliforms and Bacteroides species), although Staph. aureus is an important cause of osteomyelitis by this route also.

Clinical and diagnostic considerations

The typical manifestations of acute, haematogenous osteomyelitis include the abrupt onset of high fever and systemic toxicity, with marked redness, pain, and swelling over the bone involved. In vertebral osteomyelitis, there may be general malaise, with or without low-grade fever and low back pain. If the infection is not controlled, it may spread to produce a spinal epidural abscess, with consequent neurological symptoms.

The diagnosis of osteomyelitis is confirmed by bone biopsy. A bone scan may help to localize the site and extent of the infection. However, bone scan is simply a demonstration of increased blood supply to the affected area and cannot distinguish between infection and other causes of inflammation. A positive bone scan should be a stimulus to further investigation, whereas a negative bone scan makes the diagnosis of osteomyelitis unlikely. Magnetic resonance imaging provides additional information about the presence and location of a sequestrum. Blood cultures should be taken in addition to bone biopsy. In patients with chronic osteomyelitis, it may be misleading to base antibiotic treatment on the results of cultures of pus obtained from a draining sinus, which will often yield organisms that are secondarily colonizing the sinus. For precise bacteriological diagnosis, material must be obtained during the surgical removal of dead bone and tissue.

Guidelines for antibiotic therapy and management

It is generally agreed that acute haematogenous osteomyelitis can be cured without surgical intervention, provided antibiotics are given while the bone retains its blood supply and before extensive necrosis has occurred. In practice, this is within the first 72 h of the development of symptoms. Antibiotic therapy must, therefore, start immediately after a bone biopsy and blood cultures have been obtained. Results from a Gram-film of aspirated material may help in the initial choice of antibiotic. If no organisms are seen *Staph. aureus* is the prime suspect in any age group, and an antistaphylococcal agent should be used (flucloxacillin or clindamycin). If Gram-negative bacteria are isolated a fluoroquinolone is the drug of choice.

To ensure adequate concentration at the site of infection, high doses of antibiotics should be given parenterally. If an abscess has already formed when the patient is first seen, or there is no significant clinical improvement within 24 h of starting parenteral therapy, then surgical drainage of the abscess is essential. Combination antimicrobial therapy is often used in osteomyelitis, especially for chronic infections and those cases caused by more resistant pathogens, for example MRSA. However, recent reviews have concluded that the evidence for combination therapy is inconsistent, and is based primarily on *in vitro* and particularly animal experiments. Rifampicin may be beneficial, as part of combination treatment, in device or bone infections due to its activity against slow-growing staphylococcal cells that are found in biofilms. It should be noted that for deep seated infections such as osteomyelitis, when using combination therapy ideally the individual antibiotics should both achieve good penetration to the site of infection. If this does not happen then the bacteria may in effect only be exposed to therapeutic concentrations of one drug. This scenario increases the risk of selecting resistant strains, especially during prolonged therapy and/or with some agents known to be associated with a high risk of resistance emergence (e.g. rifampicin and fusidic acid).

It is clear that the details of treatment, including duration of intravenous therapy and total duration of treatment should be determined by specialists with experience in the management of these complex conditions.

Key points

- *Staph. aureus* is the most important cause of septic arthritis and osteomyelitis and is particularly common in children.
- The management of prosthetic joint infection requires close liaison between a specialist orthopaedic surgeon and medical microbiologists/infectious diseases physicians.
- Coagulase-negative staphylococci are frequent causes of prosthetic joint infection but are also common contaminants, and so interpretation of results is not straightforward.
- Chronic osteomyelitis is often treated with combination antibiotic therapy for prolonged periods and requires close monitoring of inflammatory markers.

Further reading

Rao N, Ziran BH, Lipsky BA (2011), 'Treating osteomyelitis: antibiotics and surgery', *Plastic Reconstructive Surgery*, 127 Suppl 1:177S–187S.

Nguyen HM, Graber CJ (2010), 'Limitations of antibiotic options for invasive infections caused by meticillin-resistant *Staphylococcus aureus*: is combination therapy the answer?', *Journal of Antimicrobial Chemotherapy*, 65: 24–36.

Chapter 28

Infections of the central nervous system

Infections of the central nervous system include meningitis, encephalitis, and brain abscess. These can be caused by viruses, bacteria, fungi, and protozoa; however, bacterial and viral causes predominate.

Infection is generally acquired from an exogenous source and spreads to the central nervous system via the bloodstream. Penetrating injuries and trauma, including neurological procedures can be complicated by infection. In the case of brain abscess, bloodstream or spread from adjacent infected sites (middle ear, sinuses) are also important. All infections of the central nervous system are serious. Many infections, notably meningitis and brain abscess, will prove fatal unless diagnosed and treated promptly.

Meningitis

Meningitis is an infection within the subarachnoid space resulting in inflammation of the membranes covering the brain and the spinal cord and the intervening cerebrospinal fluid (CSF). Infection is usually caused by bacteria, viruses, and occasionally fungi (Table 28.1). The inflammatory process in bacterial meningitis extends throughout the subarachnoid space and often involves the ventricles; the brain itself is generally not affected in immunocompetent individuals.

Viral meningitis is usually self-limiting. In the case of bacterial meningitis, which remains a relatively common and devastating disease with a mortality of 10 to 30%, the outcome is dependent upon the organism, the age of the patient, the state of consciousness on admission, the speed of diagnosis, and the timeliness of treatment. Long-term neurological sequelae in survivors are common especially in neonates, infants, and those infected with *Streptococcus pneumoniae*.

Bacterial meningitis

About 2000 cases of bacterial meningitis are notified annually in the UK; most are caused by *Neisseria meningitidis* and *Str. pneumoniae*. The introduction of a conjugate vaccine against *Haemophilus influenzae* type b in 1992 has now virtually eliminated infection with this organism. *N. meningitidis* is now the commonest cause of acute bacterial meningitis and is likely to remain so, until a suitable vaccine becomes available for strains of serogroup B, which account for over 60% of all cases of meningococcal disease in the UK. The introduction of vaccine against serogroup C meningococci has successfully controlled such infections.

The incidence of occurrence of the various forms of bacterial meningitis is strikingly age related. In the past, *Escherichia coli* and other enterobacteria dominated as agents of neonatal meningitis, but *Str. agalactiae* (Group B streptococcus) is now the leading cause. Less common causes are *Listeria monocytogenes*, enterobacteria other than *Esch. coli*, *Candida albicans*, and *Str. pneumoniae*.

N. meningitidis is an important cause of meningitis in childhood and early adult life. Household and institutional outbreaks in schools and universities occur sporadically. After the age of 40

Table 28.1 Infectious causes of meningitis (UK)

Bacteria	Viruses	Fungi
Neisseria meningitideis	Enteroviruses	Cryptococcus neoformans
Streptococcus pneumoniae	Mumps	Candida albicans
Str. agalactiae (Group B)	Herpes simplex	
Enterobacteria	HIV	
Staphylococcus aureus		
Coagulase-negative staphylococci		
Listeria monocytogenes		
Mycobacterium tuberculosis		
Treponema pallidum		

meningitis is most commonly caused by *Str. pneumoniae*. Other organisms that are occasionally encountered include *L. monocytogenes* (especially in those with underlying diseases), *Esch. coli*, *Staphylococcus aureus* (usually post-neurosurgery), and *Mycobacterium tuberculosis*.

Pathogenesis and clinical features

Str. pneumoniae and *N. meningitidis* are found as normal upper respiratory tract commensals in a proportion of the population. Meningitis most commonly follows haematogenous spread of the micro-organism from the nasopharynx. The sequence of events is believed to be mucosal colonization, passage through the mucosal epithelium, bacteraemia, penetration of the blood–brain barrier, and multiplication within the subarachnoid space. Occasionally, haematogenous spread from the middle ear, or other infected focus, may occur. Rarely, bacteria reach the CSF by direct extension from adjacent suppurative tissues or a ruptured intracranial abscess, or may be directly implanted into the subarachnoid space from the nasopharynx through dural defects of congenital or traumatic origin. Once a pathogen is introduced into the subarachnoid space, bacteria multiply rapidly because of inadequate local defences. There follows an intense inflammatory process with marked congestion, oedema, outpouring of exudate, and raised intracranial pressure. Blood vessels and nerves may be involved in the inflammatory process leading to arteritis, infective thrombophlebitis, and cranial nerve palsies, and the thick exudate may interfere with CSF circulation and absorption leading to blockage and hydrocephalus.

The clinical picture consists of signs and symptoms of systemic illness (e.g. general malaise, fever, toxicity, poor feeding, leucocytosis) increased intracranial pressure (e.g. headache, vomiting, irritability, disturbance of consciousness, seizures), and meningeal irritation (e.g. photophobia, neck pain, positive Kernig's sign). In neonates, infants, and old people the signs and symptoms may be non-specific and subtle.

The presence of a petechial or purpuric rash, predominantly on the extremities, in a patient with meningeal signs almost always indicates meningococcal disease and requires immediate antibiotic therapy and admission to hospital.

Viral meningitis

Viral meningitis is most commonly associated with enteroviruses (Coxsackie and echoviruses) (Table 28.1) and is therefore more common in the summer months. Herpes simplex meningitis, as distinct from herpes simplex encephalitis, may or may not be linked to active infection at other body sites. In the non-vaccinated, mumps meningitis is an unpleasant complication of

Table 28.2 Selected agents responsible for acute encephalitis

Viruses	Bacteria	Fungi	Protozoa
Herpes simplex	*Listeria monocytogenes*	*Cryptococcus neoformans*	*Toxoplasma gondii*
Arboviruses[a]			*Naegleria fowleri*
HIV	*Rickettsia* spp.		*Trypanosoma brucei*
Varicella zoster	*Treponema pallidum*		*rhodesiense*
Echoviruses			
Cytomegalovirus			
Coxsackie viruses			
Epstein–Barr virus			
Mumps			
Measles			
Influenza			

[a]Includes Ross River, West Nile, Japanese encephalitis, and tick-borne encephalitis viruses.

this infection. Primary HIV infection may manifest as acute central nervous system disease including meningitis and should be considered in those at risk of recent exposure. Most viral meningitides are self-limiting and without major neurological complications, although headaches may persist for several weeks.

Encephalitis

Encephalitis indicates inflammation of the brain parenchyma and is largely the result of virus infection. Some are vector borne and therefore geographically linked. However, occasionally bacteria, fungi, and protozoa are responsible (Table 28.2).

Pathogenesis and clinical features

Invasion of the brain is generally the result of bloodstream spread complicating viraemia or bacteraemia. The inflammatory reaction may be focal or generalized and is characterized by perivascular infiltration by lymphocytes and accompanying neuronal damage.

Clinically, the illness has an acute onset with fever, headache, and clouding of consciousness. Seizures may occur. The neurological findings may be either generalized or localized causing focal or global neurological deficits. The cranial nerves may also be involved.

Laboratory diagnosis

Cerebrospinal fluid examination

Examination of the CSF obtained by lumbar puncture (provided this procedure is not contraindicated; see below) is the most effective investigation for diagnosing the nature of infection of the central nervous system. In an adult at least 4–5 ml of CSF is obtained into two or three sterile bottles, which are labelled sequentially. Blood and CSF samples for the estimation of glucose are also sent for chemical assay.

Examination of the CSF should include total white blood cell (including differential) and red blood cell counts, and estimation of protein concentration. Careful examination of a prepared Gram-stained smear of the centrifuged deposit of CSF reveals the causative organism in most cases and guides appropriate initial therapy in the case of bacterial meningitis. Antibiotic treatment

Table 28.3 Typical cerebrospinal fluid changes in bacterial and viral meningitis

Property	Normal cerebrospinal fluid	Bacterial meningitis[a]	Viral meningitis
Appearance	Clear, colourless	Purulent or cloudy	Clear or slightly opalescent
Cell count (per µl)	0–5	100s or 1000s	10s or 100s
Main cell type	Lymphocytes	Polymorphs[b]	Lymphocytes[c]
Protein concentration	0.1–0.4 g/l	May be several g/l	Normal or slightly raised
Glucose concentration	≈60% blood glucose	<40% blood glucose	Unchanged
Gram-film	Negative	Positive	Negative

[a] Excluding tuberculous meningitis.

[b] Exceptions: partially treated pyogenic meningitis; tuberculous, listerial, cryptococcal, or leptospiral meningitis, in which a lymphocytic response is common.

[c] In early cases an increased polymorph count may be seen.

prior to CSF collection can alter the staining and morphological characteristics of some pathogens and requires caution in interpretation. Typical laboratory findings in bacterial and viral meningitis are shown in Table 28.3.

In patients with suspected acute meningitis or encephalitis a computed tomography (CT) brain scan is frequently obtained, especially where encephalitis is suspected, seizures occur or focal neurology is detected. Lumbar puncture is contraindicated in those with evidence of raised intracranial pressure to avoid subsequent and potentially fatal compression of the brainstem through the foramen magnum ('coning').

Other tests, such as those that detect pneumococcal capsular polysaccharide are increasingly used but rarely show diagnostic superiority over a carefully prepared Gram-stain smear and culture of CSF. In the case of viral meningitis and tuberculous meningitis (Chapter 30, p. 324) polymerase chain reaction tests are now widely used to establish a diagnosis.

Blood cultures

Blood cultures (two sets) should be collected, ideally before antimicrobial therapy is begun, from patients with suspected meningitis, since bacteraemia is present in a high proportion of patients with meningococcal or pneumococcal disease.

Therapeutic considerations

The treatment of bacterial meningitis requires prompt initiation of treatment, started on the basis of Gram-film findings (if available) and on the appreciation of certain principles and guidelines. However, if the patient is acutely ill, with a short history suggestive of meningitis, or if the CSF appears cloudy, then empirical (based on age and clinical setting) high-dose intravenous antibiotics should be given immediately, without waiting for laboratory results, since mortality is high in these patients.

Penetration of antibiotics into cerebrospinal fluid

The CSF represents an area of impaired host defence. Hence, agents are selected that are bactericidal and also penetrate into the CSF in therapeutic concentrations. Compounds entering CSF must traverse the blood–brain barrier (a lipid membrane in the brain capillary), the epithelial layer of the choroid plexus, or both. The choroid is impermeable to lipid-insoluble molecules.

The penetration of antibiotics into the CSF is enhanced by high lipid solubility, a low degree of ionization, low molecular weight, high serum concentration of the drug, low protein binding, and the presence of meningeal inflammation.

Antimicrobial agents can be divided according to their ability to penetrate into CSF:

- those that penetrate inflamed and non-inflamed meninges in standard doses: chloramphenicol, sulphonamides, trimethoprim, metronidazole, isoniazid, pyrazinamide, and fluconazole;

- those that penetrate in the presence of inflamed meninges, or when used in high doses: benzylpenicillin, ampicillin, flucloxacillin, cefotaxime, ceftriaxone, vancomycin, rifampicin, amphotericin, and flucytosine;

- those that penetrate poorly even when the meninges are inflamed: aminoglycosides, erythromycin, tetracyclines, and fusidic acid.

Choice of antimicrobial agent

The initial choice of antimicrobial agent is based on the most likely pathogen, which is determined by the age of the patient, the clinical features, the Gram-film results of the CSF, and knowledge of the local sensitivity patterns of the suspected organism. A bactericidal agent in high dose intravenously is recommended for the treatment of meningitis, since rapid killing of bacteria occurs only when the bactericidal titre of the CSF for the relevant bacteria is between one in 10 and one in 20.

Cefotaxime and ceftriaxone, exhibit excellent activity against *H. influenzae, Str. pneumoniae, N. meningitidis*, group B streptococci, *Esch. coli*, and other enterobacteria, and are agents of choice for most forms of bacterial meningitis. High-dose intravenous cefotaxime or ceftriaxone provides CSF concentrations many times those necessary to kill the organisms. Although these cephalosporins are effective in most varieties of meningitis, listerial, and staphylococcal meningitis are exceptions (see below). Chloramphenicol, which penetrates well into CSF and was formerly widely used in neonates and adults, but is now a reserve agent for the treatment of selected patients who are allergic to penicillin, owing to toxicity and lower efficacy rates.

Duration of therapy

Antibiotic treatment of meningitis varies by pathogen. Meningococcal disease responds in five to seven days; *H. influenzae* is best treated for a minimum of seven to 10 days to ensure complete eradication of the organism and prevent relapse. Antimicrobial treatment of pneumococcal meningitis should be continued for at least 10 to 14 days. In neonatal meningitis and adult meningitis due to unusual organisms, such as *L. monocytogenes*, more prolonged therapy may be indicated and each case should be reviewed in consultation with a clinical microbiologist or infectious disease specialist.

Adjunctive therapy

Despite the use of appropriate, effective, bactericidal antibiotics, mortality and morbidity in bacterial meningitis remain high. Attention has therefore focused on the possibility of modulating the complex inflammatory process within the subarachnoid space and meninges that contributes to mortality and morbidity, including sensorineural hearing loss.

Dexamethasone therapy in concert with antimicrobial agents has been shown to decrease the incidence of sensorineural hearing loss in children with *H. influenzae* meningitis, but there is no reduction in mortality and gastrointestinal bleeding occurs in some patients. With the declining incidence of *H. influenzae* meningitis in those countries that have adopted childhood immunization against this disease, the use of dexamethasone is now used selectively in the management of other forms of bacterial meningitis, such as pneumococcal meningitis where early use has reduced mortality. It should be avoided in viral meningitis and where the diagnosis of meningitis is uncertain.

It is also contraindicated in patients with septic shock complicating meningitis or in those receiving immunosuppressive therapy. Dexamethasone is the steroid of choice; it is important that it be started before the first dose of antibiotic and continued for four days.

Meningococcal disease

Infections caused by *N. meningitidis* are both endemic and epidemic. Epidemics may occur in closed institutions, such as schools, halls of residence, and military barracks. In sub-Saharan Africa epidemics occur every few years. *N. meningitidis* affects primarily infants, children, and young adults. The organism is carried asymptomatically in the nasopharynx of a small proportion of the population and this represents the reservoir of infection. The disease has a seasonal incidence with most cases occurring in winter and spring. Coexisting or antecedent viral infection may play a part in invasive meningococcal disease. The following broad clinical groups can be recognized in patients with meningococcal disease according to the presenting clinical features.

Sepsis syndrome with or without meningitis About 15 to 20% of cases of meningococcal disease are characterized by the rapid development over a period of 24 to 48 h. The symptoms include fever, rigors, myalgias, and a petechial rash. In a few patients headache, confusion, and neck stiffness may develop later, signifying the onset of meningitis. However, the onset of illness in those with fulminant meningococcal septicaemia is much more abrupt and dramatic. The duration of illness is often less than 24 h, and on admission the patient is gravely ill, shocked, and covered with a rapidly spreading purpuric rash, which may coalesce, become ecchymotic, and even proceed to tissue necrosis. Disseminated intravascular coagulation may follow and death can occur within hours. Blood cultures are invariably positive. There may be no signs of meningism, but it is not uncommon for *N. meningitidis* to be recovered from an otherwise normal CSF, implying the onset of early meningitis. Mortality is 20 to 30% in patients with meningococcal sepsis.

Meningitis with or without the sepsis syndrome This is the commonest presentation with signs and symptoms of meningitis that may occur rapidly or evolve more gradually over several days. The CSF is typically cloudy with a high polymorphonuclear leucocyte count, raised protein, and low glucose concentration. A typical petechial or purpuric rash is present in about 60% of patients; occasionally the rash may be initially maculopapular. Blood cultures are positive in about 40% of cases. With appropriate treatment, mortality is 3 to 5%.

Rarer forms of meningococcal disease Occasionally *N. meningitidis* may localize in the joints or on heart valves producing acute septic arthritis or endocarditis. Chronic meningococcal septicaemia, although uncommon, is characterized by intermittent pyrexia, rash, and arthralgia. Occasionally a diagnosis is made retrospectively because of transient positive blood cultures in children with mild, self-limiting, febrile illness. They usually recover quickly and spontaneously without the use of antibiotics.

Treatment and prophylaxis

Ceftriaxone is the drug of choice. Therapy should be started on first suspicion of meningococcal disease. Although most strains of *N. meningitidis* are highly sensitive to penicillin (minimum inhibitory concentration <0.16 mg/l), some strains of reduced sensitivity are occasionally encountered and hence the reason why ceftriaxone is the preferred agent.

To prevent secondary cases of meningococcal disease, household and secretion (kissing) contacts are offered antibiotic prophylaxis. The standard agent for prophylaxis is oral rifampicin, twice daily for 2 days (adults 600 mg; children 10 mg/kg). Rifampicin-resistant strains occur, but are presently uncommon. A single intramuscular injection of ceftriaxone (adults 250 mg; children 125 mg) or a single oral dose of ciprofloxacin (adults 500 mg) are alternative prophylactic regimens. Pregnant women should be offered ceftriaxone rather than rifampicin.

Pneumococcal meningitis

Meningitis caused by *Str. pneumoniae* may occur at any age. The mortality in children and adults is about 20 and 35% respectively. The outlook is grave in those over the age of 60 years. There is often a pre-existing focus of infection elsewhere (e.g. pneumonia, acute otitis media, or acute sinusitis), predisposing risk factor (e.g. recent or remote head trauma, recent neurosurgical procedure, CSF leak, sickle cell anaemia, an immunodeficiency state, alcoholism, or an absent spleen). *Str. pneumoniae* is the commonest cause of recurrent or post-traumatic meningitis. Patients who have had a splenectomy are at particular risk of developing overwhelming pneumococcal infection. The onset of pneumococcal meningitis may be sudden and the course rapid with death occurring within 12 h. Alterations of consciousness and focal neurological defects may occur and survivors often suffer significant neurological deficits.

Treatment

Ceftriaxone is the preferred agent to treat pneumococcal meningitis. The global spread of penicillin-resistant pneumococci has eroded the efficacy of benzylpenicillin, which was formerly the drug of choice. Strains of pneumococci that are resistant to expanded-spectrum cephalosporins such as ceftriaxone are being increasingly reported from around the world but are currently rare in the UK; rifampicin or vancomycin have been used in such cases, but are less than ideal.

The duration of treatment is at least 10 days, but is extended up to 14 days in young infants or in complicated cases.

Haemophilus meningitis

Almost all cases of meningitis due to *H. influenzae* are caused by the capsulate type b strains. Before the introduction of the highly successful conjugate vaccine, *H. influenzae* meningitis affected children under six years of age, reflecting the absence of anticapsular antibody in this age group. The mortality was about 7%. The onset of *H. influenzae* meningitis is often insidious, progressing over a period of three to five days. In some infants the illness may be limited to fever, vomiting, and diarrhoea in the early stages, making diagnosis of meningitis difficult.

Treatment and prophylaxis

Cefotaxime or ceftriaxone, which are active against β-lactamase-producing and non-β-lactamase-producing strains of *H. influenzae* are the agents of choice for treatment. Rifampicin is used as prophylaxis for all household contacts when there is an unvaccinated sibling in the house aged four years or younger.

Neonatal meningitis

The highest risk of developing meningitis in the newborn is within the first two months of life, the incidence being about 0.3 per 1000 live births. Neonatal meningitis carries a high mortality. The incidence of neurological deficits in those who survive is also depressingly high. Brain abscess is a rare complication.

Predisposing factors include prematurity, low birth weight, prolonged and difficult labour, prolonged rupture of membranes, and maternal perinatal infection. Some cases complicate congenital defects of the neuraxis.

Neonatal meningitis is usually the result of vertical transfer of pathogens from the mother *in utero* or during delivery, leading to early-onset (occurring within seven days of delivery) septicaemia or meningitis; less commonly they are acquired from the environment, leading to late-onset meningitis (occurring after seven days and occasionally up to two months after delivery). Early-onset disease often presents as overwhelming sepsis syndrome with apnoea and shock. The pulmonary manifestations may be difficult to differentiate from respiratory distress syndrome. Meningitis occurs in 30% of cases. About one in 100 newborns colonized with group B streptococci develop early-onset disease; mortality is over 50%. Late-onset disease usually presents as meningitis and mortality is about 20%.

The early signs and symptoms are often non-specific and include fever, lethargy, and refusal of feed. A bulging fontanelle, resulting from raised intracranial pressure, is a relatively late sign. A high degree of suspicion and prompt investigation with lumbar puncture is essential. Of those who survive, about half will have evidence of neurological damage.

Treatment

Neonatal meningitis is more difficult to treat, since a wide variety of organisms may be involved and their susceptibility to antibiotics can be unpredictable. The chosen therapy should be supported by appropriate laboratory tests.

Group B haemolytic streptococci The treatment of choice is high dose benzylpenicillin for at least two weeks. Some strains show enhanced killing *in vitro* when benzylpenicillin is combined with gentamicin, which may be given for the first seven to 10 days.

Escherichia coli **and other enterobacteria** The most widely used regimen is high-dose cefotaxime often in combination with gentamicin to provide synergistic bactericidal activity against *Esch. coli* or other enterobacteria. Ceftriaxone together with gentamicin is preferred for meningitis caused by salmonellae, and ceftazidime plus gentamicin for *Pseudomonas aeruginosa*. The duration of treatment should be at least three weeks.

Listeria monocytogenes This is a Gram-positive bacillus that exists as a soil saprophyte in nature. Infection is probably acquired from dairy or vegetable produce contaminated from animal sources. The organism may be carried asymptomatically in the gastrointestinal or the female genital tract. The neonate may be infected transplacentally *in utero* or from the genital tract during delivery. Bacteraemia may occur in a pregnant woman following a flu-like illness, which might result in intrauterine infection of the fetus leading to abortion and stillbirth, or the baby may develop symptoms of disseminated infection a few days after delivery. Neonatal mortality with intrauterine listeriosis is about 30%. Most cases of late-onset infection present as meningitis in a previously normal neonate.

L. monocytogenes also causes meningitis in adults, particularly in the elderly, the immunocompromised, or those with an underlying disease. Occasionally the disease occurs in previously healthy adults of all ages.

The organism is sensitive to a variety of agents, but the treatment of choice is high-dose ampicillin with or without gentamicin. In adults with a history of penicillin allergy, intravenous or oral co-trimoxazole (which is bactericidal to *L. monocytogenes*) should be substituted, with chloramphenicol as a further alternative. Cephalosporins have no useful activity against *L. monocytogenes*.

The duration of therapy should be 3 weeks since cerebritis may accompany the meningitis and requires more prolonged treatment.

A summary of current recommendations for the initial therapy of the commoner forms of bacterial meningitis is outlined in Table 28.4.

Table 28.4 Antibiotic treatment of the common types of bacterial meningitis

Age	Cerebrospinal fluid Gram-film findings	Presumptive organism	Treatment of choice Antibiotic(s)	Daily dose (interval)	Duration	Comments
<2 months	Gram-positive cocci in chains	Group B streptococci	Benzyl penicillin+ gentamicin[a]	200 mg/kg (6 h)	2 weeks	In selected patients, gentamicin may be discontinued after 7–10 days
	Gram-negative bacilli	'Coliforms' (usually *Esch. coli*)	Cefotaxime +gentamicin[a]	200 mg/kg (6 h)	3 weeks	Change to ceftriaxone if *Salmonella*, or ceftazidime if *Ps. aeruginosa*
	Gram-positive bacilli	*L. monocytogenes*	Ampicillin + gentamicin[a]	200 mg/kg (6 h)	3 weeks	Rare cause of neonatal meningitis
	No organisms seen	Any of the above	Cefotaxime ± gentamicin[a] ± ampicillin	200 mg/kg (6 h) 200 mg/kg (6 h)	Variable[b]	Ampicillin added if *L. monocytogenes* strongly suspected
2 months- 6 years	Gram-negative diplococci	*N. meningitidis*	Benzylpenicillin	300 mg/kg (4 h)	7 days	Cefotaxime if allergic to penicillin
	Gram-positive diplococci	*Str. pneumoniae*	Benzylpenicillin	300 mg/kg (4 h)	10 days	Cefotaxime or ceftriaxone if allergic to penicillin[c]; in young infants and complicated cases treatment may be extended up to 2 weeks
	Gram-negative coccobacilli	*H. influenzae*	Cefotaxime or ceftriaxone	200 mg/kg (6 h) 80 mg/kg (24 h)	10 days	Chloramphenicol in patients with severe cephalosporin allergy
	No organisms seen	Any of the above 3	Cefotaxime or ceftriaxone	200 mg/kg (6 h) 80 mg/kg (24 h)	Variable[b]	Change as appropriate according to culture result
>6–40 years	Gram-negative diplococci	*N. meningitidis*	Benzylpenicillin	Child: as above Adult: 14.4 g (4 h)	7 days	As above
	Gram-positive diplococci	*Str. pneumoniae*	Benzylpenicillin	As above	10 days	As above[c]
	No organisms seen	Either of the above 2	Ceftriaxone	80 mg/kg (24 h)	Variable[b]	

(continued)

Table 28.4 (Cont'd)

Age	Cerebrospinal fluid Gram-film findings	Presumptive organism	Treatment of choice Antibiotic(s)	Daily dose (interval)	Duration	Comments
>40 years	Gram-positive diplococci	*Str. pneumoniae*	Benzylpenicillin	14.4 g (4 h)	10 days	As above
	Gram-positive bacilli	*L. monocytogenes*	Ampicillin + gentamicin	12 g (4 h)	2–3 weeks	Co-trimoxazole if the patient allergic to penicillin
	Gram-negative bacilli	*Esch. coli*, etc.	Cefotaxime + gentamicin	12 g (4 h)	3 weeks	Or ceftriaxone (4 g once daily) + gentamicin
	No organisms seen	Pneumococci or listeria	Ampicillin	12 g (4 h)	Variable[b]	Add flucloxacillin for neurosurgical patients; change as appropriate according to culture result
Any age	Gram-positive cocci in clusters	Staphylococci (usually *Staph, aureus*)	Flucloxacillin + Rifampicin (oral)	Adult: 12 g (4 h) Child: 200 mg/kg (4–6 h) Adult: 600 mg (12 h) Child: 20 mg/kg (12 h)	3–4 weeks	If shunt-associated removal of shunt usually necessary; vancomycin instead of flucloxacillin if: –patient penicillin allergic –MRSA –*Staph. epidermidis* isolated

MRSA, meticillin resistant *Staph. aureus.*

[a] In neonates with normal renal function, the unit dose is based on the body weight (usually 2.5 mg/kg) but the interval between the doses varies with the gestational age and the postnatal age (gestational age <28 weeks, 24 h; 29–35 weeks, 18 h; 36–40 weeks, 12 h; >41 weeks, 8 h).

[b] Duration will depend on the organism isolated.

[c] Use cefotaxime or ceftriaxone also in areas of high prevalence of pneumococci with reduced susceptibility to penicillin.

Viral and parasitic encephalitis

The treatment of herpes simplex encephalitis and African trypanosomiasis are discussed in Chapters 32 and 35 respectively.

Rarer forms of meningitis

Staphylococcus aureus

Meningitis due to *Staph. aureus* may occur in patients with fulminating septicaemia secondary to pneumonia or endocarditis, or as a complication of penetrating head injury, recent neurosurgical procedures (including insertion of shunts), and ruptured cerebral or epidural abscess. Mortality is high and neurological sequelae are common in survivors.

Most *Staph. aureus* strains are resistant to penicillin. For meticillin-sensitive strains high-dose flucloxacillin (at least 12 g daily) combined with oral rifampicin (600 mg daily) is recommended in adults. In patients who are allergic to penicillin or in meningitis due to meticillin-resistant strains, treatment is even more problematic. Parenteral vancomycin (1 g every 12 h) combined with oral rifampicin is recommended. However, since penetration of vancomycin into the CSF is limited, daily intraventricular vancomycin should also be considered. Intraventricular vancomycin is also warranted in meningitis with meticillin-sensitive strains if the CSF is persistently positive despite flucloxacillin and rifampicin, and in patients with shunt-associated meningitis. The duration of treatment for *Staph. aureus* meningitis should be at least three weeks.

Shunt-associated meningitis

In patients with hydrocephalus the ventricular CSF is diverted to other compartments of the body (usually the peritoneal cavity) with a silastic catheter (shunt). Unfortunately, 15–25% of these patients develop meningitis at some point in the life of the shunt. *Staph. epidermidis* accounts for about half and *Staph. aureus* for about a quarter of shunt infections. Among many other micro-organisms associated with such infections are *Propionibacterium acnes*, diphtheroids, enterococci, and Gram-negative bacilli. Most infections are believed to be due to colonization of the shunt at the time of surgery; occasionally organisms may reach the CSF and shunt through the bloodstream or by retrograde spread. Examination of the CSF obtained by needle aspiration of the reservoir is essential and yields an organism in over 90% of cases. It is not unusual to isolate bacteria from an otherwise normal CSF. Blood cultures are positive only if meningitis is associated with a ventriculo-atrial shunt.

Some patients who develop meningitis due to *N. meningitidis, H. influenzae,* or *Str. pneumoniae* are treated with appropriate antibiotics, without shunt removal. However, many infections will fail to be controlled unless there is complete removal of the shunt.

Since *Staph. epidermidis* is commonly resistant to flucloxacillin, therapy should be commenced with parenteral vancomycin combined with oral rifampicin and daily intraventricular vancomycin. High-dose flucloxacillin should be substituted for parenteral vancomycin if the isolate proves sensitive. Treatment should be continued for two to three weeks before a new shunt is inserted.

Mycobacterium tuberculosis

Tuberculous meningitis can affect any age. It is uncommon in developed countries and cases can be missed unless the physician is aware of the possibility and the laboratory is willing to exclude tuberculous meningitis in all cases in which abnormal clinical or CSF findings (increased lymphocytes, raised protein, low CSF glucose) have not been satisfactorily explained. The treatment of tuberculous meningitis is described in Chapter 30.

Cryptococcal meningitis

Cryptococcus neoformans is a saprophytic encapsulated fungus commonly found in soil and pigeon droppings. It is an uncommon cause of meningitis, occurring mainly in patients who are immunocompromised due to disease or drugs. Cryptococcal meningitis is reported to occur in about 4% of AIDS patients in the UK and up to a third of African patients with AIDS. It is probably transmitted via the respiratory tract. Most patients present with features of a subacute meningitis or meningo-encephalitis.

The treatment of cryptococcal CNS disease consists of an initial two week induction phase with intravenous amphotericin, with or without flucytosine (by mouth or intravenously). Flucytosine is associated with more rapid sterilization of the CSF and fewer failures or relapses. Following induction, a consolidation phase with fluconazole is adopted. Lipid formulations of amphotericin are increasingly being used as an alternative to amphotericin. The total duration of treatment is determined by clinical response, monitoring levels of cryptococcal antigen in the blood and CSF and central nervous system imaging where appropriate. In those with underlying HIV infection and low CD4 counts fluconazole is used long term as chemoprophylaxis to prevent recurrent infection.

Culture-negative pyogenic meningitis

About 40% of patients presenting with meningitis will already have received antimicrobial therapy before lumbar puncture and this may lead to failure to isolate the organism. Prior therapy does not seriously alter cell counts or protein and glucose concentrations and it is usually still possible to differentiate between bacterial and viral meningitis. In about 10% of cases the aetiology remains unknown.

Although prior therapy may confuse the clinical picture it is not detrimental to the individual patient who has as good a prognosis as those who are untreated. 'Best guess' therapy should be aimed at common bacterial pathogens; ceftriaxone (or cefotaxime) with or without gentamicin for seven to 14 days is a reasonable choice. The duration of therapy should be determined by clinical response and repeat CSF examination where appropriate. In the presence of an obvious meningococcal rash seven days treatment is sufficient.

All patients in whom there is no history of previous antibiotic to account for the negative results must be investigated further to exclude conditions such as tuberculous or cryptococcal meningitis, superficial brain abscess, or other parameningeal infections.

Brain abscess

Brain abscess is a localized collection of pus within the brain parenchyma. It is a life-threatening condition, although the mortality has been reduced to less than 10% by the introduction of CT and magnetic resonance imaging, leading to earlier diagnosis and more precise localization; by improvements in surgical and bacteriological techniques; and by the use of appropriate antibiotics. About four to 10 cases a year are seen in neurological units of developed countries. Brain abscess in children accounts for less than 25% of all cases and, except in neonates, it is rare in those under 2 years of age.

Pathogenesis

Brain abscesses develop most commonly by spread of infection from an adjacent cranial site (e.g. paranasal sinuses, middle ear, mastoid, or teeth), following a penetrating cranial trauma or neurosurgery, or by haematogenous spread from a distant site (e.g. lung abscess, bronchiectasis, or endocarditis). Blood-borne spread often leads to multiple abscess formation. In about 20% of cases the primary focus of infection remains unrecognized—so-called cryptogenic abscess.

The organisms isolated usually reflect those found in the primary focus of infection. With proper attention to microbiological culture techniques, the role of anaerobes and polymicrobial infection has become apparent. Brain abscess in association with sinusitis is usually located in the frontal lobe and is most commonly caused by *Str. milleri* with or without anaerobes. In contrast, brain abscess following chronic suppurative otitis media or mastoiditis is usually located in the temporal lobe or cerebellum. The infection is invariably polymicrobial, and the pus obtained may yield a variety of anaerobic and aerobic bacteria. *Staph. aureus* is usually isolated in pure culture from brain abscess that has followed trauma or neurosurgery, or is secondary to a haematogenous spread from infective endocarditis, whereas *Str. milleri* together with anaerobes and other respiratory pathogens should be suspected in brain abscess complicating pyogenic lung abscess. Rare causes include *M. tuberculosis, L. monocytogenes, Nocardia asteroides, Toxoplasma gondii, Cryptococcus neoformans*, and other fungi.

Treatment

Although some patients with early cerebritis, or small, deep, or multiple abscesses have been treated successfully with antimicrobial therapy alone, most require surgical drainage. CT-guided stereotaxic aspiration allows more accurate drainage with minimal interference to the surrounding normal brain. Lumbar puncture is unhelpful in diagnosis and may be hazardous. Blood cultures may be positive and should be taken.

Pus obtained after any of these procedures requires prompt microscopy and culture. Because mixtures of aerobic and anaerobic bacteria are likely, antimicrobial therapy should cover both possibilities. Cefotaxime or other similar agents (ceftriaxone, ceftazidime) are recommended. When used in high doses these antibiotics penetrate well into brain abscess pus, and they are bactericidal against many of the organisms commonly encountered, including *Str. milleri, Actinomyces* spp., and enterobacteria. However, cephalosporins are not reliably bactericidal against all anaerobes, and for this reason metronidazole should also be used. This agent is bactericidal for almost all anaerobes and therapeutic concentrations are achieved in the brain.

The initial choice of empirical antimicrobial therapy in brain abscess depends on the site of the abscess, any predisposing factors, and the results of the Gram-film examination of pus, if available. Therapy may be modified, if required, once the culture results are available.

Frontal lobe abscess of sinus origin should be treated with high (meningitic) doses of benzylpenicillin in combination with metronidazole, since *Str. milleri*—with or without anaerobes—is a frequent pathogen. Temporal lobe or cerebellar abscess of otogenic origin is treated with a combination of high-dose ceftriaxone and metronidazole. Gentamicin may be added to this regimen if coliform organisms are seen on the Gram-film or are grown in culture. For brain abscesses secondary to trauma or a neurosurgical procedure, or when *Staph. aureus* is strongly suspected or grown, high-dose flucloxacillin in combination with oral rifampicin should be used, and in the case of MRSA, vancomycin.

The duration of antimicrobial therapy remains unsettled. It is our practice to administer antibiotics parenterally for at least three weeks to all surgically treated patients, often followed by appropriate oral therapy for four to six weeks.

Key points

- Bacterial meningitis is a life threatening disease and requires rapid diagnosis and treatment.

- *Streptococcus pneumoniae* and *Neisseria meningitidis* are the lead causes of bacterial meningitis. In the neonate, *Escherichia coli* and Group B streptococci predominate.

- Treatment requires high dose parenteral antibiotic such as penicillin or ceftriaxone that can penetrate the CSF; treatment is tailored to the particular pathogen.

- Abscesses of the brain vary by site; their microbiology is often mixed and reflects the predisposing condition. Their management requires coordination of radiological, neurosurgical and antibiotic expertise.Other causes of CNS infections include mycobacteria, viruses (meningitis and encephalitis) and rarely fungi and parasites.

Further reading

Quagliarello V, Scheld WM (1992), 'Bacterial meningitis: pathogenesis, pathophysiology, and progress', *New England Journal of Medicine*, **327** (12): 864–72.

Finch RG, Greenwood D, Norrby SR, Whitley RJ (2010), 'Bacterial infections of the central nervous system', in *Antibiotic and chemotherapy: anti-infective agents and their use in therapy* (9th edn), London: Elsevier Saunders, 633–649.

Finch RG, Greenwood D, Norrby SR, Whitley RJ (2010), 'Viral infections of the central nervous system', in *Antibiotic and chemotherapy: anti-infective agents and their use in therapy* (9th edn), London: Elsevier Saunders, 650–658.

Chapter 29

Skin and soft tissue infections

General considerations

At birth the skin of the baby rapidly becomes colonized with bacteria from the mother, other handlers, and the environment. Some of these essentially non-pathogenic microbes, including coryneforms, coagulase-negative staphylococci, micrococci, and propionibacteria become established as the resident flora of the normal skin. In intact skin, these micro-organisms usually prevent potential pathogens such as *Staphylococcus aureus* and *Streptococcus pyogenes* (haemolytic streptococci of Lancefield group A) from becoming established. However, if the skin is broken by accidental or surgical trauma, burns, a foreign body, or a primary skin disease (psoriasis, atopic dermatitis), these pathogens may not only become established as resident organisms; they may also give rise to infection of the skin and subcutaneous tissue.

Other bacteria from, for example, faeces or the environment can briefly colonize the skin as transient flora; they are readily removed by washing, whereas resident organisms will persist in moderate numbers despite even the most thorough skin disinfection. If introduced through, for example, a dirty wound or compound fracture, transient micro-organisms can also give rise to skin and soft-tissue infection. Such infections are often polymicrobial (mixed).

The general condition of the patient, including factors such as underlying immunodeficiency, diabetes mellitus, or systemic or topical treatment with corticosteroids, can also predispose to skin infection. Treatment with broad-spectrum antibiotics, which disrupts the resident flora, can give rise to cutaneous candidiasis (thrush). In one of the commonest skin infections—a boil or furuncle—there is usually no evident breach in the skin nor any other predisposing factor.

Many different micro-organisms, including bacteria, fungi, and some viruses, may be involved in skin and soft-tissue infections. However, by far the commonest bacterial causes are *Staph. aureus* and *Str. pyogenes*. Thrush is usually caused by the yeast *Candida albicans*, and cold sores by the virus herpes simplex.

Skin and soft tissue infections are common (Fig. 29.1) and frequently severe (Table 29.1). In European hospitals skin, soft tissue, bone, and joint infections account for 19% of all antibiotic treatments, second only to respiratory tract infections (Fig. 29.1) Nearly a quarter of hospital inpatients with skin and soft tissue infection have sepsis and a third of patients with severe sepsis die (Table 29.1).

Common clinical presentations

Impetigo

Impetigo consists of discrete purulent lesions on the exposed areas of the body, especially the face and extremities. It is nearly always caused by *Str. pyogenes* or *Staph. aureus*. Impetigo is most common in tropical countries but is also prevalent in more temperate zones especially during the summer. It is most common in children aged two to five years but can occur in older children or adults. The prevalence is strongly related to personal hygiene and impetigo is much commoner in socially deprived communities.

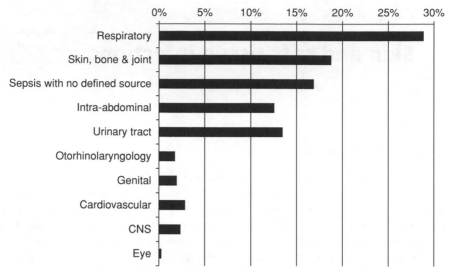

Fig. 29.1 Anatomical sites recorded for antibiotic treatment of 2760 patients in 20 European hospitals. Drawn from data in Table 2 of Ansari, F, Erntell, M, Goossens, H, Davey, P (2009) The European surveillance of antimicrobial consumption (ESAC) point-prevalence survey of antibacterial use in 20 European hospitals in 2006. *Clinical Infectious Diseases* **49**(10): 1496–1504.

The lesions of impetigo start with papules that evolve into pustules and then form a characteristic thick crust over 4–7 days. The lesions are sometimes bullous. Antibacterial treatment can be either topical or systemic (Table 29.2).

Pustular lesions

Such lesions of the skin are by far the commonest bacterial infection in man and include:

◆ folliculitis (pimples), where the infection is confined to hair follicles and does not involve the surrounding skin or subcutaneous tissue; such infections are usually mild and self-limiting, and do not need medical attention;

Table 29.1 Appropriateness of antibiotic treatment and mortality by severity of sepsis for 189 hospital inpatients with skin and soft tissue infection. From data in Marwick, C, Broomhall, J, McCowan, C, Philips, G, Gonzalez-McQuire, S, Akhras, K, Merchant, S, Nathwani, D, Davey, P (2011) Severity assessment of skin and soft tissue infections: cohort study of management and outcomes for hospitalised patients. *Journal of Antimicrobial Chemotherapy* **66**(2): 387–397

Severity of sepsis	Number (% total)	Treatment classification by comparison with UK guidance			Mortality
		appropriate treatment	over-treatment	under-treatment	
No sepsis	144 (76%)	27%	63%	24%	6%
Sepsis without organ impairment	33 (18%)	30%	30%	39%	18%
Severe sepsis	12 (6%)	8%	0%	92%	33%
All	189	26%	43%	31%	10%

◆ furuncles (boils), where the folliculitis has spread deeper and is surrounded by an area of cellulitis;

◆ carbuncles, where several furuncles have coalesced and extended into subcutaneous fat to form a large, indurated, painful lesion that contains loculated pus with multiple drainage points.

Antibiotics are rarely required for these lesions unless they are recurrent (Table 29.2). Acne is discussed in Chapter 22.

Cellulitis and erysipelas

These are both diffuse, spreading skin lesions. Cellulitis, which is much more common, occurs in the deeper layers of the skin and subcutaneous tissues. The obviously affected area is red and hot but the demarcation between this and the normal skin is gradual and there is no palpable raised margin. It is more common if there is obstruction to venous or lymphatic drainage or gross obesity, which make the skin more fragile and local host defences less effective. In contrast erysipelas occurs in the superficial layers of the skin, which results in a very clear, abrupt line of demarcation between the affected and normal skin, with a palpable lesion that is raised above the level of the normal skin. Cellulitis may be caused by *Str. pyogenes* or *Staph. aureus*, whereas erysipelas is almost always caused by *Str. pyogenes*. Erysipelas usually occurs on the face or on the legs, whereas cellulitis can occur anywhere on the body although it is commonest on the legs. Both types of lesion are usually preceded by a break in the skin. Meticillin-resistant *Staph. aureus* (MRSA) is increasingly incriminated in community-acquired cellulitis in some countries.

Signs of spreading infection include extension of the line of demarcation, lymphangitis (infection spreading up the lymph vessels with a characteristic thin streak of erythema running up to a lymph node), and painful tender lymph nodes distal to the lesion. Systemic inflammatory response means that the patient has sepsis and is at risk of progressing to severe sepsis or septic shock (see Chapter 26). Blood cultures should be taken from patients with sepsis arising from cellulitis, as about 50% are positive.

Both cellulitis and erysipelas can be treated with an antistaphylococcal penicillin. In theory erysipelas could be treated with penicillin V, but it is not worth taking the risk that the cause may be *Staph. aureus*. There is a belief that an antistaphylococcal penicillin should be combined with benzylpenicillin or penicillin V, since the latter are much more active against *Str. pyogenes*. However, provided antistaphylococcal penicillins are given in adequate dosage they are just as effective alone.

Prevention of recurrent cellulitis requires enhancement of host defences by preventing breaks in the skin (e.g. dry thoroughly between the toes after washing), or wearing compression stockings to reduce oedema. If these measures fail then long-term prophylactic antibiotics are unfortunately not usually effective. It is preferable to give the patient a course of antibiotics to start as soon as symptoms begin.

Cellulitis following animal or human bites

Infections following animal bites are polymicrobial, often including anaerobic bacteria and unusual organisms such as *Pasteurella multocida*, a human pathogen that is part of the normal oral flora of cats. Human bites are often associated with greater damage to the skin and soft tissues and are also polymicrobial with aerobic and anaerobic bacteria. Co-amoxiclav is an effective treatment for all these infections (Table 29.2).

Diabetic foot infections

Infections of the feet are particularly common in diabetics because several important host defences, including circulation and sensation, are compromised. This enables minor injuries to progress to advanced stages of infection rapidly and with very few symptoms. Consequently it is

Table 29.2 Most likely bacterial causes and antibacterial treatment for common skin infections

Clinical diagnosis	Most likely causes	Antibacterial treatment
Impetigo	*Str. pyogenes*	Topical: fusidic acid or mupirocin; reserve for patients with a limited number of lesions
	Staph. aureus	
		Systemic: antistaphylococcal penicillin (e.g. flucloxacillin), clindamycin, or a tetracycline
Pustules, furuncles and carbuncles	*Staph. aureus*	Small lesions: no treatment is required in most cases
		Larger lesions: incision and drainage. Antibiotics required only if there are signs of spreading cellulitis or systemic inflammation
		Recurrent lesions: topical mupirocin to the nose for the first 5 days of each month. If this fails try clindamycin 150 mg once daily dose for 3 months
Uncomplicated cellulitis and erysipelas	*Str. pyogenes,* *Staph. aureus*	Antistaphylococcal penicillin (e.g. flucloxacillin), clindamycin, or a tetracycline
		See Figure 29.2 for management of severe infections
Animal bites	Bacteria from the animal's normal mouth flora (e.g. *Pasteurella multocida*)	Co-amoxiclav. For penicillin-allergic patients doxycycline plus metronidazole
Human bites	Mixed aerobic and anaerobic mouth flora	Co-amoxiclav. For penicillin-allergic patients clindamycin plus a fluoroquinolone
Diabetic foot infections	*Str. Pyogenes, Staph. Aureus,* Gram-negative aerobic bacteria, anaerobic bacteria	Co-amoxiclav. For penicillin allergic patients clindamycin + a fluoroquinolone unless at high risk of *C. difficile* infection

vital to educate patients with diabetes about how to avoid trauma to the feet and how to recognize infection early. Patients with diabetes also have impaired healing so that chronic ulcers are common.

Chronic ulcers without spreading cellulitis do not require antibiotic treatment, even if there is some purulence in the exudate as this simply indicates bacterial colonization of the ulcer. If there is cellulitis spreading up to 2 cm from the margin of the ulcer the infection is likely to respond to oral antibiotics, but if the infection spreads more widely or is associated with signs of sepsis then referral to hospital for intravenous treatment should be considered. Taking swabs from chronic ulcers is not helpful because they will be colonized with possibly harmless bacteria; even if infection is present the bacteria cultured are not always the ones that are responsible. Meaningful cultures can be obtained only by debriding the ulcer and then obtaining tissue specimens from the base of the lesion by curettage (scrapings with a sterile blade). Empirical treatment should cover both aerobic and anaerobic pathogens (Table 29.2).

Because of the combination of impaired circulation and sensation diabetic foot infections are particularly likely to progress to osteomyelitis because they may be present for weeks before the patient seeks medical attention. Osteomyelitis should be considered as a potential complication of any deep or extensive ulcer, especially if it is overlying a bony prominence or contains visible bone particles. Management of osteomyelitis is considered in Chapter 27.

Miscellaneous infections

Viral infections of the skin, such as herpes simplex and varicella zoster, are discussed in Chapter 32. Superficial fungal infections usually respond to topical therapy (Chapter 22), although dermatophyte infections of finger- or toenails may require oral treatment with terbinafine for up to 3 months, or with griseofulvin for a year or more. These agents are deposited in newly formed keratin and the prolonged treatment is needed to allow healthy nail to replace the diseased tissue. Even so, treatment of chronic infections of toenails may be unsuccessful, although terbinafine is more reliable in this respect than griseofulvin.

Severe skin and soft tissue infections

Necrotising fasciitis and toxic shock syndrome have received considerable media attention. However both of these problems are rare in comparison with severe sepsis associated with cellulitis. In comparison with pneumonia relatively little attention has been given to auditing and improving the management of severe skin and soft tissue infection. The principles of treatment are not complex (Table 29.1 and Fig. 29.2):

1 Oral, narrow spectrum therapy for uncomplicated cellulitis.

2 Intravenous narrow spectrum therapy for sepsis without organ impairment.

3 Broad spectrum intravenous therapy for patients with severe sepsis or evidence of necrotising fasciitis. This should include clindamycin both for cover against anaerobic bacteria and because clindamycin reduces toxin production by bacteria.

However, studies of the management of skin and soft tissue infection show that most antibiotic treatment is inappropriate, with under treatment of severe infections as well as over treatment of uncomplicated infections (Table 29.1). In this cohort study 35 different antibiotic regimens were used for initial treatment of skin and soft tissue infections, whereas the protocol in Fig. 29.2 contains six regimens that should cover all eventualities. Hospitals need to audit and improve their management of these common infections.

Necrotising skin and soft tissue infections: These are rapidly spreading and life-threatening forms of cellulitis that involve the deeper fascial and/or muscle compartments in addition to skin and subcutaneous tissue. Infection usually arises following a break in the skin after trauma or elective surgery. Most cases are caused by *Str. pyogenes* either alone or in combination with other bacteria, including *Staph. aureus*, coliform bacilli, and anaerobes. *Staph. aureus* strains that produce the PVL (Panton Vallentine Leukocydin) toxin are also associated with necrotising infections. Many variations of necrotising skin and soft tissue infections have been described according to the tissues involved, the anatomical site of the infection and the microbial causes, but the basic principles of management are the same. The key is early distinction between a cellulitis that will respond to antibacterial treatment and a deeper necrotising infection that is likely to require surgical debridement as well. The following clinical features indicate the possibility of necrotising infection:

♦ severe, constant pain that is disproportionate to the visible inflammation in the skin;

♦ bullae on the skin, which occur because of occlusion of deep blood vessels that cross the fascia or muscle compartments;

♦ skin necrosis or bruising;

♦ gas in the soft tissues detected by palpation or imaging;

♦ oedema that extends beyond the margin of erythema;

♦ cutaneous anaesthesia;

♦ systemic toxicity, manifested by signs of severe sepsis (see Chapter 26);

♦ rapid spread of infection despite appropriate antibiotic therapy.

Blood cultures are often positive and streptococci can also be isolated from the bullous lesions. The management of these rare conditions is primarily surgical, with radical debridement of all necrotic tissue, intensive life-support therapy, and the treatment of shock. Antimicrobial therapy

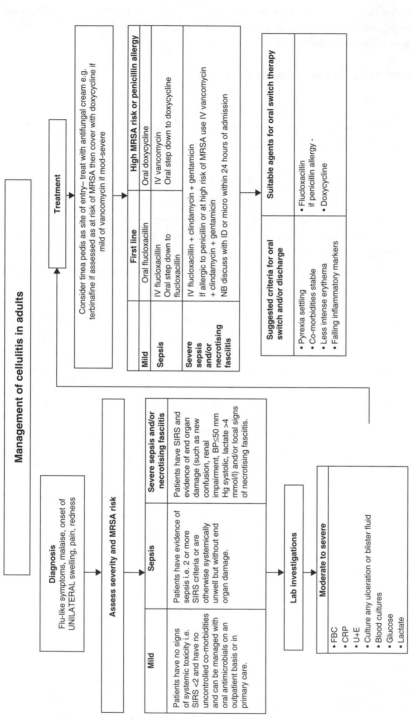

Fig. 29.2 Protocol for management of cellulitis in adults in hospitals. Adapted from NHS Tayside Antibiotic Policy http://www.nhstaysideadtc.scot.nhs.uk/TAPG%20html/MAIN/Front%20page.htm.

must be directed against aerobic Gram-positive and Gram-negative bacteria and against anaerobic bacteria until the results of cultures are available. Clindamycin is active against aerobic Gram-positive and anaerobic pathogens, it also suppresses toxin production by group A streptococci and may be superior to penicillins for these infections. Gentamicin should be added initially to treat Gram-negative aerobic pathogens.

Gas gangrene: Gas gangrene (clostridial myositis) is a life-threatening, invasive infection that can be caused by several species of *Clostridium*, principally *C. perfringens*. These bacteria are part of the normal intestinal flora of man and animals, and clostridial spores are common in soil. Gas gangrene develops when impaired blood supply, tissue necrosis, or the presence of foreign bodies produce a low oxygen tension in the tissues and thus create conditions in which the spores can germinate. Extensive soft-tissue injury contaminated with soil or dirt carries an increased risk of gas gangrene. Gas gangrene may rarely complicate surgical wounds, particularly after intestinal or biliary surgery, or be a complication of septic abortion. Clostridial anaerobic cellulitis occurs under similar circumstances, but exploration of the wound usually reveals that the muscle is spared.

A clinical diagnosis is made on the basis of palpable (crepitus) or radiological signs of a spreading, gas-producing infection in a toxic patient with the above risk factors. Immediate and extensive surgical excision of all involved tissues and the removal of any foreign body are essential, and may mean hysterectomy (after septic abortion), excision of subcutaneous tissue and muscle of the abdominal wall, or even amputation of a limb. Parenteral benzylpenicillin should also be given promptly in high dosage. For patients allergic to penicillin, metronidazole may be used. Despite these desperate and mutilating measures, the mortality remains high.

Toxic shock syndrome

Certain phage types of *Staph. aureus* and *Str. pyogenes* produce toxins that cause a multisystem disease characterized by the sudden onset of fever, myalgia, vomiting, diarrhoea, hypotension, and an erythematous rash: the toxic shock syndrome. Staphylococcal toxic shock syndrome was originally thought to affect only menstruating women who used a particular type of tampon; it is now known to be a rare sequel of any type of staphylococcal infection. An antistaphylococcal penicillin (e.g. flucloxacillin) or clindamycin should be given, but antibiotic therapy is secondary to systemic support. Clinical results with intravenous immunoglobulin are inconsistent, probably because different batches of immunoglobulin contain variable quantities of neutralizing antibodies to some of these toxins.

MRSA infections and PVL toxin

MRSA is most likely to cause skin and soft tissue infections in hospital patients and the risk of MRSA colonization increases with duration of hospitalization. However, patients may present from the community with MRSA infection despite having no contact with hospitals or healthcare. Strains of MRSA that cause community-acquired infection are genetically and phenotypically distinct from hospital-acquired MRSA. They typically resemble some strains of meticillin-susceptible *S. aureus* (MSSA) in being susceptible to a wider range of anti-staphylococcal antibiotics (some are resistant only to β-lactams), and often produce PVL, a toxin that destroys white blood cells and is a staphylococcal virulence factor. In the UK both community-acquired MRSA infection and infection with PVL producing strains of *Staph. aureus* are rare. The overall prevalence of *Staph. aureus* strains that carry the gene for PVL production is believed to be <2.0%, and these are mainly MSSA. PVL toxin-related infection should be suspected in patients with recurrent boils or abscesses or with necrotising skin infection or with community-acquired necrotising or haemorrhagic pneumonia.

Key points

◆ Many different micro-organisms, including bacteria, fungi, and some viruses, may be involved in skin and soft-tissue infections. However, by far the commonest bacterial causes are *Staph. aureus* and *Str. pyogenes*.

◆ Skin and soft tissue infections are common and may be severe. In European hospitals skin, soft tissue, bone, and joint infections account for 19% of all antibiotic treatments, second only to respiratory tract infections. Nearly a quarter of hospital inpatients with skin and soft tissue infection have sepsis and a third of patients with severe sepsis die.

◆ Many skin infections are localized (impetigo, pustules, and abscesses). However, spreading cellulitis indicates invasive infection with risk of progression to sepsis.

◆ The principles of treatment are simple so it is disturbing that both over-treatment of mild cases and under-treatment of severe cases are common.

1 Oral, narrow-spectrum therapy for uncomplicated cellulitis.

2 Intravenous narrow-spectrum therapy for sepsis without organ impairment.

3 Broad-spectrum intravenous therapy for patients with severe sepsis or evidence of necrotising fasciitis. This should include clindamycin both for cover against anaerobic bacteria and because clindamycin reduces toxin production by bacteria.

Further reading

Lipsky BA, Berendt AR, Deery HG, Embil JM, Joseph WS, Karchmer AW, LeFrock JL, Lew DP, Mader JT, Norden C, Tan JS (2004), 'Diagnosis and treatment of diabetic foot infections', *Clinical Infectious Diseases*, **39**: 885–910.

Nathwani, D, Morgan, M, Masterton, RG, Dryden, M, Cookson, BD, French, G, Lewis, D (2008) 'Guidelines for UK practice for the diagnosis and management of meticillin-resistant Staphylococcus aureus (MRSA) infections presenting in the community', *Journal of Antimicrobial Chemotherapy*, **61**(5): 976–994.

Stevens DL, Bisno AL, Chambers HF, Everett ED, Dellinger P, Goldstein EJ, Gorbach SL, Hirschmann JV, Kaplan EL, Montoya JG, Wade JC (2005), 'Practice guidelines for the diagnosis and management of skin and soft-tissue infections', *Clinical Infectious Diseases*, **41**: 1373–1406.

Chapter 30

Tuberculosis and other mycobacterial diseases

Tuberculosis

Tuberculosis (TB) is one of the most widespread human infections. The World Health Organization (WHO) estimates that a third of the world's population harbour *Mycobacterium tuberculosis*, and every year more than eight million people develop new clinical disease. The pulmonary form was described by Hippocrates, and characteristic lesions of TB of the spine have been demonstrated in the mummies of ancient Egypt. The disease attacks both man and animals, affects all ages and every organ in the body, and ranges from latent to hyperacute (the 'galloping consumption' of Victorian times), killing young and old alike, the famous and the unknown. This reservoir of infected persons is made up of those with infectious pulmonary TB (sputum-smear positive) who can infect between 10 and 15 people every year. Co-infection with human immunodeficiency virus (HIV) is the most potent risk factor for the development of active TB: according to the WHO over 40 million people are co-infected.

The last 60 years have seen enormous progress in the understanding of the epidemiology, prevention, and treatment of TB and, although far from eradicated, this age-old killer of man has become a preventable and curable disease. The prevalence in a population is linked to a number of socio-economic factors, notably poverty, malnutrition, social exclusion, and poor health services. Furthermore, the HIV pandemic has magnified the impact of TB, particularly in sub-Saharan Africa, where co-infection rates are greatest. Prisoners and migrants from resource-poor countries are also vulnerable. The control of TB is a global healthcare priority and cannot be successful unless HIV prevention and control become parallel priorities.

Immune response

Immunity in TB is cell mediated; the key to restriction of intracellular growth of the bacillus is co-operation between macrophages and sensitized lymphocytes. Humoral reactions are thought to play little part. The generation of clones of antigen-specific T cells initiates the immune response, which is depressed in HIV-positive patients. T-cell clones may facilitate elimination of the pathogen by macrophage activation and granuloma formation or by cytotoxic action; or they may interact with B cells to produce specific antibodies, which, in conjunction with phagocytic cells or complement, also act as an effector arm. The mechanism by which mycobacteria survive inside activated macrophages is unknown and may be oxygen dependent or oxygen independent. A genetic predisposition to tuberculous disease has been sought. Certain HLA-haplotypes have been associated with heightened susceptibility.

Principles of management

TB can affect many organs and tissues (Table 30.1). However, the pulmonary form of the disease is most common (65%) and accounts for its spread. The effective management of pulmonary TB

Table 30.1 Tuberculosis: presenting infections

Common	Less common	Uncommon
Pulmonary	Meningitis	Pericardial
Lymph node	Intra-abdominal	Skin
Genito-urinary	Bone	

therefore remains the greatest priority in controlling this disease. The key components of management are:

- rapid detection of active disease;
- reliable microbiological diagnosis;
- supervised treatment with combination chemotherapy;
- notification of cases and contact tracing;
- monitoring for drug-resistant disease;
- continuous reporting and surveillance.

Vaccination is included in this strategy by some countries, including the UK. The vaccine is based on a laboratory-modified strain of *M. bovis*, which is administered as BCG (bacille Calmette-Guérin—named after the two French originators of the vaccine). However, the efficacy of this vaccine has proved highly variable in published studies. Furthermore, it requires pre-immunization Mantoux test screening of the recipients using tuberculin (an extract of *M. tuberculosis*) to distinguish between previously infected (positive tuberculin test) and non-infected (negative tuberculin test) persons. Because of the logistics of testing, and the occasional difficulty in interpreting the skin test outcome, together with the fact that the vaccine sensitizes recipients to tuberculin thus reducing its value in skin testing to identify at-risk persons, many countries have not adopted this approach. In the UK BCG immunization is now restricted to babies and older people who are most at risk of TB, such as those living in areas with a high rate of TB or whose parents or grandparents were born in countries with a high prevalence of the disease and children less than 16 exposed to a case of respiratory tuberculosis.

Clinical diagnosis

Symptoms of persistent cough, often with minimal sputum production, occasional coughing up of blood (haemoptysis), weight loss, and sweats (often at night) should all raise suspicions for pulmonary TB. A chest X-ray will often show evidence of diffuse upper lobe streaking and consolidation. More advanced disease results in cavity formation.

Microbiological diagnosis

Specimens, notably sputum from patients with suspected pulmonary TB, should be examined microscopically using either a fluorescent stain (auramine) or the more traditional Ziehl-Neelsen stain. The microscopic detection of bacilli with the typical appearances of *M. tuberculosis* permits early diagnosis. Such a patient is classified as 'smear-positive' and managed as if they have 'open' (contagious) TB.

Other samples for diagnosis include biopsy material (lymph node, bone marrow, other tissues). Culture of *M. tuberculosis* is slow and may take three to six weeks to confirm the diagnosis. More rapid semi-automated broth-based cultures are being increasingly adopted. Susceptibility testing of anti-TB drugs adds to the length of this process. Rapid methods of identification are becoming more widely available, including rapid tests of susceptibility to isoniazid and rifampicin.

Table 30.2 Recommended first line treatment regimens for tuberculosis in adults

Drug	Initial phase (2 months)	Continuation phase (4 months)	Major side effects
Standard regimen			
Rifampicin	10 mg/kg/day (450–600 mg/day)	10 mg/kg/day (450–600 mg/day)	Hepatitis; gastrointestinal upsets
Isoniazid[a]	5 mg/kg/day (200–300 mg/day)	5 mg/kg/day (200–300 mg/day)	Peripheral neuropathy; hepatitis
Pyrazinamide	30 mg/kg/day (1.5–2 g/day)		Gastrointestinal upsets; gout
Ethambutol	15 mg/kg/day		Retrobulbar neuritis
Intermittent regimen (3 times weekly)			
Rifampicin	10 mg/kg	10 mg/kg	As above
Isoniazid	15 mg/kg	15 mg/kg	
Pyrazinamide	50 mg/kg		
Ethambutol	30 mg/kg		

[a] Or streptomycin (15 mg/kg/day or 0.75–1 g/day for 2 months if resistant to isoniazid).

Treatment

The chemotherapy of human TB has depended almost entirely on large prospective controlled trials of different regimens, which have helped define the current recommendations for the treatment and prevention of the disease. There is still no *in vitro* or animal model that can reliably predict the response to treatment in man.

Standard first-line treatment for TB requires compliance with a multidrug regimen for a minimum period of six months. Rifampicin and isoniazid are potent anti-TB agents and are administered throughout the six months. Pyrazinamide is added for the initial two months. A further drug, such as ethambutol is also included for the first two months if there are concerns about drug-resistant disease, with streptomycin as a further alternative (Table 30.2).

The rationale for this multidrug regimen is to provide effective therapy while avoiding the emergence of naturally occurring low frequency drug-resistant mutant strains of *M. tuberculosis*, which may cause relapse of the disease following the eradication of the susceptible strains. The initial three to four drug regimen is effective in preventing this from happening. Under normal circumstances, culture and sensitivity information should be available by two months to permit the safe transfer to rifampicin and isoniazid for the final four months of treatment.

Multidrug-resistant TB, defined as resistance to both isoniazid and rifampicin, is increasing worldwide. It currently accounts for less than 5% of isolates in the UK but has reached very high levels (>35%) in parts of Russia and some eastern European countries. This is of major concern since laboratory facilities to support the clinical management of TB in resource-poor countries are often inadequate and coincide with highest incidence rates of disease, including that caused by multiresistant TB. Second-line agents for treating TB (Table 30.3) are not only less active but often more toxic than first-line drugs. Treatment must also be prolonged for periods of up to 18–24 months.

Treatment of TB requires expert supervision and should be under the direction of a specialist in respiratory medicine or infectious diseases and supporting staff. The key factors to a successful outcome are compliance with the regimen, an assured supply of medication, avoidance of interactions

Table 30.3 Second-line drugs for the treatment of tuberculosis in adults

Drug	Usual adult dose	Toxicity
Amikacin	7.5 mg/kg every 12 h[a]	Nephrotoxicity, ototoxicity, rash, neuromuscular blockade, eosinophilia
Capreomycin	1 g/day	Nephrotoxicity, ototoxicity, hypersensitivity
Ciprofloxacin[b]	750 mg every 12 h	Gastrointestinal intolerance, crystaluria, tremor, convulsions, rash, hepatitis, renal failure
Cycloserine	250 mg every 12 h or every 8 h	Seizures, psychoses, various central nervous system effects
Ethionamide (protionamide)	0.5–1.0 g/day (divided dose)	Gastrointestinal intolerance, hepatitis, hypersensitivity, convulsions, depression, alopecia
Kanamycin	15 mg every 12 h[a]	Nephrotoxicity, ototoxicity, hypersensitivity
Para-aminosalicylic acid	12 g/day (divided doses)	Gastrointestinal intolerance, hypersensitivity, hypothyroidism, crystaluria
Thiacetazone	150 mg daily	Gastrointestinal intolerance, Stevens–Johnson syndrome, bone marrow depression, ototoxicity, hepatitis

[a] Peak drug levels should be less than 3 mg/dl (30 mg/l) and trough less than 1 mg/dl (10 mg/l).
[b] Alternatives include: ciprofloxacin and levofloxacin.

with any other concomitant medicines, early detection of drug toxicity and dose adjustment for weight and renal function, since these may alter during the period of treatment.

TB is a notifiable disease in many countries. This ensures that there is not only close supervision of the infected person but that household and other contacts can be assessed for evidence of infection (a positive tuberculin skin test) or active disease based on symptoms and a positive chest X-ray. Outbreaks continue to occur, emphasizing the importance of notification and contact tracing.

Factors involved in the response to chemotherapy

In pulmonary TB, most of the tubercle bacilli are found on the walls of cavities in the lungs open to the bronchi. Here the pH is relatively high, at least on the alkaline side of neutrality. The oxygen tension is also high and the bacilli are actively multiplying. In addition, there is another smaller population of bacilli, dormant in closed cavities, or in caseating tissue, or inside macrophages, where the pH and oxygen tension are both low, and bacterial multiplication is slow.

The drugs available for the treatment of TB differ in their activity against tubercle bacilli under different conditions. For example, rifampicin acts against both extracellular and intracellular organisms, and also on those dormant in caseous nodules, while streptomycin and isoniazid are bactericidal against actively multiplying bacteria under alkaline conditions. Pyrazinamide acts largely on intracellular organisms in an acid medium. Bactericidal activity against actively multiplying bacteria largely determines the early response of the sick patient to chemotherapy, while sterilizing activity against the dormant 'persisters' in the bacterial population is most important when considering the risk of relapse after cessation of treatment.

First-line antituberculosis drugs

Isoniazid (isonicotinic acid hydrazide; INH)

Isoniazid is an important anti-TB drug being highly potent and bactericidal. Primary resistance in *M. tuberculosis* in the UK is uncommon (<5%) but increasing. However, resistance develops quickly with single-drug therapy and is avoided by a combined drug regimen. Together with rifampicin, isoniazid is the most widely used drug in the treatment of TB. It penetrates rapidly into all tissues and lesions and, its activity is not affected by pH. It is also well tolerated and cheap. It is given as a single daily oral dose as it is more important to achieve a high peak concentration than it is to maintain a continuously inhibitory level. Following oral absorption, plasma concentrations are good and cerebrospinal fluid (CSF) penetration is about 50–80% of the serum levels. Urinary concentrations are high. In intermittent regimens, increased doses can be used and higher peak levels attained.

Isoniazid is metabolized mainly by acetylation in the liver, at a rate which is genetically determined. Patients can be divided into two groups—rapid and slow inactivators. This is usually of little clinical importance in patients treated daily, or even twice weekly, but with intermittent regimens in which the drug is given only once a week, rapid inactivators (within 1 h) fare less well than slow inactivators (within 3 h), and there is some practical value in determining to which group a patient belongs when an intermittent regimen is contemplated.

Adverse reactions are uncommon but include hypersensitivity rashes and hepatitis (0.1%). The latter is potentially serious and the risk increases with age. It can be easily managed by prompt withdrawal of treatment. A sharp rise in serum transaminases at the outset of treatment is relatively common and may be enhanced by the concomitant use of rifampicin, but is usually of little significance. Liver function tests should be checked before starting treatment as a yardstick to measure any subsequent adverse reactions. Isoniazid interferes competitively with pyridoxine metabolism by inhibiting the formation of the active form of the vitamin and hence often results in peripheral neuropathy, which can be prevented by co-administration of pyridoxine. It also tends to raise plasma concentrations of warfarin, diazepam, phenytoin, and carbamazepine by inhibiting their metabolism in the liver. Overdosage may give rise to vomiting, dizziness, blurred vision, and slurring of speech.

Rifampicin and other rifamycins

Rifampicin is one of the most important of the anti-TB drugs, possessing high potency and efficacy in the treatment of primary and relapsing infection. It has been successfully used for decades in TB. Resistance rates remain low in the UK but are increasing. However, resistance rates of 10–20% are found in certain parts of the world, notably Thailand, the Dominican Republic, Russia, and some eastern European countries of the former USSR; such strains may be multiresistant. Rifampicin may be given daily or as part of an intermittent regimen. However, rifampicin is not available in some developing countries because it is expensive.

Side effects such as hepatitis and cutaneous reactions require expert supervision. Curiously, side effects are more common on intermittent regimens than when the drug is taken daily. They typically begin 2–3 h after the single morning dose when symptoms described as 'flu-like' develop. Once-weekly regimens are more toxic than twice-weekly ones. With daily regimens, side effects are uncommon and often trivial. An exception is the occurrence of purpura, which is an indication to stop the drug and not give it again. Drug interactions with rifampicin are common and require careful management.

Rifampicin is also key to the drug treatment of leprosy (see later) and is sometimes used in the treatment of life-threatening staphylococcal infections and in the prophylaxis of meningococcal and *Haemophilus influenzae* meningitis. There is no evidence that these occasional uses of rifampicin have jeopardized the value of its use in the treatment of TB.

Three other rifamycins—rifabutin, rifapentine, and benzoxazinorifamycin—are active against *M. tuberculosis*. They are somewhat more active than rifampicin, accumulate within macrophages and exhibit longer half-lives, but have not achieved widespread use in the treatment of TB.

Rifabutin has found use in the prophylaxis of *Mycobacterium avium* complex in patients with HIV and low CD4 lymphocyte counts.

Pyrazinamide

Pyrazinamide is particularly effective against intracellular tubercle bacilli in acid conditions and has therefore found an important place in short-course chemotherapy to prevent relapse at the end of treatment. It is given orally, produces high serum levels and penetrates freely into CSF. Adverse reactions are rare, but include anorexia, nausea, and flushing; hepatic toxicity has been a problem; hypersensitivity reactions and photosensitivity of the skin also occur.

Treatment for longer than two months is not recommended. Drug interactions occur with allopurinol, causing hyperuricaemia with attacks of gout, and with oral antidiabetic agents, causing a further fall in blood sugar. The dose should be reduced in renal impairment and avoided in patients with severe liver damage or a history of gout.

Ethambutol

Ethambutol is active against *M. tuberculosis* and many atypical mycobacteria. It has a primarily bacteristatic action on proliferating bacteria. Resistance develops slowly during therapy, but primary resistance occurs in less than 4% of strains of *M. tuberculosis*. It is rapidly absorbed after oral administration and high serum levels are found after 2 h, with even higher levels inside erythrocytes. Adequate levels are found in the CSF. Ethambutol is excreted in the urine both unchanged and as inactive metabolites.

Dose-dependent optic (retrobulbar) neuritis can result in impairment of visual acuity and colour vision. Early changes are usually reversible, but blindness can occur if treatment is not discontinued promptly. It is unusual at currently recommended doses, but it is recommended that the patient's visual acuity be tested before ethambutol is first prescribed and monitored during treatment.

Streptomycin

This was the first effective drug against human TB. Like all aminoglycosides it is not absorbed when given orally, and must be administered as an intramuscular injection. It is more bactericidal during the proliferative phase than in the resting phase of bacterial growth. Adequate concentrations are attained in lung, muscle, uterus, intestinal mucosa, adrenals, and lymph nodes. Diffusion into bone, brain, and aqueous humour is poor. Little normally enters the CSF, although penetration increases when the meninges are inflamed. The deep intramuscular injections are painful and must be administered daily for up to two months.

Ototoxicity is the most serious adverse reaction. Vestibular damage occurs in about 30% of cases while cochleotoxicity is less common. The plasma half-life is normally 2–3 h, but is considerably extended in the newborn, in the elderly, and in patients with severe renal impairment. Serum levels need to be monitored in patients over 40 years of age. The dose is adjusted for age and renal function. Hypersensitivity reactions in the form of fever and skin rashes may develop.

Second-line drugs

Thiacetazone

Thiacetazone is one of the earliest anti-TB drugs, and is cheap to manufacture. It is bacteristatic against *M. tuberculosis* and is sometimes used in combination with isoniazid to inhibit the emergence of resistance, particularly in the continuation phase of long-term regimens. It is well absorbed from the gastrointestinal tract and plasma levels are sustained for long periods of time. Side effects include nausea, vomiting, diarrhoea, skin rashes, and bone marrow depression. Rare cases of fatal exfoliative dermatitis and acute hepatitis failure have been reported.

Ethionamide and protionamide

Because of its gastrointestinal side effects—anorexia, salivation, nausea, abdominal pain, and diarrhoea—ethionamide is one of the most unpleasant of all anti-TB drugs to take and is no longer recommended. Protionamide is closely related in structure, and is better tolerated. It is absorbed quickly when given by mouth with good tissue and CSF levels. It is bacteristatic at therapeutic concentrations but bactericidal at higher concentrations. Contraindications include pregnancy, severe liver damage, and gastric complaints; care should be exercised in epilepsy and in psychotic patients. Combinations with isoniazid, cycloserine, or alcohol should be avoided.

Cycloserine, amikacin, kanamycin, and capreomycin

These are four rather weak drugs used as reserves for the treatment of TB resistant to the first-line agents. Capreomycin, amikacin, and kanamycin all need to be given by injection. Primary resistance is rare but resistance can develop rapidly.

Fluoroquinolones

Several fluoroquinolones are active against *M. tuberculosis*. They include ciprofloxacin, ofloxacin, levofloxacin, and moxifloxacin. They are bactericidal, orally administered, and well tolerated. They are increasingly being used in the treatment of drug-resistant TB.

p-Aminosalicylic acid

This was formerly used in combination regimens to prevent the emergence of drug-resistant organisms. Up to 10–12 g a day were given orally, in two or three doses. The drug tastes most unpleasant, and gastrointestinal intolerance was common. *p*-Aminosalicylic acid is no longer used and is included here for historical reasons only.

Short course and intermittent therapy

The discovery that both pyrazinamide and rifampicin are active against dormant as well as actively dividing tubercle bacilli prompted the investigation of shorter periods of treatment. Based on clinical trials, it has been shown that all regimens containing two of the three drugs, isoniazid, pyrazinamide, and rifampicin cure more than 90% of patients in six months and virtually all in nine months. The limitations of treatment are those of cost and of patient compliance. In developing countries, short course intermittent therapy permits supervised mass treatment at a cost the communities can afford.

Affluent countries have slightly different aims. These countries require highly effective unsupervised regimens for use where patient motivation is high and compliance good. The standard regimen of treatment recommended by the British Thoracic Society is an initial phase of two months treatment with rifampicin, isoniazid, plus pyrazinamide and ethambutol, then a continuation phase of treatment with isoniazid and rifampicin for a further four months (Table 30.2). The regimen of three or four drugs during the initial intensive phase of treatment is important in bringing the acute illness under control as rapidly as possible.

Intermittent regimens have become popular in developing countries for ease of administration. Rifampicin in standard dose, together with isoniazid and pyrazinamide at doses higher than the standard regimen are given on three days of the week, again for a total of six months (Table 30.2).

Directly observed therapy

To ensure compliance with medication and to avoid the risk of relapsing disease and drug-resistant TB, directly observed therapy, whereby a healthcare provider or other responsible person observes the ingestion of medication, has been employed. This policy is widely adopted in many developing countries and can be used selectively in developed countries where there are concerns over compliance. Supervised treatment can be given in the patient's home, place of employment, or school. It is effective in improving clinical cure rates and in decreasing rates of drug resistance. Use of fixed drug combinations (e.g. Rifinah: rifampicin + isoniazid; Rifater: rifampicin + isoniazid + pyrazinamide) reduces the risk of inappropriate monotherapy. Although such combinations may not contain exactly the same concentration as individual drugs, clinical results are favourable. It is important not to make mistakes in prescribing and dispensing because of the similarity of names.

Effective chemotherapy rapidly reduces the population of viable bacilli (sputum smears may be positive but cultures remain negative) and consequently reduces the risk of transmission, often within two weeks. Hospital care should be kept as short as possible since most patients can be managed in the community.

Non-antimicrobial treatment

Steroids have a limited place in the routine management of TB, but are of value in treating patients with pericarditis, pleural effusion, tuberculous meningitis, and severe miliary TB with dyspnoea when administered as short courses.

Surgical resection is rarely necessary except for rare situations such as severe repeated haemoptysis or resection of extensive disease of a lobe or lung in those with multidrug-resistant or poorly responsive TB.

Monitoring the therapeutic response

Inadequate compliance is by far the most important cause of therapeutic failure. Most cases of chronic or relapsing TB are the result of irregular, inadequate administration of prescribed drugs or the use of less potent regimens, and often result in the selection of resistant strains. The clinical response to treatment requires monitoring weight changes, fever, and symptoms of cough and shortness of breath. Where resources permit, cultures and smears can be examined for acid-fast bacilli. Fixed-dose combinations that include rifampicin can be detected by observing the red-orange discoloration of body fluids, especially urine.

Pregnancy and lactation

Treatment should not be interrupted or postponed if TB is diagnosed during pregnancy. Because of risk to the fetus, aminoglycosides such as streptomycin and fluoroquinolones should be avoided. Patients can breast feed normally while taking anti-TB drugs.

Tuberculosis and HIV infection

HIV infection results in progressive depletion and dysfunction of CD4 lymphocytes and impaired macrophage and monocyte function. Because CD4 cells and macrophages are essential to the host response to TB, HIV exerts an enormous influence on *M. tuberculosis* infection. Higher rates of reactivation disease occur (7–10% per year, compared with 5–8% per lifetime for HIV-negative patients). There are also much higher rates of acute disease (including extrapulmonary TB), skin anergy (producing a false-negative TB test), and possible malabsorption of anti-TB medications owing to enteropathy. The presenting features of pulmonary TB also differ according to the stage of HIV infection. In early disease, conventional presentations with cavitation are usual. However, in advanced disease chest X-ray changes may be atypical or absent. Serious drug-drug interactions can occur, especially between rifamycins, protease inhibitors, and non-nucleoside reverse transcriptase inhibitors used to treat HIV.

The treatment of TB in HIV-positive patients is therefore problematic and requires expert knowledge of both anti-TB and antiretroviral drugs. Treatment regimens may need to be prolonged. Multiresistant strains are more common in AIDS patients; in parts of Africa resistance to all first-line drugs is not uncommon. The microbiological diagnosis of TB in HIV-positive individuals may also be difficult, owing to concurrent infection with *Pneumocystis jiroveci* (*P. carinii*), cytomegalovirus, or fungi. Atypical mycobacteria (see below) are also more frequent.

Chemoprophylaxis against tuberculosis

Chemoprophylaxis of HIV-infected persons who are found to be tuberculin skin test positive is widely practised in the USA but is less commonly used in the UK. Isoniazid is used alone as prophylaxis because it is effective, cheap, acceptable, and has few side effects. Fears that isoniazid-resistant organisms would emerge have so far proved unfounded and largely reflects the lower bacillary load compared with that associated with clinical disease.

Drug-resistant tuberculosis

Current recommended drug regimens are designed to prevent the emergence of drug resistance. However, control of TB is threatened by the worldwide emergence of drug resistance in *M. tuberculosis*. Outbreaks of multiresistant TB have occurred in hospitals, centres for the care of patients with AIDS, and prisons, posing considerable clinical and public health problems. In the UK, the incidence of resistance to isoniazid alone is presently below 6%; resistance to isoniazid and rifampicin (with or without resistance to other drugs) is less than 1.5% but has been increasing steadily. However, with the emergence of multidrug-resistant and extensively drug-resistant (resistance to both isoniazid and rifampicin as well as two or more second line agents) tuberculosis in many countries worldwide, enhanced surveillance is essential.

Molecular genetic methods that allow the rapid detection of isoniazid- and rifampicin-resistant strains are available in reference centres and are helpful in modifying therapy or prompting patient isolation (see below). Likewise, genotyping helps to differentiate re-infection from reactivation and can be used to characterize cross-infection among close contacts of infectious cases.

Hospital transmission of multiresistant *M. tuberculosis*

Healthcare workers are at risk from TB from patients with unsuspected pulmonary TB, or during the period required for chemotherapy to render them non-infectious.

Infection control measures require early detection of patients with smear positive TB, especially those with multiresistant *M. tuberculosis*. They should be cared for in isolation rooms. Negative air pressures should be maintained in these rooms. To prevent transmission, high-efficiency particulate air (HEPA) filters may have to be fitted if there is difficulty in exhausting contaminated air from buildings. Filter masks should be worn by staff and visitors to reduce the risk of inhaling infectious airborne particles.

Extrapulmonary tuberculosis

Tuberculous meningitis

This form of tuberculous infection is invariably fatal if untreated, and appropriate chemotherapy is vital. It is a frequent complication of untreated miliary TB, and may vary from an abrupt and severe illness resembling other acute bacterial meningitis to a subtle and chronic disease extending over several weeks. The diagnosis is made on the basis of CSF examination. Treatment should be given promptly and include isoniazid and rifampicin. During the first intensive phase, these drugs should be accompanied by pyrazinamide and ethambutol. After about 2 months, these can be discontinued, but the isoniazid and rifampicin should be continued for at least a further 10 months. Intrathecal antibiotics are unnecessary, but additional treatment with corticosteroids should be used in severe cases especially in those with raised intracranial pressure or cranial nerve palsies.

Other forms of tuberculosis

TB can affect any system in the body including, in decreasing order of frequency, superficial lymph nodes, bone and joints, the genito-urinary tract, the abdomen, the breast, and skin. Patients with non-respiratory TB can be regarded as non-infectious. Generally, the principles described for the treatment of pulmonary TB are also appropriate for the treatment of other forms, although few regimens have been subject to controlled clinical trials. Surgical intervention is sometimes necessary to establish the diagnosis, or to drain large abscesses, relieve pressure from tuberculous masses, or repair damage from scar tissue, but is no longer the mainstay of treatment.

Opportunistic (atypical) mycobacteria

The so-called opportunistic or 'atypical' species of mycobacteria, also known as 'mycobacteria other than TB', that can cause human disease include *M. kansasii*, *M. marinum*, *M. avium*, *M. intracellulare*, *M. fortuitum*, and several others. The isolation of atypical mycobacteria does not prove that disease is present unless the organism is isolated from a normally sterile body site; colonization with these organisms is not uncommon. Nevertheless, disease caused by these organisms may be indistinguishable from true TB. Atypical mycobacteria are usually more resistant to the standard anti-TB agents than is *M. tuberculosis*.

Atypical mycobacteria of the *M. avium* complex have also come into prominence since the appearance of AIDS. Patients with AIDS seem particularly prone to develop infection with these mycobacteria, and the disease may be associated with a severe 'wasting syndrome'. These mycobacteria are also usually highly resistant to the common anti-TB drugs and alternative regimens are recommended (see p. 333).

Leprosy

This is a chronic communicable tropical disease caused by infection with *M. leprae*, which mainly affects the skin and peripheral nerves causing anaesthesia, muscle weakness, paralysis, and consequent injury and deformity. Currently, the disease is restricted to some six countries as a result of a WHO eradication programme. Over the centuries, those with leprosy have often been ostracized and excluded from society, despite the fact that it is not very contagious. Transmission is caused by respiratory droplet spread from close contact. There is a spectrum of disease determined by the extent of cell-mediated immune response by the host. This not only distinguishes the major types of the disease but also has implications for treatment (Fig. 30.1).

Two major types are described: lepromatous and tuberculoid leprosy. In lepromatous leprosy there is diffuse involvement of skin and mucous membranes, with ulceration, iritis, and keratitis; scrapings of skin or mucous membranes contain numerous acid-fast bacilli. The tuberculoid form is more localized, but nerve involvement occurs early; only scanty bacilli are present. In both forms, progress of the disease is slow. The tuberculoid form may heal spontaneously in a few years. Death is usually due to other causes.

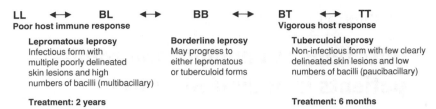

Fig. 30.1 The spectrum of leprosy as determined by host response and bacillary load and its implications for treatment. LL, lepromatous leprosy; BL, borderline lepromatous; BB, borderline leprosy; BT, borderline tuberculoid; TT, tuberculoid leprosy.

The approach to leprosy control includes early case detection, adequate treatment with a combination of dapsone, rifampicin, and clofazimine, and the prevention of disabilities and rehabilitation of sufferers. Paucibacillary (tuberculoid) disease is cured in 6 months with dapsone and rifampicin while multibacillary (lepromatous) disease requires at least 2 years' treatment with dapsone, clofazimine, and rifampicin. Dapsone (diaminodiphenylsulphone) resistance is avoided by the use of triple therapy. Rifampicin is more rapidly bactericidal than dapsone, but resistance may arise if it is used alone. Clofazimine is effective, but some patients develop discoloration of the skin that may prove unacceptable. The treatment of leprosy requires specialist expertise.

With such long and complicated regimens, patient compliance is naturally a problem, particularly in areas of the world where leprosy is most prevalent. Second-line agents include minocycline, ofloxacin, and clarithromycin. Furthermore, a single-dose triple combination of rifampicin, ofloxacin, and minocycline has been successful in lepromatous leprosy and provides a further alternative. If confirmed, this offers an attractive regimen for use in endemic areas.

It should be remembered that patients with leprosy might also have TB; regimens used for leprosy treatment are inadequate for treating TB.

Key points

♦ Tuberculosis is increasing worldwide and is acquired by droplet spread.

♦ Respiratory disease predominates but TB may also affect any body site such as bone, kidney, gut, and meninges.

♦ Pulmonary TB is diagnosed by sputum examination and culture and chest X-ray findings.

♦ Treatment requires a prolonged multidrug regimen with isoniazid, rifampicin, pyrazinamide with or without ethambutol for 2 months, followed by a further 4 months isoniazid and rifampicin for pulmonary tuberculosis.

♦ Compliance with medication is key to success.

♦ Tuberculosis is a notifiable disease. Contacts should be assessed.

Further reading

Ormerod L Peter (2010). 'Tuberculosis and other mycobacterial infections', in *Antibiotic and Chemotherapy*. Finch RG, Greenwood D, Norrby SR, Whitley RJ (eds), London: Elsevier Saunders, 752–770.

Chapter 31

Infections in immunocompromised patients including HIV/AIDS

The care of the immunocompromised patient is an increasingly important and challenging aspect of medicine that encompasses individuals suffering from a variety of underlying disease states which render them especially vulnerable to microbial challenge. The term immunocompromised describes patients who have immunodeficiency states or those who are immunosuppressed.

Immunodeficiency

Immunodeficiency may be congenital or acquired and can affect particular aspects of humoral, cell-mediated, or phagocytic cell function (Table 31.1). In general such states are relatively rare in medical practice. However, the advent of the HIV pandemic significantly altered this situation. It is now estimated that more than 59 million people have been infected worldwide, which includes 20 million who have died to date, making HIV infection the commonest cause of acquired immunodeficiency. The primary deficiency in HIV infection is one of an inexorable decline in cell-mediated immune function as a result of the human immunodeficiency virus targeting CD4-positive T cells, which have a central role in orchestrating the immune system and cells of the monocyte/macrophage series.

Immunosuppression

In contrast to immunodeficiency states, immunosuppression affects patients whose immune defences are impaired, either as a result of an underlying disease or its management by cytotoxic, immunosuppressive, or radiation therapy. The immunosuppressed patient often has an underlying malignant disease, or has undergone organ or bone marrow transplantation. In both situations, part of the therapeutic strategy involves temporary suppression or ablation of host immune functions.

In general the state of immunosuppression is finite, unlike immunodeficiency disorders, which are generally permanent or progressive; once the immunosuppressive regimen is reduced or withdrawn, the host defences can recover. The compromised defences include not only the humoral, phagocytic, and cell-mediated components of the immune system, but also skin and mucous membranes, the integrity of which may be impaired by cytotoxic drugs. The vulnerability of the patient to infection may be compounded by the use of intravascular catheters, bladder catheters, and in the case of ventilated patients, endotracheal tubes. These either interfere with pharyngeotracheal clearance mechanisms (respiratory tract) or connect a normally sterile body site (bladder, vascular compartment) with the external environment.

The major features of immunosuppression associated with various malignant conditions are summarized in Table 31.2. Such patients are often cared for in high-dependency or intensive care facilities that provide opportunities for cross-infection and the acquisition of hospital-associated, and therefore frequently antibiotic-resistant, pathogens.

Table 31.1 Examples of immunodeficiency states associated with an increased frequency of severity of infection

Congenital immunodeficiencies
B-cell deficiencies
Selective IgA deficiency
X-linked hypogammaglobulinaemia
Common variable immunodeficiency
IgG subclass deficiency
T-cell deficiencies
DiGeorge anomaly
Wiskott–Aldrich syndrome
Ataxia telangiectasia
X-linked hyper-IgM syndrome
Combined T and B cell defects
Severe combined immunodeficiency
Congenital deficiency of phagocytosis
Congenital neutropenia
Chronic granulomatous disease
Leucocyte adhesion deficiency
Acquired immunodeficiencies
AIDS
Cytotoxic and immunosuppressive therapy
Lymphoproliferative and myeloproliferative disorders
Hypersplenism
Autoimmune neutropenia
Splenectomy

Microbial complications in the immunocompromised host

A wide variety of infections may occur in immunocompromised patients. These arise from either exogenous (external source) or endogenous (host derived) micro-organisms. The distinction between exogenous and endogenous infections is not always clear-cut, since in hospital the bacterial flora of the skin and mucous membranes often alters.

In the case of virus infections, the herpesvirus group predominates and may represent primary infection or reactivation of latent virus; these infections are often more severe than those in the immunocompetent host and carry the risk of dissemination. Adenovirus and para-influenza virus infections of the lung are also observed in profoundly neutropenic patients.

Fungal infections can be particularly severe. Candidosis of the mouth and upper gastrointestinal tract is particularly common and from time to time may be complicated by candidaemia, with spread to other organs. *Cryptococcus neoformans*, a yeast that was an uncommon cause of meningitis until the AIDS pandemic, occasionally complicates organ transplantation and malignant lymphoma.

Table 31.2 Examples of immunosuppressive states associated with an increased frequency or severity of infection according to altered host defences

Disease	Mucosal surfaces	Phagocytosis	Humoral immunity	CMI
Acute lymphoblastic leukaemia	+	++	−	+
Acute myeloblastic leukaemia	+	++	−	+
Chronic lymphocytic leukaemia	−	−	++	+
Hodgkin, non-Hodgkin lymphoma	−	−	−	+
Solid tumours	++	−	−	+
Multiple myeloma	−	−	++	−

CMI, cell-mediated immunity. −, association absent; +, definite association; ++, marked association.

Among the filamentous fungi, *Aspergillus* spp. are the most common pathogens. Their ubiquitous spores are normally harmless to the immunocompetent, but in the immunocompromised patient they can cause serious lung infection that may disseminate throughout the body. This risk is greatest in patients with profound neutropenia. Aspergillosis is not only difficult to treat but is also difficult to diagnose, especially in the early stages of infection.

Pneumocystis jiroveci (carinii) has emerged as the leading opportunistic infection complicating HIV infection. It primarily affects the lung where it produces a severe progressive pneumonia, which may be fatal unless treated early. Pneumocystosis may also occur in patients undergoing organ transplantation and in those with lymphoblastic leukaemia or malignant lymphoma; profound impairment of cell-mediated immunity characterizes all these conditions. *P. jiroveci*, although a fungus, has a pattern of susceptibility to chemotherapeutic agents that is more in keeping with a protozoon. Other parasitic infections in the immunocompromised host include toxoplasmosis and in endemic regions, leishmaniasis. There are also a variety of gut infections such as giardiasis, cryptosporidiosis, microsporidiosis, and strongyloidiasis. The latter can progress to a state of hyperinfection with extensive larval invasion of the body.

Principles of chemotherapeutic control

The vulnerability of the immunocompromised patient to infection has been emphasized. Not only is the range of possible infections broad, but, because of the state of immunosuppression, the presentation may be atypical and the course fulminant. A specific clinical and microbiological diagnosis can be difficult to establish; the therapeutic management of such patients is consequently based on a set of principles that has evolved to meet their particular needs.

It is essential that the patient is thoroughly examined at the earliest suspicion of infection. Particular attention should be paid to the skin, perineum, entry sites for catheters, the mouth, lungs, and abdomen. Appropriate microbiological samples should be collected and necessary radiographic investigations obtained. Timely biopsy of lymph nodes, bone marrow, cutaneous or intrapulmonary lesions is appropriate in selective cases. The approach to the chemotherapeutic management of the immunocompromised patient is particularly well demonstrated in:

- patients with haematological malignancies undergoing cytotoxic chemotherapy or bone marrow transplantation, especially during episodes of profound neutropenia;
- patients with AIDS;
- those with specific immunological defects such as hyposplenism.

Neutropenic patients

In the neutropenic patient infection can develop rapidly over a matter of hours, and if untreated can prove fatal. If fever above 38°C persists for 2 h or more, broad-spectrum antibiotic therapy should be administered promptly by the intravenous route. However, documentation of infection can be difficult: about 15% of infections will be documented by blood culture, a further 20% by other microbiological investigations, and a further 20% by clinical criteria. In the remainder, infection may only be strongly suspected without supporting clinical or laboratory evidence; non-microbial causes such as drug reactions, blood or platelet transfusions, or the underlying disease state may be responsible for the febrile episode.

Treatment regimens

The variety and relative frequency of bloodstream pathogens in the neutropenic patient are summarized in Table 31.3. There has been a striking increase in Gram-positive infections in recent years, which in part relates to the widespread use of vascular catheters for drug administration, as well as the selective pressure arising from the use of broad-spectrum antibiotics, notably β-lactam and quinolone agents.

In general the antibiotic regimens have been based on a combination of a β-lactam antibiotic and an aminoglycoside, which together are active against most of the likely pathogens. Among the β-lactam agents, a broad-spectrum cephalosporin such as ceftazidime has been most widely used, although the ureidopenicillin piperacillin, in combination with tazobactam, is also popular. An aminoglycoside such as gentamicin or amikacin is administered simultaneously since both are active against Gram-negative bacilli, including *Pseudomonas aeruginosa*. Some centres have adopted the use of a single agent such as ceftazidime or imipenem, but the combined regimen offers synergistic activity that may be useful, especially when dealing with serious *Ps. aeruginosa* bacteraemia. Increasing drug resistance to β-lactams such as ceftazidime, adds further complexity to the choice of initial empirical therapy.

The increase in Gram-positive infections caused by staphylococci, enterococci, and viridans streptococci is compounded by a relative antimicrobial weakness in the above regimens; as a result a glycopeptide, such as vancomycin or teicoplanin, may be needed, especially in patients who have recently undergone bone marrow transplantation in whom a neutropenic febrile

Table 31.3 Distribution of the more common bloodstream isolates complicating neutropenic states

Micro-organism	Approximate percentage
Gram-positive bacteria	
Staphylococcus epidermidis	28
Staph. aureus	10
Corynebacterium spp.	5
Streptococci	12
Gram-negative bacteria	
Gram-negative enteric bacilli	28
Pseudomonas aeruginosa	7
Others	7
Fungi	
Candida spp.	3

episode can be particularly serious. However, increased use of glycopeptides is being accompanied by infections caused by glycopeptide-resistant enterococci.

Candida infection is best treated with intravenous amphotericin or caspofungin with the azole fluconazole as a reserve agent. Amphotericin is a toxic drug and careful dosaging and monitoring of renal function is essential to avoid serious nephrotoxicity. Lipid formulations of amphotericin are less nephrotoxic and increasingly used but much more expensive.

Cryptococcal yeast infections are managed with a combination of amphotericin with or without the addition of flucytosine (see Chapter 28, p. 304). Filamentous fungal infections, notably *Aspergillus* infection, are best treated with intravenous voriconazole. Amphotericin provides an alternative choice. For unresponsive disease, caspofungin is used as salvage therapy.

Chemoprophylaxis

The seriousness of infections in the severely immunosuppressed neutropenic patient has led to the use of chemoprophylactic drug regimens, particularly in patients undergoing cytotoxic chemotherapy for haematological malignancies and in bone marrow transplant recipients. Regimens are directed at those micro-organisms likely to result in bacteraemic disease.

The varied choice of prophylactic regimen reflects different views on the pathogenesis of infection in these patients. One view is that oral, non-absorbable antibiotics are desirable in that their effect is confined to the gastrointestinal tract, which is the major source of invasive micro-organisms. These regimens are now much less widely used than in the past, but have included agents active against *Candida* spp., because of the frequency and severity of upper gastrointestinal candidosis, together with framycetin and colistin, which are non-absorbed agents. Other variations have included neomycin, colistin, and nystatin; or gentamicin, vancomycin, and nystatin. One important problem with these regimens is that their bitter taste leads to poor patient compliance. Moreover, evidence that they reduce the frequency and severity of bacteraemic infections has been difficult to obtain.

As an alternative to these regimens, other agents have been adopted which have systemic antibiotic effects. Co-trimoxazole has been widely used for its activity against many Gram-negative enteric bacilli and Gram-positive pathogens. It is also active against *P. jiroveci*. However, the emergence of drug-resistant strains, poor activity against *Ps. aeruginosa*, and the danger of bone marrow suppression in bone marrow recipients make this antifolate compound less than ideal.

Fluoroquinolones provide broad-spectrum activity, high potency, and a systemic antibiotic effect and achieve significant drug concentrations within the gut. There is strong evidence to indicate that these drugs achieve a reduction in serious Gram-negative bacteraemia, although the relative weakness of the quinolones against Gram-positive pathogens has also been clearly demonstrated. Ciprofloxacin has been the most widely used agent. When given by mouth it provides a cost-effective approach in high-risk patients, especially those undergoing bone marrow transplantation.

Selective decontamination of the digestive tract

As well as patients rendered neutropenic by chemotherapy or disease, the ventilated patient on the intensive care unit is at considerable risk of infection, in particular from pneumonia from aspiration of oropharyngeal flora. One approach adopted in some centres has been to use a topical antibiotic regimen, applied to the mouth in the form of paste and given in liquid form via a nasogastric tube into the stomach and hence the gastrointestinal tract. The aim is to suppress the flora of the gastrointestinal tract, which is largely made up of aerobic and anaerobic micro-organisms. One widely studied regimen is a combination of polymyxin, gentamicin, and amphotericin, often supplemented for the first few days with intravenous cefotaxime. The pathogens targeted by this regimen include *Staphylococcus aureus, Escherichia coli, Proteus* spp., *Klebsiella* spp., and *Candida* spp., which are among the more common causes of infection in such patients. Studies have shown a reduction in bacterial counts in the mouth, stomach, and colon. There is also evidence that nosocomial pneumonia can be reduced. This is more readily achievable, in young, relatively fit patients who have sustained major trauma than in the elderly or those with chronic lung disease. Among other populations of ventilated patients the cost–benefit of this procedure in terms of reduced mortality and length of stay in hospital has proved difficult to establish.

AIDS

The clinical impact of HIV infection lies in its persistent nature and the accompanying progressive immunodeficiency which gives rise to a range of complicating infections and malignancies. These target many organs as well as producing systemic illness. Table 31.4 summarizes the more important complicating infections.

In contrast to their effects in the immunocompetent host, these infections often present atypically and with heightened severity. Furthermore, many of the infections recur after treatment in those with advanced HIV disease. Thus, in the HIV-infected patient the initial course of treatment must be more intensive than in the immunocompetent host, and for many conditions long-term suppressive therapy is needed to prevent relapse. In addition, by controlling the underlying HIV infection, the frequency and severity of opportunistic infections can be reduced, as well as the risk of recurrent opportunistic infection.

The introduction of combination antiretroviral therapy (cART, previously referred to as highly active antiretroviral therapy, HAART), in which three-drug regimens of two nucleoside analogues with a protease inhibitor or a non-nucleoside reverse transcriptase inhibitor are used, has permitted

Table 31.4 Common opportunist pathogens complicating HIV disease

Site	Micro-organism
Gastrointestinal tract	*Cryptosporidium parvum*
	Salmonella enterica serotypes
	Mycobacterium avium complex
	Cytomegalovirus
	Herpes simplex virus
	Candida spp.
Respiratory tract	*Pneumocystis jiroveci (carinii)*
	Streptococcus pneumoniae
	Mycobacterium tuberculosis
	Cytomegalovirus
Central nervous system	*Toxoplasma gondii*
	Cryptococcus neoformans
	Cytomegalovirus
	Herpes simplex virus
	Varicella zoster virus
	JC polyoma virus

cessation of primary prophylaxis against *P. jiroveci* in selected patients. These regimens are discussed in Chapter 34. They are generally well tolerated and, provided the patient is compliant with the medication, have a major impact on the quality of life. Although they all act in a suppressive manner to delay disease progression, none is curative.

The chemotherapeutic approach to selected opportunistic infections is discussed in order to emphasize the principles and associated problems that arise.

Pneumocystis jiroveci (P.carinii)

Among the many opportunistic infections that complicate HIV infection, *P. jiroveci* predominates. The primary site of infection is the lung. Clinical disease represents reactivation of endogenous infection usually acquired in childhood. Typical symptoms include progressive shortness of breath with or without a relatively unproductive cough, progressive hypoxaemia, and diffuse bilateral chest radiograph infiltrates. The diagnosis has been greatly facilitated by the availability of a fluorescent antibody to *P. jiroveci*, which can be applied to expectorated sputum or to a saline lavage obtained by bronchoscopy. Genome amplification techniques have also contributed to enhanced diagnosis, as *P. jiroveci* DNA may be detectable in peripheral blood.

The treatment of choice is high-dose co-trimoxazole, by mouth or intravenously, for 3 weeks. The risk of hypersensitivity to the sulphonamide component is greatly increased in HIV disease and alternative regimens, such as intravenous pentamidine or oral atovaquone, or a combination of clindamycin and primaquine may be necessary.

Once the patient has recovered it is necessary to continue with secondary prophylaxis with low-dose co-trimoxazole for as long as CD4 counts remain below 200 cells/μl. Alternative agents that can be used in those intolerant of the standard regimens include dapsone and atovaquone. Nebulized pentamidine given once monthly as an aerosol inhalation provides another choice. In view of the seriousness of *P. jiroveci* pneumonia, patients with HIV infection are now offered primary prophylaxis when their CD4 lymphocyte counts fall below 200 cells/μl in order to prevent infection. The choice of agent and frequency of administration is the same as for secondary prophylaxis.

Toxoplasmosis

The protozoon *Toxoplasma gondii* can cause serious disease in people with HIV infection. This may occur as a primary infection, although it more usually represents reactivation of dormant parasites. The disease presents most frequently as a space-occupying lesion of the brain with focal neurological features. The diagnosis is based on clinical suspicion and computed tomography scan. Serodiagnosis is difficult. The presence of tachyzoites in brain biopsy is confirmatory. However, it is more usual to carry out a trial of chemotherapy in the first instance since this can avoid potentially dangerous neurosurgery.

Toxoplasmosis is treated with pyrimethamine and sulfadiazine in high dosage for six weeks before reducing to a maintenance dose. This regimen often results in bone marrow suppression or is complicated by an allergic skin eruption. Alternative drugs include high-dose clindamycin or the azalide azithromycin in combination with pyrimethamine, which also exhibits useful activity. Atovaquone plus pyrimethamine provides a further option. The principles of treatment are similar to those for controlling *P. jiroveci* pneumonia in that initial control is followed by continuous maintenance therapy, until immune system function is restored following antiretroviral therapy. There is evidence that co-trimoxazole given as prophylaxis for *P. jiroveci* may also be suppressive for toxoplasmosis.

Cytomegalovirus infection

Cytomegalovirus infection is extremely common. In those with HIV infection, reactivation is associated with a range of manifestations, which may involve the gastrointestinal tract, lung, liver, and in particular the eye, where a progressive retinopathy may lead to loss of vision or total blindness. Treatment with ganciclovir, valganciclovir, foscarnet, or cidofovir is suppressive but not curative (see Chapter 34).

Mycobacteriosis

Patients with HIV infection are at increased risk of mycobacterial infection. This may be newly acquired but is more usually the result of endogenous reactivation as cell-mediated immunity steadily declines. *Mycobacterium tuberculosis* is the commonest infecting organism, but disease may present atypically owing to altered host immunity. In many parts of the world drug-resistant tuberculosis has emerged as an important problem, and there have been instances of spread within prisons and hospitals (see p. 315). Where there is good evidence for previous tuberculosis, chemoprophylaxis with isoniazid is recommended for one to two years.

Infection with organisms of the *Mycobacterium avium* complex is a common problem in patients with AIDS. Disease presents with fever, sweats, weight loss, and diarrhoea. Patients are frequently bacillaemic and have high bacterial loads within the gut and bone marrow. The organisms are extremely resistant to conventional antituberculosis regimens and a combination of clarithromycin with rifabutin and ethambutol is recommended. Response to treatment may, unfortunately, be short-lived. Attempts have therefore been directed at preventing disease with rifabutin, alone or in combination with azithromycin.

Hyposplenism

The spleen is an important site of host defences, rich in lymphoid follicles and phagocytic cells. In its absence the patient is at increased risk of infection, including fulminating bacteraemia. Apart from splenectomy, a variety of medical conditions can cause hyposplenism. These include hereditary conditions such as sickle cell anaemia and hereditary spherocytosis. The risk of serious infections is greatest in early childhood but declines with age, although the risk remains throughout life. Among the fulminant infections are those caused by *Streptococcus pneumoniae, Haemophilus influenzae, Esch. coli, Neisseria meningitidis,* and a rare pathogen of man, *Capnocytophaga canimorsus.* Hyposplenic or asplenic patients should be alerted to their increased risk and recommended to seek early medical attention in the presence of symptoms suggestive of severe infection. Immunization against pneumococcal infections is possible in those over 2 years of age and is the best form of prevention. Likewise, children should be immunized against *H. influenzae* and group C meningococcal infection. Long-term chemoprophylaxis with phenoxymethylpenicillin (penicillin V) is of proven benefit in children with sickle cell disease. However, the additional benefit of life-long prophylaxis in those who have been actively immunized is marginal. Compliance with lifelong penicillin V prophylaxis is a further problem, as is the steady increase in resistance to penicillin among pneumococci, especially in parts of Europe and North America.

Further reading

Gazzard BG, on behalf of the BHIVA Treatment Guidelines Writing Group (2008), 'British HIV Association guidelines for the treatment of HIV-1-infected adults with antiretroviral therapy 2008. British HIV Association Guidelines', *HIV Medicine,* **9**: 563–608.

Wey E, Kibbler CC (2010), 'Infections associated with neutropenia and transplantation', in *Antibiotic and Chemotherapy* (9th edn), Finch RG, Greenwood D, Norrby SR, Whitley RJ (eds), London: Saunders Elsevier, 502–523.

Davies JM, Barnes R, Milligan D (2002), 'Update of guidelines for the prevention and treatment of infection in patients with an absent or dysfunctional spleen', *Clinical Medicine* September/October Vol 2, **5**: 440.

Chapter 32

Viral infections

Diseases caused by viruses are extremely common and range from trivial coughs and colds to life-threatening infections. Most viral infections are self-limiting, although some that normally cause relatively minor problems can be serious in immunosuppressed patients or neonates. Some viruses nearly always cause severe disease regardless of the initial status of the host. Rabies, human immunodeficiency virus (HIV), and several of the viruses causing haemorrhagic fevers fall into this category. Furthermore, long-term complications may arise from viral infections of the central nervous system (Chapter 28) or liver (Chapter 34).

Most success in the control of serious virus infections has been achieved by immunoprophylaxis, and to a lesser extent immunotherapy, notably to manage rabies and hepatitis B virus infections, rather than by the use of specific antiviral chemotherapy. However, there is an ever-increasing list of useful antiviral drugs (see Chapters 4 to 6) and, as knowledge of the molecular biology of viral replication increases, more potential targets are being identified. In general, the most widely treated virus infections comprise herpes viruses, respiratory tract infections (both dealt with in this Chapter), HIV infection (see Chapter 33) and viral hepatitis (Chapter 34).

Herpesvirus infections

All eight herpesviruses that infect man (Table 32.1) exhibit the phenomenon of latency. Following acute infection, virus is not eliminated from the body, but viral DNA remains quiescent without causing any apparent damage to the latently infected cells. Later, virus may be reactivated; the virus replicates, and disease may re-emerge. Herpesvirus infections can therefore be classified as primary, the host's first encounter with the virus, or secondary, due to reactivation of latent virus. Alternatively, secondary infection may arise from exogenous reinfection with a distinct strain of virus. The clinical features of primary and secondary herpesvirus infections are often very different.

Aciclovir is very active against certain herpesviruses and was the first truly selective antiviral agent. Two more oral antiherpetic drugs have subsequently been developed: valaciclovir (an oral pro-drug of aciclovir) and famciclovir (a pro-drug of penciclovir) (pp. 52–54). These newer agents exhibit greater oral bioavailability than aciclovir, which allows an easier dosing schedule.

Herpesviruses differ in their sensitivity to aciclovir and penciclovir (Table 32.1). Cytomegalovirus (CMV) and human herpesvirus type 6 do not possess thymidine kinase, and cannot activate the drugs efficiently. In practice, these drugs are useful only in the treatment of herpes simplex virus (HSV), in varicella-zoster virus infection, and in certain unusual manifestations of Epstein–Barr virus infection. Clinical trials in various manifestations of herpes simplex and varicella-zoster infection have shown the two compounds to be equipotent. Aciclovir is the only agent licensed for intravenous use, and thus must be used in life-threatening diseases necessitating intravenous therapy. For oral therapy, the choice between aciclovir, valaciclovir, and famciclovir may depend on considerations of relative costs and convenience of dosing.

Herpes simplex virus infections

Although most HSV infections are asymptomatic, there can be a wide range of clinical manifestations.

Table 32.1 Human herpesviruses

Name	Usual abbreviation	Sensitivity to aciclovir
Herpes simplex type 1	HSV1	Very sensitive
Herpes simplex type 2	HSV2	Very sensitive
Varicella-zoster virus	VZV	Fairly sensitive
Epstein–Barr virus	EBV	Poorly sensitive
Cytomegalovirus	CMV	Insensitive
Human herpesvirus type 6	HHV6	Insensitive
Human herpesvirus type 7	HHV7	Not known
Human herpesvirus type 8	HHV8	Insensitive

Primary orolabial infection

Symptomatic primary infection, which usually occurs in children, presents with extensive painful blistering and ulceration of the lips, tongue, and mucous membranes of the mouth, sometimes with marked cervical lymphadenopathy and fever. Left untreated, the infection is self-limiting with complete healing in two to three weeks. Oral anti-herpes therapy reduces the manifestations of systemic disease, the formation of new lesions, the period of virus excretion, and the time to healing; it is of unquestioned therapeutic benefit.

Recurrent orolabial infection

Resolution of primary disease is followed by the establishment of latency of HSV within the trigeminal nerve ganglion. This virus can be reactivated in later life and track back down the nerve to reach the mouth. The manifestations of reactivated disease in an immunocompetent host are much milder: there is no systemic upset, only a few lesions (cold sores), localized to a small area on the lips; the inflammatory response is less, with less pain and swelling, and the lesions heal in about five to six days. Aciclovir therapy enhances resolution of lesions by about 24 h. Given the mild nature of recurrent disease (as compared with primary infection), and the marginal benefit of aciclovir, routine systemic treatment of cold sores is not recommended.

Eczema herpeticum

Intact skin is a very efficient barrier to the spread of viruses. However, in patients with chronic dermatitis or eczema, this barrier is not intact, and virus can spread freely. Eczema herpeticum is a severe complication of primary or secondary orolabial HSV infection in patients with eczema. Lesions extend to large areas on the face, neck, and upper chest. Virus may also gain access to the bloodstream through cracks in the skin, putting the patient at risk of death from disseminated HSV infection. Antiviral therapy is mandatory. Patients should be given supplies of valaciclovir or famciclovir so that they can self-medicate in the early stages of recurrent disease.

Ocular herpes simplex virus infection

HSV is the commonest infectious cause of blindness in the UK. Children are particularly prone to self-inoculating the eye with virus-infected oral secretions. Spread of virus to the cornea results in keratitis and may lead to severe inflammation and repeated reactivations predispose to chronic ulceration. Management should include systemic and topical aciclovir (together with consideration of the use of steroids to damp down the damaging host inflammatory response) and prompt referral for specialist ophthalmological assessment.

Genital herpes

The clinical manifestations and management of primary and secondary genital herpes are analogous to those of orolabial disease. Thus primary infection may result in extensive bilateral, painful ulceration with spread to adjacent skin, inguinal adenopathy, and fever, lasting two to three weeks. Lesions close to the urethral meatus may give rise to pain when passing urine. Cervicitis with profuse discharge is common in women. Oral anti-herpes therapy is of proven benefit. Recurrent disease is much more localized, with no systemic upset, and shorter-lasting; oral anti-viral therapy is of marginal value.

Some unfortunate individuals may suffer severe recurrent attacks of genital herpes as frequently as once a month. The immunological basis for this debilitating and depressing condition is not understood. One approach to the management of these patients is to give them continuous pro-phylactic anti-herpes therapy. This results in a considerable decrease in the frequency of attacks and rarely gives rise to significant side effects.

Neonatal herpes

Pregnant women with genital herpes are at risk of passing on the infection during childbirth. Neonatal HSV infection is a potentially devastating disease, as virus readily disseminates to internal organs, and such babies may die of HSV hepatitis, pneumonitis, or encephalitis. Survivors are almost invar-iably left with severe neurological sequelae. Although mortality from neonatal herpes has improved with the use of intravenous aciclovir, overall morbidity has scarcely been affected, presumably because by the time the diagnosis is made, and therapy initiated, the damage has already been done.

Herpes simplex encephalitis

Herpes simplex encephalitis is the commonest form of sporadic viral encephalitis (Chapter 28), with an annual incidence of about one case per million population. Most cases occur in individu-als with evidence of prior infection with HSV. Thus the disease is usually a manifestation of secondary infection, although the route by which virus gains access to the brain is not clear. Untreated, mortality is high, and survivors suffer severe long-term damage. Diagnosis is difficult but should be suspected in all patients with features of acute encephalitis with focal signs, espe-cially when confirmed by computed tomography scans or magnetic resonance imaging of the brain. The cerebrospinal fluid usually shows a pleocytosis, but it is very rare to succeed in isolating the virus from cerebrospinal fluid. HSV DNA can be detected in cerebrospinal fluid during the acute stage by the polymerase chain reaction. Intravenous aciclovir, in high dosage, improves the prognosis dramatically, provided therapy is started as soon as the diagnosis is suspected, without waiting for laboratory confirmation.

Immunocompromised patients

Patients who are immunocompromised for whatever reason are at risk of severe primary or secondary HSV disease. All HSV infections in this group of patients should be treated promptly with aciclovir, if necessary by the intravenous route. In bone marrow transplant recipients, prophylactic aciclovir is recommended because of the potentially severe and life-threatening nature of such infections.

Varicella-zoster virus

Chickenpox

The primary manifestation of infection with varicella-zoster virus is chickenpox. This is usually a trivial disease of children, despite the dramatic rash. The most important complication is varicella pneumonia, which can be life-threatening. This is considerably more common in adults than in children, and seems to be more common in pregnant women. Adults with chickenpox are thus at risk of severe pneumonitis and should be referred promptly to hospital for intravenous aciclovir therapy if evidence of respiratory involvement occurs.

It has been suggested that all children, with chickenpox should be given aciclovir. The arguments in favour of this blanket approach are economic rather than medical. Aciclovir allows resolution of the disease 24–48 h earlier than would otherwise be the case, enabling adults, or carers of sick children to return to work that much sooner. Primary infection in adults is usually a more disabling disease than in children, and consideration of aciclovir therapy in this instance is reasonable.

Neonatal chickenpox

Pregnant women who develop chickenpox in late pregnancy may pass this infection on to their baby if it is born within a week of onset of the maternal rash since there is insufficient time to allow the mother to generate protective antibodies that can be transferred across the placenta. Neonatal chickenpox is a feared disease, and babies at risk should be given passive immunization with hyperimmune zoster immune globulin. It is also reasonable to give such babies prophylactic aciclovir by mouth, although some withhold the drug until the baby develops signs of disease.

Immunocompromised patients

Chicken-pox in a patient who is immunocompromised may be life-threatening, especially if the immunodeficiency is in cell-mediated immunity (e.g. HIV positive patients, transplant recipients on immunosuppressive drugs, patients on high dose steroids). Such individuals should be tested for their immune status with regard to varicella zoster virus, and if susceptible, should report all contacts with either chicken-pox or herpes zoster, so that varicella-zoster immunoglobulin can be administered. Treatment of the disease itself in such individuals should be with high-dose intravenous aciclovir, no matter how trivial the disease appears to be when first seen.

Herpes zoster

The site of latency of varicella-zoster virus (VZV) is the dorsal root ganglion. The systemic nature of varicella infection means that dorsal root ganglia up and down the spinal cord become latently infected. Reactivation of infection results in virus travelling down the dorsal nerve route in question, to reach the dermatome supplied by that nerve. This accounts for the characteristic rash of shingles, or herpes zoster, the clinical manifestation of reactivated VZV infection. The onset of rash is often preceded by pain or abnormal sensation in the distribution of the dermatome. The rash usually heals uneventfully, but pain in the area of the rash may persist long after the rash itself has resolved. This post-herpetic neuralgia is more likely to occur in elderly patients, and can be extremely debilitating.

Other complications of secondary VZV infection occasionally occur: reactivation of virus in the ophthalmic branch of the trigeminal nerve may result in keratitis and damage to the cornea; facial nerve involvement may cause a form of Bell's palsy; motor nerve damage may also be evident in zoster affecting the limbs; involvement of sacral ganglia may result in urinary and anal retention.

A prolonged or atypical attack of herpes zoster may be the presenting feature of a number of diseases in which host immune responses are impaired. These include malignancy of the reticuloendothelial system and HIV infection. In any immunocompromised patient with zoster, dissemination of the virus in the bloodstream may occur, with the appearance of lesions beyond the initial dermatome. This spread of virus also puts the patient at risk of life-threatening internal organ infection.

The aims of antiviral therapy include alleviation of the pain and discomfort of the rash, and the prevention of complications, including post-herpetic neuralgia and dissemination. Antiviral therapy given early in the course of zoster reduces the incidence of post-herpetic neuralgia and accelerates the resolution of pain. It is therefore logical to use antiviral therapy (aciclovir or its congeners) in the following types of zoster, provided this is started within 72 h of onset of the rash (or longer for immunocompromised patients):

◆ any form of zoster in an immunocompromised patient, no matter how mild the attack appears to be on first presentation;

◆ ophthalmic zoster;

◆ zoster involving motor nerves, including the facial nerve;

◆ sacral zoster;

◆ zoster occurring in patients at 50 years of age or above who are therefore at increased risk of post-herpetic neuralgia.

Epstein–Barr virus

Considerably larger doses of aciclovir are necessary to inhibit Epstein–Barr virus replication than herpes simplex or varicella-zoster virus *in vitro*. This presumably reflects the differing efficiency of the phosphorylation of the drug by these viruses. The results of clinical trials of aciclovir in patients with infectious mononucleosis have been disappointing. The only manifestation of Epstein–Barr virus infection in which aciclovir is useful is oral hairy leukoplakia. This unusual disease arises only in immunocompromised patients, most commonly those with HIV infection. It presents as a whitish coating on the tongue or buccal mucosa, which may resemble candidiasis. The lesions are packed with replicating virus. The lesions may respond to aciclovir therapy, but reappear when treatment is stopped, so that long-term use of the drug may be necessary.

Cytomegalovirus

Primary infections

Primary CMV infections of immunocompetent individuals are usually asymptomatic, although a small minority result in the infectious mononucleosis syndrome (glandular fever). Reactivation of latent virus fails to induce any recognizable disease in the individual concerned. There are two groups of patients, however, in whom the virus is a significant pathogen: babies infected *in utero*, and immunocompromised patients.

Congenital infection

Transfer of CMV across the placenta may arise from both primary and reactivated maternal infection. Congenital infection affects about one in 300 live births in the UK. Most of these babies develop normally, but about 5 to 10% are born with so-called cytomegalic inclusion disease, which has a poor prognosis. A further 5 to 10% are normal at birth, but later develop abnormalities such as deafness, impaired neurodevelopment, or learning difficulties. Controlled clinical trials of twice daily intravenous ganciclovir for six weeks in congenitally infected neonates with symptoms related to the central nervous system have shown significant benefit in terms of hearing outcome, and this has therefore become the standard of care for such neonates. Trials of oral valganciclovir for either six weeks or six months, and in neonates with manifestations other than those restricted to the central nervous sytem, are now in progress. There is currently no effective strategy for the prevention of congenital infection, although experimental vaccines have shown some promise in protecting susceptible individuals from infection. It may therefore be possible to protect women who reach child-bearing age without having had CMV infection from acquiring it during pregnancy.

Immunocompromised patients

Symptomatic CMV disease may arise from primary or secondary infection in immunocompromised patients, including transplant recipients and those infected with HIV. In these patients, active CMV infection is a multisystem disease. In transplant recipients, it often presents with fever and leucopenia; other complications include hepatitis, myositis, and pneumonitis. In HIV-infected patients, retinitis is the commonest manifestation, accounting for 85% of all CMV disease in patients with AIDS, but infection may also involve any part of the gastrointestinal tract, the brain, lungs, liver, adrenals, and peripheral nerves. Diagnosis is dependent upon clinical suspicion, virus isolation from normally sterile body samples, biopsy, and quantitative measurements of CMV viraemia. As management of HIV infection itself has improved significantly over the years, manifestations of CMV disease in HIV-infected patients have become less common.

Treatment

Although several drugs are now available, the goal of a safe, easily administered, and effective therapy for CMV infection has yet to be attained. Ganciclovir, foscarnet, and cidofovir must all be given by intravenous infusion, but fomivirsen is administered by intraocular injection. Side effects may be serious: bone marrow suppression (ganciclovir), nephrotoxicity (foscarnet and cidofovir), and painful penile ulceration (foscarnet) are the most notable.

Ganciclovir or valganciclovir (administered orally) are the drugs of first choice, with foscarnet as an alternative. Experience with cidofovir and fomivirsen is so far restricted to the management of CMV retinitis. Not all complications of CMV infection respond equally well to therapy. Drugs can save the sight of patients with retinitis, and infections of the bowel and liver also respond well, but treatment of CMV pneumonitis in bone marrow transplant recipients is often unsuccessful because immune responses to the virus may also contribute to the disease process.

Therapy does not eliminate the virus, and in patients who remain immunosuppressed, CMV disease often recurs when therapy is stopped.

Prophylaxis

Avoiding transplantation of material from latently infected donors to uninfected recipients can significantly reduce serious CMV disease in solid organ transplant recipients. In contrast, bone marrow recipients most at risk of life-threatening CMV disease are those who are seropositive themselves, but receive marrow from a seronegative donor. However, matching of CMV serostatus between donor and recipient in order to prevent the risk of disease is not a practicable solution to the problem. If recipients are deemed to be at risk, administration of CMV prophylaxis is appropriate. The exact regimen is a matter of debate, but trials in different transplant settings have demonstrated the benefit of CMV immunoglobulin, oral valganciclovir, and, surprisingly, oral aciclovir or valaciclovir. Serum levels of aciclovir in these patients are well below the concentrations necessary to inhibit CMV replication, but sufficiently high levels may be achieved inside infected cells.

Human herpesviruses 6, 7, and 8

Human herpesvirus type 6 is the causative agent of roseola infantum, one of the many rashes of childhood. Occasional cases are associated with hepatitis or encephalitis. The virus is sensitive *in vitro* to ganciclovir, but not aciclovir; however, the value of treatment is unknown. No disease has yet been associated with either primary or secondary infection with human herpesvirus type 7.

Human herpesvirus type 8, also known as Kaposi's sarcoma-associated herpesvirus, is the causative agent of all forms of Kaposi's sarcoma. Management of this malignant disease involves chemotherapy, and a role for antiviral drugs remains to be defined.

Respiratory tract infections

Upper respiratory tract infections

Infections of the upper respiratory tract with rhinoviruses (of which there are over 100 serotypes), corona-, entero-, adeno-, respiratory syncytial, and para-influenza viruses are extremely common, but, fortunately, result in very little serious morbidity or mortality. Despite considerable effort, no specific antiviral therapy has been successfully developed for treatment or prevention of these infections. Intranasal interferon spray is effective in the treatment and prophylaxis of common colds that are caused by rhinoviruses, but patients experience nasal stuffiness, irritation, and bleeding, which negates any possible therapeutic benefit. This approach to the management of the common cold has now been abandoned.

Lower respiratory tract infections

Viral infection of the lower respiratory tract is potentially much more dangerous. The commonest viral infections giving rise to bronchiolitis and pneumonia are those due to respiratory syncytial and influenza viruses. Varicella pneumonia and CMV pneumonitis have been referred to above. In addition, giant cell pneumonia is a rare and fatal complication of measles, usually in leukaemic children who escaped vaccination.

Respiratory syncytial virus infection of infants

Bronchiolitis and pneumonia due to respiratory syncytial virus infection are relatively common in infants under 1 year of age. Ribavirin reduces viral shedding, hastens resolution of fever, improves respiration, and shortens stay in hospital. The main difficulty is that the drug needs to be administered by use of a small particle aerosol generator. Moreover, for maximum benefit, the infant must breathe nebulized drug for at least 12 h each day. Thus, ribavirin is not usually used in otherwise uncomplicated infection in an immunocompetent host. In babies with congenital immunodeficiency or heart or lung defects, where mortality from acute RSV infection may exceed 50%, ribavirin can be life saving.

Influenza

The preferred drugs for the management of influenza virus infections are the neuraminidase inhibitors (e.g. zanamivir, oseltamivir). Controlled trials have shown a shorter time to the resolution of symptoms and lower usage of antibiotics among patients treated with these drugs. However, they must be given within 48 h of onset of symptoms for maximum benefit—a timeframe not often met by patients suffering influenzal symptoms. Zanamivir has poor oral bioavailability, is not licensed for children under five years of age and has to be given by oral or nasal inhalation. Oseltamivir, in contrast, can be administered by mouth in capsules and a five day course is standard. Currently in the UK, it is recommended that neuraminidase inhibitors be used for the treatment of an influenza-like illness in an 'at-risk' individual when influenza is circulating in the community. 'At-risk' individuals comprise those with chronic respiratory, heart, renal, liver, or neurological disease, or diabetes mellitus, together with the immunocompromised and those aged 65 years or older.

These drugs can also be used, in the same target population groups, for post-exposure prophylaxis (PEP), assuming those individuals are not effectively protected by prior influenza vaccination. Such PEP is appropriate following exposure to someone suffering from an influenza-like illness in the same household or residential setting, when influenza is known to be circulating in the community.

The influenza pandemic of 2009 was the first in history to occur at a time when effective anti-influenza drugs were available. Most governments had stockpiled millions of doses of neuraminidase inhibitors (mostly oseltamivir) for just such an eventuality. When the pandemic first emerged, most use of the drugs was as prophylaxis for close contacts of laboratory-proven cases, in order to try and reduce the spread of disease (the containment phase). Once the infection was widespread in the community, the strategy switched to a treatment phase, where the drugs were used primarily as therapy for those with proven infection. It is difficult to assess how successful these tactics were, as, fortunately, the causative pandemic virus was of relatively low virulence. Stockpiling as part of pandemic preparedness plans will continue, and may prove to be of great benefit should a highly pathogenic virus, such as avian influenza A H5N1 virus, which has been circulating at low levels in humans since 1997, adapt to become a human pandemic strain in the future.

Extensive use of the neuraminidase inhibitors, as treatment for both influenza A H5N1 and for pandemic influenza A H1N1 has, perhaps inevitably, been associated with the emergence of resistant variants. A single point mutation (H275Y) in the neuraminidase gene induces considerable resistance to oseltamivir. Resistance to zanamivir is less common, and, indeed, oseltamivir resistant strains may still be sensitive to zanamivir. For severely ill patients with oseltamivir resistance, zanamivir can be administered intravenously. There are also new neuraminidase inhibitors in the pipeline, such as peramivir, which can be administisired via this route.

Some influenza A viruses are susceptible to the uncoating blockers amantadine and rimantadine. Clinical trials in boarding schools and other places in which large numbers of individuals are crowded together have shown that amantadine is effective in the treatment and prophylaxis of influenza A. Those treated with the drug have a milder, shorter-lasting infection. About 70% of contacts given the drug are protected from infection. However, amantadine is unpopular in the elderly, who suffer the brunt of serious influenza, because of its stimulatory actions on the central nervous system. Patients become confused and agitated, and may be unable to sleep. Rimantadine, a derivative of amantadine, is said to be equipotent in its anti-influenzal properties but less prone to side effects. However, it is not currently licensed in the UK. Viral resistance emerges rapidly in patients treated with either of these drugs.

Other infections

Warts

Papillomavirus infections (warts) are amenable to physical (cryotherapy, surgery) and chemical (podophyllin and derivatives, salicylic acid) therapies. Interferons may have a place in the management of recalcitrant warts. About 50% of warts disappear following intralesional or intramuscular interferon, but they often recur. Topical application of imiquimod, a new imidazoquinoline that stimulates interferon and other cytokines, appears to be modestly effective.

More serious consequences of HPV infection include cancer of the uterine cervix. New vaccines, containing the surface proteins of the commonest high risk HPV types (16 and 18) are now licensed for the prevention of this malignancy. Most countries have adopted a policy of targeting the vaccine at teenage girls.

Polyomavirus infections

Progressive multifocal leucoencephalopathy, a disease that occurs almost exclusively in HIV-positive and other immunosuppressed patients, is a manifestation of reactivation of a polyomavirus in the brain. Treatment is difficult, but there are reports that cidofovir (p. 55) may be useful.

Lassa fever

Ribavirin, taken orally, is very effective in the treatment and prophylaxis of Lassa fever, a haemorrhagic virus infection with a high mortality rate encountered in certain parts of West Africa.

Diarrhoea

The treatment of viral gastroenteritis is considered in Chapter 25.

Key points

- ◆ Aciclovir and derivatives (valaciclovir, famciclovir) are effective against infections with HSV-1, HSV-2 and VZV.

- ◆ Antiviral therapy is therefore recommended for all primary HSV infections (oropharyngeal or genital); eczema herpeticum; herpetic keratitis (primary or secondary); suspected herpes simplex encephalitis; neonatal HSV infection. It may also be useful as prophylaxis against recurrent herpetic disease in heavily immunocompromised individuals.

- ◆ Antiviral therapy is also recommended for primary VZV infection (chicken-pox) in adults (including pregnant women if required); in any immunocompromised individual; and in neonatal varicella. In reactivated infection (herpes zoster or shingles), therapy is recommended for ophthalmic zoster; zoster involving motor nerves (e.g. facial palsy); any zoster in an immunocompromised patient; zoster in anyone over the age of 50.

- ◆ Treatment of CMV infection with (val)ganciclovir, cidofovir, or foscarnet is less satisfactory owing to drug toxicities, but may be life- or sight-saving in immunocompromised patients (e.g. HIV infection, solid organ or bone marrow transplant recipients).

- ◆ Influenza virus infections can be treated with neuraminidase inhibitors. Ideally, therapy should be initiated within 72 hours of onset of symptoms. These drugs are targeted at those individuals at high risk of serious complications should they acquire influenza virus infection, although in the setting of an emerging pandemic, they may be offered universally either for prophylaxis or therapy.

Further reading

Yin MT, Brust JCM, Tieu HV, Hammer SM (2009), 'Antiherpesvirus, anti-hepatitis virus, and anti-respiratory virus agents', in *Clinical Virology* (3rd edn). Richman DD, Whitley RJ, Hayden FG (eds). Washington DC: ASM Press, 217–264.

Gupta R, Warren T, Wald A (2007), 'Genital herpes'. *Lancet*, **370**: 2127–2137.

Wareham DW, Breuer J. (2007), 'Herpes zoster—clinical review'. *British Medical Journal* **334**: 1211–5.

Chapter 33

Management of HIV infection

There have been many significant advances in our understanding and management of HIV infection within the 30 years or so since the first appearance of patients with the acquired immunodeficiency syndrome. Improvements in drug design and in understanding the replication cycle of HIV have led to the development of an increasing number of antiretroviral agents (see Table 5.1, p. 62). Moreover, application of molecular biological techniques allows accurate monitoring of the amount of HIV RNA in peripheral blood (viral load) in individual patients. Treatment regimens and management protocols are becoming ever more complex. In order to achieve optimization and standardization of clinical practice, bodies such as the British HIV Association publish consensus guidelines for antiretroviral treatment of HIV-seropositive individuals. Such is the pace of change that these guidelines need regular revision. It is nevertheless possible to discern some important underlying principles governing the appropriate use of antiretroviral therapy, although their detailed application may vary from place to place and over time.

Natural history of HIV infection

The natural history of HIV infection is relatively straightforward. The virus infects CD4-positive T cells and cells of the monocyte/macrophage series. Infection results in cell death. Initially, dying cells can be replenished, but over a prolonged period of time, there is an inexorable decline in the circulating CD4 T cell count. These cells play an integral role in the orchestration of adaptive immune responses, and their loss is accompanied by ever-increasing clinically evident immunodeficiency, culminating in the acquired immunodeficiency syndrome (AIDS). Whilst there are differences in the rate of progression of disease between individuals, nevertheless, the vast majority of untreated patients will eventually die from the disease.

Following initial infection, which may or may not be associated with a 'seroconversion illness' about 4–6 weeks after infection, patients enter an asymptomatic phase. During this period, the viral load is a relatively stable marker within an individual patient—this is referred to as the viral load 'set-point'. This is a reflection of the turnover of virus replicating within cells, which in turn will reflect the rate of CD4 cell death, and it is therefore not surprising that the viral load set-point is the strongest predictor of how long it will take an individual patient to reach the clinical end point of AIDS.

Disease progression can therefore be monitored by regular measurement of both the circulating CD4 T cell count, and the viral load. The primary aim of therapy is to suppress the viral load to as low as possible—preferably to levels which are undetectable using modern ultrasensitive assays which can detect down to around 40 copies of viral RNA per ml of blood. Suppression of viral replication will halt the decline of the CD4 T cell count, and indeed will be followed by an increase in CD4 T cell numbers. The returning CD4 T cells are functional, and thus there is, to a greater or lesser extent, a reconstitution of the damaged host immune system. As the immunodeficiency recedes, then the risk of those complications of HIV infection that define AIDS also recede. As a consequence, it is possible to discontinue prophylaxis against infections such as pneumocystis, toxoplasmosis, and cryptococcosis in patients responding successfully to therapy.

Table 33.1 When should combination anti-retroviral therapy be initiated?

Symptomatic HIV disease
History of an AIDS-defining illness
CD4 T cell count below 350/μl
Pregnancy
Co-infection with HBV/HCV

When to treat?

Given that there are now drugs available that can substantially decrease the viral load within an individual patient, and that this can be monitored, the question arises as to when antiretroviral therapy should be started. This decision is an important one. It requires commitment from the patient to take the medication for a prolonged period, usually for life. This may incur both physical and psychological morbidity, disadvantages that have to be weighed against the potential therapeutic benefits to be gained. At present, UK guidelines recommend starting therapy in any patient with symptomatic HIV infection or AIDS regardless of their viral load or CD4 count. In those who are asymptomatic the CD4 count is the major determinant for starting therapy. All those with counts <350 cells/μl should be offered therapy (Table 33.1). Those with counts between 350 and 500 cells/μl are evaluated further for viral load, rate of CD4 decline, evidence of coexisting conditions and patient preference. Currently, treatment is deferred for those with CD4 counts above 500 cells/μl, although such patients could be enrolled into ongoing 'when to start' clinical trials. Evidence for long-term survival benefit of early treatment of primary HIV infection is currently lacking, and this should only be considered as part of a clinical trial to address this question. Management of HIV infection in pregnancy is a further specialist issue (see below).

What to treat with?

The history of drug development in HIV infection demonstrates very clearly that successful therapy must consist of multiple drugs given in combination. Initially zidovudine (AZT) was the only option available. However, monotherapy with AZT invariably led to the selection of mutations in the error-prone reverse transcriptase gene, rendering the virus resistant to the drug after around 6 months. Thus, it is essential to model the treatment of HIV infection on that used for the treatment of tuberculosis: use of multiple agents to reduce the chances that the virus will become resistant to all of the drugs simultaneously. This principle has now been validated for a variety of combination therapies and has become the standard of care.

Triple drug combinations are highly effective in reducing viral load, both in degree and in duration of the effect. With the choice of agents including nucleoside and non-nucleoside inhibitors of reverse transcriptase, inhibitors of the viral protease and, integrase enzymes, and entry and fusion inhibitors (Table 5.1, p. 62), there are numerous possible triple drug combinations. The continuing emergence of new agents will complicate this even further. It is clearly not possible to test each one of these combinations in full-scale clinical trials, but several regimens have proved to be highly effective. Such combination therapies are now collectively referred to as 'combination antiretroviral therapy' (cART), having formerly been known as 'highly active antiretroviral therapy' (HAART).

Regimens recommended in the UK include two nucleoside reverse transcriptase inhibitors plus either a non-nucleos(t)ide reverse transcriptase inhibitor or a protease inhibitor (Table 33.2). The reason for not selecting one drug of each category, which might appear intuitively to be the best

Table 33.2 Recommended Initial cART Regimens

1st choice: −2 NRTIs +1 NNRTI

    Preferred NRTIs: Coformulations, i.e

                         Truvada (Tenofovir/Emtricitabine) or

                         Kivexa[1] (Abacavir/Lamivudine)

    Preferred NNRTI: Efavirenz

2nd choice: −2 NRTIs +1 ritonavir boosted PI

    Preferred PI: Darunavir/Atazanavir/Lopinavir/Fosamprenivir

[1] Must ensure patient is HLA-B*5701 negative.

idea, is to reserve some classes of drugs for the time when (if) initial therapy begins to fail. At this time, the virus present within the patient may have acquired a number of mutations conferring resistance to the drugs contained within his/her regimen, but the virus should remain fully sensitive to drugs in the unused classes. In the absence of such 'class-sparing', the options for salvage therapy in the event of treatment failure are much reduced, as cross-resistance between drugs of the same class is common.

The exact choice of drugs for an individual patient depends on a number of variables. It cannot be assumed that virus in a patient who has received no previous antiretroviral therapy will be sensitive to all drugs, as the patient may have been infected with a resistant strain. Such primary drug resistance now affects more than 10% of newly diagnosed patients in the UK. Thus, virus from newly diagnosed patients should be sent for resistance testing prior to initiation of therapy. Moreover, adverse events are often unpredictable and regimens may need tailoring to individual patients. Clearly, the more drugs a patient takes, the greater the risk of adverse reactions. For example, there is particular concern about the long-term safety of protease inhibitors, owing to their effect on lipid metabolism. Adverse events associated with the antiretroviral drugs are listed in Table 33.3.

As outlined above, antiretroviral therapy is monitored by serial viral load measurements. Viral load should decline significantly, and usually to undetectable levels, within three months of onset of cART. Regular monitoring at three monthly intervals thereafter is standard, as failure of treatment, for whatever reason, will first become apparent due to a rise in viral titres. Patients stabilized on cART are also reviewed frequently for CD4 T cell count, clinical assessment, lipid analysis, and evidence of organ or bone marrow toxicity arising from treatment or complications of their HIV infection.

Treatment failure: non-compliance and resistance

Should viral load start to rise, then consideration must be given to understanding the reasons for treatment failure. The two most important are non-compliance with therapy, and emergence of drug resistance.

Drugs are only effective for as long as their concentration in the tissues is high enough. Failure to take the requisite regular doses of an antiviral drug leads to a fall in tissue levels, with a consequent risk of escape of the virus from inhibition of replication, and an increased likelihood of mutation to resistance. It is important, therefore, that patients adhere to the prescribed regimens. The more doses that are missed, the faster resistant virus will emerge.

Compliance is a significant problem, especially with multidrug regimens, in which some tablets should be taken with food and others on an empty stomach; some twice a day, others three or four

Table 33.3 Major adverse events associated with antiretroviral agents

Drug class	Drugs	Main adverse effects
Reverse transcriptase inhibitors		
(i) Nucleos(t)ide analogues		
	Abacavir (ABC)	Hypersensitivity reactions in HLA B5701-positive patients
	Didanosine (ddI)	Peripheral neuropathy, pancreatitis
	Emtricitabine	Pruritus
	Lamivudine (3TC)	
	Stavudine (d4T)	Fat redistribution, peripheral neuropathy
	Tenofovir (TDF)	Increased serum phosphate, renal dysfunction
	Zidovudine (AZT)	Macrocytic anaemia, fat redistribution
(ii) Non-nucleoside Analogues		
	Efavirenz	CNS toxicity, teratogenic – avoid in pregnancy
	Etravirine	Rash
	Nevirapine	Rash, may cause severe hepatotoxicity
Protease inhibitors		
	Atazanavir	Most PIs are metabolised by the P450 CYP3A system and may cause drug-drug interactions. Most PIs are associated with hyperlipidaemia and possibly insulin resistance. Many PIs are associated with gastrointestinal disturbance (e.g. diarrhoea)
	Darunavir	
	Fosamprenivir	
	Indinavir	
	Lopinavir	
	Nelfinavir	
	Ritonavir	
	Saquinavir	
	Tipranavir	
Fusion inhibitors		
	Enfuvirtide	Must be given by subcut injection, very expensive
CCR5 inhibitors		
	Maraviroc	
Integrase inhibitors		
	Raltegravir	No toxic effects yet reported

times a day. By combining drugs in fixed dose formulations, compliance can be increased and this is now the preferred treatment approach, with the aim being 'one tablet, once a day'. Patients may also be on a variety of other agents (e.g. for prophylaxis against pneumocystis pneumonia or recurrent herpes simplex disease). Moreover, in any disease, and HIV infection is no exception, adherence to treatment is poorer in patients with symptom-free disease. Failure to take the tablets must always be considered as an explanation for a sudden rise in viral titre.

If non-compliance is ruled out, then the possible emergence of drug-resistant virus must be assessed. Resistance testing is performed in reference laboratories, and is mostly based around sequencing of the target viral genes, and comparison of those sequences against an extensive database of possible resistance mutations. Identification of which mutations are present in which viral genes will allow determination of which drugs within the cART regimen are failing, and therefore rational decision-making about how to change the cART regimen. This may involve replacing one, two, or even all three of the drugs. Drug-resistance genotyping is expensive but has become integral to defining initial therapy and for identifying resistance arising during treatment. Comparative trials have shown that genotypic resistance testing confers a significant benefit on the virological response when choosing therapeutic alternatives.

Pregnancy

A special consideration is the use of antiretroviral drugs in pregnancy. In the absence of any interventions, around 25% of babies of infected mothers will acquire HIV infection themselves. However, mother-to-baby transmission of HIV is almost entirely preventable with appropriate interventions. As such interventions can only be applied to pregnant women who are known to be infected with HIV, it is imperative that HIV testing is routinely instituted for all pregnant women. Such a policy of universal screening for HIV infection in pregnancy was introduced in the UK some years ago.

There is compelling evidence that the risk of vertical transmission of HIV from mother to baby is proportional to the maternal viral load during pregnancy. Reduction of maternal viral load by use of antiretroviral agents significantly reduces the risk of transmission. Thus, viral load should be determined in all HIV-infected pregnant women, and appropriate regimens of antiretroviral therapy offered dependent on the starting viral load and the patient's past history of antiretroviral usage. Delivery by caesarian section may also reduce the risk of transmission, especially if the maternal viral load is above 50 copies/ml, although the benefit in women with undetectable viral load is minimal. Post-exposure prophylaxis should be given to the neonate—the precise regimen is dependent on maternal therapy and viral load at delivery. Breast feeding is not advised, as this doubles the risk of transmission.

Co-infection with hepatitis B or C viruses

As management of HIV infection has improved, co-infected patients have started to survive long enough to develop life-threatening liver disease arising from their chronic viral infection. It is therefore important that all HIV-infected patients be tested to determine if they are co-infected with HBV or HCV. If they are, then appropriate management of both their HIV and HBV/HCV infections must be instituted. If monotherapy is considered for the HBV co-infection, care must be taken to choose a drug (e.g. adefovir) which will not induce resistance mutations within the HIV, or alternatively, a specific cART regimen may be chosen because it also has effective anti-HBV activity (e.g. tenofovir/emtricitabine as the NRTI backbone). In HCV co-infection, it may be necessary to treat the HIV infection in a patient who would not otherwise be offered it, purely for the purposes of enhancing the chances of successful anti-HCV therapy.

Conclusions

The complexity of HIV disease and its attendant complications, most notably of opportunistic infections (Chapter 31), requires specialist management over many years. While cART has substantially improved the survival and quality of life of those affected by HIV/AIDS, the disease remains incurable. New therapeutic approaches are needed, with novel modes of action and fewer side effects. This will remain the situation until an effective vaccine is developed, which despite an enormous research effort, remains an elusive goal.

HIV-positive patients are at risk of a wide range of serious infections. These are discussed in Chapter 31.

Key points

- The aim of antiretroviral therapy is to prevent (or halt or reverse) immunological damage arising from HIV infection and so avert the associated risks of opportunistic infections and other morbidities associated with the acquired immunodeficiency syndrome.

- HIV management is best delivered by a multidisciplinary team with appropriate experience. Combination antiretroviral therapy (cART) is essential in order to avoid the emergence of drug resistance.

- cART should be considered for patients displaying symptomatic disease; having an AIDS-defining illness; having a CD4 count less than 350 cells/μl. Additional considerations are pregnancy, and co-infection with HBV or HCV.

- Drug resistance testing should be performed prior to initation of therapy as patients may be infected de novo with resistant strains.

- Recommended initial cART regimens include 2 NRTI plus an NNRTI or 2 NRTI plus a PI. Response should be monitored by regular viral load testing.

- Compliance is essential but may be difficult. All antiretrovirals may give rise to adverse events, both short- and long-term. It may be necessary to try different regimens to find one that an individual patient can tolerate.

Further reading

Volberding PA, Deeks SG (2010), 'Antiretroviral therapy and management of HIV infection', *Lancet* **376**: 49–62.

The British HIV Association website contains a number of authoritative guidelines for the management of HIV infection, available at: http://www.bhiva.org/PublishedandApproved.aspx.

Gazzard BG, on behalf of the BHIVA Treatment Guidelines Writing Group (2008), 'British HIV Association guidelines for the treatment of HIV-1-infected adults with antiretroviral therapy 2008', *HIV Medicine* **9**: 563–608.

Chapter 34

Treatment of chronic viral hepatitis

With over 500 million individuals chronically infected with either hepatitis B or C viruses, all of whom are at risk of development of end-stage liver disease and hepatocellular carcinoma, chronic viral hepatitis creates a huge health and economic burden worldwide. The outlook for such patients has dramatically improved in the last 10–15 years with a number of antiviral therapies being shown in appropriately controlled clinical trials to be effective (see Chapter 6).

Hepatitis B

Natural history of chronic HBV infection

Chronic infection with hepatitis B virus is defined as the persistence of hepatitis B surface antigen (HBsAg) in the peripheral blood for more than six months. However, HBsAg-positive individuals can be subdivided further into those in whom HBeAg (a breakdown product of the viral core antigen) can be detected, and those with antibodies to this antigen, anti-HBe. HBeAg is a surrogate marker of active viral replication in hepatocytes. HBe antigen seroconversion is therefore associated with a significant decline in the viral load detectable in peripheral blood.

Hepatitis B virus itself is not cytopathic—it is the immune response (especially that mediated by cytotoxic T cells) to infected hepatocytes which induces liver cell death. The intrahepatic response to liver cell injury is the laying down of fibrous tissue. Thus, the end result of the inflammatory hepatitis induced by chronic HBV infection is cirrhosis of the liver. However, liver disease progression is not linear over time, and a number of pathologically distinct phases of chronic infection are now recognized (see Table 34.1). Soon after the establishment of chronic infection, there is extensive virus replication within hepatocytes, with no apparent immune response. This is the immunotolerant phase. The patient will be HBeAg positive (a marker of active virus replication), the peripheral blood viral load will exceed 10^6 copies per ml, but the serum alanine aminotransferase level (ALT, a marker of liver cell death) will be normal. When, eventually, an immune response is mounted to the virus, there may be extensive hepatocyte death and an intense intrahepatic inflammation which may result in severe liver damage. This phase is referred to as immune clearance or 'e' seroconversion. During this phase, the ALT levels will be raised, indicating ongoing inflammation. Eventually, as the bulk of infected cells are killed, resulting in loss of replicating virus, HBeAg is lost from peripheral blood, the viral load declines to levels below 10^3, and eventually anti-HBe is detectable in the peripheral blood. The patient then enters a quiescent phase of low or non-detectable virus replication. The intrahepatic inflammation has died down, and therefore ALT levels return to normal. This has previously been referred to as an inactive carrier state, but this terminology is perhaps slightly misleading, as virus is still present within the liver, and replication may recommence as the patient enters the reactivation phase. Such reactivation occurs with virus that has acquired mutations in its genome such that it is no longer able to synthesize HBeAg—such mutants are referred to as precore mutants. Virus reactivation is associated with increased viral loads and inflammatory responses despite the patient being anti-HBe positive, resulting in raised ALT and the propensity to cause progressive liver damage.

Table 34.1 Natural history of chronic hepatitis B virus infection

Phase	Intrahepatic viral replication	Viral load (copies/ml) in peripheral blood	HBeAg/anti-HBe status	Serum ALT	Active liver damage
Immunotolerant	High	$>10^6$	HBeAg +ve	Normal	No
Immune clearance	Declining	Declining	Seroconverting	High	Yes
Low/non-replicative	Low	$<10^3$	Anti-HBe +ve	Normal	No
Reactivation	Flares of high activity	$>10^4$	Anti-HBe +ve	High	Yes

Note that patients remain HBsAg positive throughout all phases of infection.

Progression through these phases of chronic infection is dependent on a number of factors including:

◆ age at infection. Neonates who acquire infection at birth from their carrier mothers enter a prolonged immunotolerant phase which may last up to 30 years. In those who acquire infection as adults, this phase may only last for a year or two;

◆ immune function, for obvious reasons;

◆ HBV genotype. The ease with which the virus can acquire the key pre-core mutations resulting in a replication competent strain which cannot synthesise HBeAg is dependent on the starting wild-type sequence, which differs between viral genotypes.

Which patients should be treated?

Therapy should be directed at those patients most at risk of progressive liver disease. Several learned societies (e.g. the European Association for the Study of the Liver, EASL, or the American Association for the Study of Liver Disease, AASLD) have issued extensive guidance on selection of patients for therapy. The fundamental principles are that the risk of progressive liver disease is highest in the immunoclearance and reactivation phases of infection, and high viral loads are an important prognostic indicator of long-term development of liver disease. Assessment of an individual patient for therapy therefore requires knowledge of:

◆ their HBeAg/anti-HBe status;

◆ the viral load;

◆ the ALT (a marker of liver cell death/inflammation).

If in doubt, it may also be helpful to perform a liver biopsy and thereby obtain a histological assessment of disease activity. Patients most likely to warrant therapy will therefore be those who are:

◆ HBeAg positive with high viral loads (HBV DNA >2000 IU/ml), high ALT (above the upper limit of normal), and/or histological evidence of active liver disease (immunoclearance phase);

◆ anti-HBe positive with high viral loads (as above), high ALT (again), and/or histological evidence of active liver disease.

What should patients be treated with?

As outlined in Chapter 6, there are two strategies for the treatment of chronic HBV infection—immunomodulation with pegylated interferon, and viral suppressive therapy with nucleos(t)ide analogue polymerase inhibitors. Both modalities have their advantages and disadvantages.

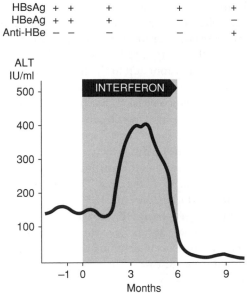

Fig. 34.1 Treatment of chronic hepatitis B infection with interferon showing the change in alanine aminotransferase (ALT) levels, loss of hepatitis B e antigen (HBeAg), and the appearance of antibody to HBe (anti-HBe). Hepatitis B surface antigen (HBsAg) is not eliminated.

Interferon enhances the expression of human leucocyte antigen (HLA) class I molecules on the surface of infected hepatocytes resulting in the efficient elimination of these cells by circulating cytotoxic T lymphocytes. This in turn reduces the amount of virus in the liver, and the production of infectious virions, with a consequent reduction in viral load.

In a patient who is HBeAg positive, a typical response to interferon is shown in Fig. 34.1. At the onset of therapy, the patient is HBsAg and HBeAg positive, and has a raised alanine aminotransferase level, which indicates an active inflammatory response as part of the immune clearance phase. Some weeks after the initiation of interferon therapy, there is a marked rise in alanine aminotransferase. Paradoxically, this indicates a good therapeutic response, since it shows that hepatocytes now express sufficient HLA Class I molecules to allow recognition and destruction by cytotoxic T lymphocytes. At the end of therapy, liver function returns to normal and the patient is now anti-HBe positive. Note that the patient remains HBsAg positive. Thus virus has not been completely eliminated, but passage through the period of immune clearance has been speeded up and the subsequent risk of ongoing liver damage is much reduced. The patient is also much less of an infection risk to sexual partners and family members. After a number of years, some patients do in fact eventually lose HBsAg.

Interferon is administered for a standard period of 48 weeks. Not all carriers will respond. Those who have been carriers of the virus from birth (the vast majority worldwide) and patients who are immunocompromised (including those with HIV infection, in whom carriage of hepatitis B virus is common, as the routes of transmission of the two viruses are similar) respond poorly. In HBeAg positive patients, anti-HBe seroconversion rates are of the order of 30%. In anti-HBe positive patients in the reactivation phase, interferon may also be useful in guiding patients back into a non-replicative phase. Therapy in these patients can only be monitored by viral load and ALT measurement, as they are already anti-HBe positive.

Nucleos(t)ide analogue therapy has become more widely adopted in the last five years or so. First-line therapy should be with a highly potent drug with a high barrier to resistance (i.e. tenofovir or entecavir) although lamivudine is still widely used in many countries because it is cheaper. These drugs suppress viral replication, and monitoring should therefore be via viral load measurement. Around 30% of HBeAg positive patients will seroconvert to anti-HBe positivity on such therapy, and again, the hope is that in time, patients will also lose HBsAg. Cessation of therapy may lead to recurrence of viral replication, up to the pretreatment level, so knowing when to stop therapy is difficult. For HBeAg positive patients, a rule of thumb is to consider stopping therapy 6 months after anti-HBe seroconversion. For patients who are already anti-HBe positive, therapy may have to be very prolonged, which carries an increased risk of the emergence of resistant virus.

Co-infection with HIV and hepatitis B virus is increasingly recognized and requires specialist management. The danger here is that monotherapy for HBV infection with a drug also active against HIV will generate HIV resistance to the drug. Thus, the management of HBV should be undertaken either with adefovir, which has no anti-HIV activity, or only as part of combination antiretroviral therapy potent enough to bring HIV replication under control.

Another area in which these newer agents have shown promise is in the prophylaxis and treatment of hepatitis B positive patients undergoing liver and other forms of transplantation. There is a reduction in risk of severe disease in the case of a grafted liver and a reduced rate of virus reactivation associated with other procedures.

Hepatitis C

Which patients should be treated?

The primary diagnostic test to determine if a patient has been infected with HCV is to look for anti-HCV antibodies in serum. Anti-HCV positivity, however, is only a marker of past infection, and a further test, looking for the presence of HCV RNA in serum, should then be performed to determine if the patient is still infected with the virus. Around 25% of infected patients will clear their infection spontaneously (i.e. without intervention). The remaining 75% become chronically infected and are at risk of progressive liver disease. Factors which increase that risk include older age at the time of infection, being male, drinking alcohol (which acts synergistically with HCV in inducing liver damage), and underlying immunodeficiency, including HIV co-infection. EASL and AASLD guidelines recommend that any patient with chronic HCV infection be considered for therapy, regardless of the degree of underlying liver damage at the time of diagnosis, and this is reflected in the National Institute for Health and Clinical Excellence (NICE) guidelines in the UK. Possible contra-indications to therapy include active injecting drug use (although most clinicians will treat active injectors), heavy alcohol intake, and chaotic lifestyle—all of which might mitigate against adherence to therapy over a prolonged period of time.

Which drugs should be used?

The current standard of care for HCV-infected patients is combination therapy with pegylated interferon (PEG, subcutaneous injection once weekly) and oral ribavirin (RV), although this is likely to change soon with the advent of directly acting antivirals (see Chapter 6). The mechanism of action of interferon in hepatitis C infection appears to be different from that in hepatitis B, as response is not accompanied by a rise in alanine aminotransferase levels. For patients infected with genotype 1 (or 4) virus, the recommended course is for 12 months. For those with genotype 2 or 3 infection, only six months therapy is required. PEG/RV therapy gives rise to a number of adverse effects (see Chapter 6) and is not easy to tolerate. Patients require extensive support to get them through a tough regimen, which is usually provided by specialist hepatitis nurses. Even so,

Table 34.2 Factors which influence the response to PEG/RV therapy in chronic HCV infection

Factor	Good prognostic indicator	Poor prognostic indicator
Viral genotype	2, 3	1, 4
Pretreatment viral load	Low (<800 000 iμ/ml)	High (>800 000 iμ/ml)
Gender	Female	Male
Age at onset of therapy	Younger	Older
Liver disease severity	No or mild fibrosis	Significant fibrosis
IL-28B genotype	Responder allele homozygosity	Non-responder homozygosity or responder/non-responder heterozygosity

a significant number of patients may not be able to complete their allocated therapy—most clinical trials have drop out rates of the order of 10-15%. Some of this is due to patient intolerance, but also some patients develop adverse reactions, such as neutropaenia, thrombocytopaenia, suicidal ideation (all due to PEG), or haemolytic anaemia (due to RV) which make it dangerous to continue.

Likelihood of response to therapy

Several factors influence the likelihood of patients achieving viral clearance with PEG/RV therapy (see Table 34.2). The genotype of the infecting virus is the dominant viral factor—cure rates for patients with genotype 1 infection are around 45%, whereas for genotype 2 infection, this approaches 90%. The molecular basis for the differing sensitivities of the different viral genotypes to therapy is unknown. However, this fundamental property is reflected in the different treatment regimens recommended for each genotype (see above). Response rates are also related to pre-treatment viral load. With regard to host factors, much interest has been generated by recent genome-wide association studies which have identified a cluster of single nucleotide polymorphisms on chromosome 19, near the gene encoding interleukin-28B (IL-28B, also known as interferon-lambda 3), which segregate with response/non-response to therapy. Again, the molecular basis for these observations is not clear, but it raises the possibility that particular therapeutic regimens may be selected for individual patients based on their IL-28B genotype.

		ANTI VIRAL THERAPY				
	Pretreatment	12 weeks	24 weeks	48 weeks	72 weeks	
HCV RNA	+	+	+	+	+	Non-responder
	+	–	–	–	+	Responder-relapser
	+	–	–	–	–	Sustained virological responder

Fig. 34.2 Patterns of response to PEG/RV therapy in chronic HCV infection.

Monitoring of therapy

Response to therapy is best monitored by measurement of the circulating HCV RNA load using quantitative real-time PCR assays. Viral load may be assessed at different times after initiation of therapy, with several definitions of response:

- Rapid virological response (RVR). Assessed at four weeks of therapy. Must be HCV RNA-negative in an assay capable of detecting down to 30 IU/ml;
- Early virological response (EVR). Assessed at 12 weeks of therapy. Complete EVR (cEVR) means viral RNA is undetectable. Partial EVR (pEVR) means there has been at least a 2-log drop in viral load, but not to negativity;
- End of treatment response (EoTR);
- Sustained virological response (SVR). Defined as HCV RNA negativity at 6 months after EoT.

Overall treatment responses are classified (Fig. 34.2) as

- SVR (see above). This equates to cure—almost 100% of individuals who reach SVR remain virus-free when tested five years later;
- Non-response (NR)—viral RNA remains detectable throughout therapy;
- Relapser-responder (RR)—viral RNA becomes undetectable during therapy, but reappears within six months of cessation of therapy.

Achievement of RVR is the best predictor that an SVR will be attained. Indeed, if patients with genotype 1 infection, and a low pretreatment viral load (defined as less than 800 000 iμ/ml) achieve RVR, then they can be treated for just six months (as opposed to 12 months) without reducing their chances of an SVR. Similarly, a shortened course of therapy (e.g. to 16 weeks) is possible for genotype 2 and 3 patients with a low pretreatment viral load who achieve RVR.

Patients who have detectable viraemia after four weeks of therapy should be retested at 12 weeks. If an EVR has not been achieved, then there is very little chance that an SVR will eventuate, and there is little point in continuing therapy beyond this point. Such patients are non-responders.

Most patients do achieve an EVR and continue through to the end of treatment. However, a significant percentage will relapse in the subsequent six months (almost always within three months) with reappearance of viraemia (responder–relapsers).

Hepatitis C virus infection is an important co-morbidity in patients with HIV infection. As management of the immunodeficiency has improved (see Chapter 33) and therefore infected patients are surviving longer, it has become apparent that development of endstage liver disease is a real threat in co-infected patients. Treatment of chronic HCV infection in co-infected patients requires specialist selection and supervision. The timing of treatment of hepatitis C in relation to the stage of HIV infection is crucial. Overall, SVR rates in co-infected individuals are less than in immunocompetent patients, but nevertheless treatment is worthwhile.

Future prospects for the treatment of chronic HCV infection

A number of directly acting antiviral agents developed for the treatment of chronic HCV infection (see Chapter 6) are currently in late stage clinical trials. The first of these, telaprevir and boceprevir, both NS3 protease inhibitors, are now licensed for clinical use. These particular agents work only against genotype 1 virus, but given in combination with PEG and RV, they enhance SVR rates from around 45% to over 65%, a significant improvement. It is also apparent that for triple therapy, there is no additional benefit to extending therapy beyond six months even for genotype 1-infected patients, thereby saving the costs of six months PEG and RV therapy.

The next DAAs likely to make it to the clinic are the NS5b polymerase inhibitors. With the advent of multiple drugs acting at different targets within the viral life cycle, there is a realistic prospect that future therapy will not be dependent on a backbone of PEG and RV. Given the difficulties of persevering with several months of PEG/RV therapy, this will be another major step forward in the management of this condition.

Key points

- Chronic hepatitis B infection proceeds through a number of distinct phases. Liver damage is most likely to occur during the immunoclearance and reactivation phases.

- The need for therapy in chronic HBV is determined by measurement of HBeAg/anti-HBe status, HBV DNA, ALT, and, if necessary, histological assessment of liver biopsy.

- Therapeutic options comprise a time-limited course of pegylated interferon (acting as an immunomodulatory agent), or long-term nucleos(t)ide inhibitors of the viral polymerase. Tenofovir and entecavir are the first choice agents in this category, due to high potency and high genetic barrier to resistance.

- Therapy should be monitored by viral load assessment, and HBeAg to anti-HBe seroconversion where appropriate.

- All patients with chronic HCV infection are eligible for therapy. Current standard of care is combination therapy with pegylated interferon and ribavirin.

- Likelihood of response is dependent on viral genotype, viral load, age, gender, pre-existing liver disease, and host IL-28B genotype.

- Duration of therapy depends on viral genotype, pretreatment viral load, and the rate of on-treatment response to therapy. Overall cure rates are around 50% (45% for genotype 1, 70–80% for genotypes 2 or 3).

- Future therapy for chronic HCV infection is likely to involve combinations of directly acting antiviral agents.

Further reading

Cooke GS, Main J, Thursz MR (2010), 'Treatment for hepatitis B', *British Medical Journal* **340**: 87–91.

EASL Clinical Practice Guidelines (2009), 'Management of chronic hepatitis B', *Journal of Hepatology* **50**: 227–242.

EASL Clinical Practice Guidelines (2011), 'Management of hepatitis C virus infection', *Journal of Hepatology* **55**: 245–264.

Nash KL, Bentley I, Hirschfield GM (2009), 'Managing hepatitis C virus infection', *British Medical Journal* **339**: 37–42.

Chapter 35

Parasitic diseases

The organisms considered as 'parasites'—that is, the protozoa, helminths, and arthropods that have an obligatory relationship to human beings or other animals—tend to cause chronic disease and many individuals, once infected, remain so for long periods. This ensures that in the warmer countries of the world, where poorer standards of hygiene often prevail, there is a high prevalence of infection and a continual high incidence of new cases. The areas with the highest parasitic burden tend to have the poorest medical care because of poverty, a legacy of inadequate facilities, and the logistics of reaching people living in scattered rural communities. In many countries the total annual health care budget would not be sufficient to treat a fraction of their population even if it were all spent on antiparasitic drugs.

Parasitic diseases are, however, far from being restricted to the tropics. Some parasites such as *Trichomonas vaginalis* and threadworm are at least as common in developed countries. Moreover, the speed and extent of international travel ensures that infections acquired in the tropics may present therapeutic challenges to medical practitioners everywhere.

Therapeutic difficulties

One of the peculiarities of treating parasitic infections is the varied relationship between man and microbe. The life cycles often ensure that at some stage the organism is not susceptible to a particular drug because it is either in a resting phase or in an inaccessible site. In many cases the host and parasite reach a steady state of co-existence with no symptoms at all. Parasites restricted to the gut lumen such as the protozoon *Giardia lamblia* (also known as *G. intestinalis*) or many helminths often reach this stage and the intruder is only discovered when stools are examined. In other cases, for example filariasis, the disease becomes 'burnt-out' after years. All these late asymptomatic cases may be diagnosed by chance during routine investigations or as part of mass screening campaigns. The contribution of the parasite burden to overall health is usually impossible to estimate and if the only available drug is potentially toxic the decision to treat an apparently healthy individual is difficult to make.

Another factor in making such a decision is the likelihood of re-infection from the community or environmental reservoirs. Intestinal parasites are found in over 70% of the population in some tropical countries and a child living in a rural environment will inevitably be quickly in contact with the parasite again. Treatment of an individual asymptomatic case without taking care to prevent re-infection is wasting resources and is not good practice. Moreover, many of the remedies for the major parasitic infections are potentially toxic and it is always necessary to weigh the consequences of iatrogenic disease against the benefit of therapy that might not always be able to effect a complete cure. Even though relatively safe compounds are now available for some parasitic diseases these considerations must still be borne in mind. If the drug is non-toxic and inexpensive there is some justification in treating asymptomatic individuals, especially if the infection may at some stage cause further problems.

Accurate laboratory diagnosis is essential if antiparasitic therapy is to be useful, since treatment of most parasitic infections is specific to the pathogen. Acute malaria is a medical emergency and demands immediate laboratory confirmation where facilities exist. Although various rapid diag-nostic tests are available, microscopic diagnosis still remains the gold standard. Some intestinal protozoa such as *Entamoeba coli* are innocuous commensals. If they are misidentified in stool microscopy as *Entamoeba histolytica* the patient may be subjected to unnecessary treatment and the risk of side effects.

Any therapy of extended duration in relatively healthy individuals in the community will be difficult to monitor and compliance may be a problem, especially if the drug is unpleasant to take and has conspicuous side effects. This can occur even with well-educated travellers taking antimalarials.

Protozoan infections

Malaria

Malaria is the most important of all parasitic diseases in terms of mortality. Although indigenous malaria is now virtually restricted to the tropics and subtropics, it is commonly imported into many temperate countries because of the rapid increase in international business travel and tourism to Africa or other tropical destinations. About 2000 cases of imported malaria are recorded in the UK each year—a figure likely to be an underestimate because of considerable under-reporting. Each year preventable fatalities from malaria occur in countries that are other-wise free of the disease. However, this is insignificant compared with the damage malaria inflicts on the populations of the tropical world, particularly in parts of Africa where many children die of falciparum malaria before they reach the age of five.

Acute malaria

After the Second World War chloroquine replaced the traditional remedy quinine as the drug of choice for the treatment of acute malaria. These agents are active against the blood forms of the parasite, which is important in the symptomatic stage of the disease when rapidly dividing schizonts cause red cell lysis; it is particularly important in falciparum malaria when infected erythrocytes block small cerebral blood vessels to give rise to the rapidly fatal form of cerebral malaria. In such cases urgent parenteral therapy is necessary in spite of the hazards of infusion.

In its time, chloroquine revolutionized the treatment and prophylaxis of malaria, but extensive use led to the appearance of resistant strains of *Plasmodium falciparum* in most areas in which the parasite occurs. Many chloroquine-resistant strains are also resistant to alternative drugs such as the combinations of pyrimethamine with sulphonamides or dapsone. Surprisingly for such an ancient remedy, resistance to quinine remains quite rare and the drug returned to favour for severe falciparum malaria but has now replaced by artemusan because of greater effectiveness. Because of the possibility of reduced susceptibility to quinine, treatment with doxycycline or clindamycin, antibacterial antibiotics that also exhibit antimalarial activity, is also usually included. Species of *Plasmodium* other than *P. falciparum* generally retain susceptibility to chlo-roquine and it still remains the drug of choice in benign tertian and quartan malarias.

Derivatives of a Chinese herbal remedy, qinghaosu (artemisinin) are increasingly being used for the treatment of malaria in the tropics and since April 2011 the WHO recommends artemesun for treatment of severe malaria (Table 35.1) in children and adults because clinical trials have shown 25% reduction in mortality in comparison with quinine. Although animal experiments revealed a potential for neurotoxicity, extensive trials, and increasing clinical experience have shown these compounds to be relatively. Various formulations, including artesunic acid (artesunate), artemotil (β-arteether), and artemether are used for intravenous or intramuscular administra-tion. Artesunate can also be given by mouth. Suppository formulations are also available and are

Table 35.1 Spectrum of activity of drugs used in the treatment of intestinal helminthiasis

Drug	Ancylostoma duodenale	Necator americanus	Ascaris lumbricoides	Strongyloides stercoralis	Trichuris trichiura	Enterobius vermicularis
Piperazine	–	–	+++	–	–	+++
Levamisole	++	++	+++	–	–	–
Pyrantel pamoate	++	++	+++	+	++	+++
Albendazole	+++	++	+++	++	++	+++
Mebendazole	++	++	+++	+	++	+++
Tiabendazole	++	++	++	++	–	++

+++, Highly effective; +, poorly effective; –, no useful activity.

particularly useful in children. Artemisinin derivatives are now also recommended as the drugs of choice in uncomplicated falciparum malaria, since they are more rapidly effective than any other drug. Because of the risk of encouraging the development of resistance, is the WHO strongly recommends that artemisinin derivatives should be used together with other antimalarial drugs: artemether with lumefantrine can be given orally if the patient is able to swallow and retain the medication. Alternatively combinations with amodiaquine, mefloquine, or sulphonamide–pyrimethamine are sometimes used, though the possibility of resistance to these agents should be borne in mind.

Mefloquine, a quinolinemethanol derivative, is usually active against chloroquine-resistant strains and has been successfully used for treatment. However, resistance to mefloquine emerges readily and there are fears that widespread use will quickly negate its value. Moreover, mefloquine use has been associated with neuropsychiatric side effects that may persist for some time owing to the very long plasma half-life of the drug. Halofantrine has a shorter half-life (one to four days, compared with two to four weeks) and fewer adverse reactions, but concern has been expressed over possible cardiotoxicity. The related lumefantrine is safer, but is available only in a combination product with artemether.

The Coma Acidosis Malaria (CAM) score is a simple method for assessment of severity of malaria in hospitalized patients and decision making about transfer of patients to high dependency care (Table 35.2).

Recurrent malaria

To effect a radical cure in recurrent malarias with a latent exo-erythrocytic phase—benign tertian malaria caused by *P. vivax* or *P. ovale*—it is necessary to use the 8-aminoquinoline primaquine. An accurate diagnosis should first be made by examining thin and thick blood films, and the acute erythrocytic attack is treated with chloroquine before primaquine is administered. Importantly, patients must be screened for glucose-6-phosphate dehydrogenase deficiency. Low levels of this red blood cell enzyme occur in many populations in endemic areas and administration of primaquine to such individuals may lead to an acute haemolytic crisis worse than the original malaria. Primaquine should not be used during pregnancy.

Reactions to primaquine have given the drug a bad name in India, where *P. vivax* infection and glucose-6-phosphate dehydrogenase deficiency are both common. To overcome this problem a primaquine analogue, bulaquine, has been developed in India and marketed there in a combination product with chloroquine for the treatment and radical cure of malaria caused by *P. vivax*.

Table 35.2 The Coma Acidosis Malaria (CAM) Score for predicting risk of mortality in patients hospitalized with malaria. A score of 0–4 is calculated from two variables: the Glasgow Coma Score (GCS) plus EITHER base deficit OR bicarbonate score OR respiratory rate score Based on Table 1 in: Hanson J, Lee SueÂ J, Mohanty S et al. (2010), 'A Simple Score to Predict the Outcome of Severe Malaria in Adults', *Clinical Infectious Diseases* **50**: 679–85

	Score		
Variable	0 (normal)	1 (deranged)	2 (very deranged)
Score up to 2 points from the Glasgow Coma Score			
Glasgow Coma Score	15	>10 to 14	≤10
Score up to 2 points from ONE of these indicators of acidosis			
Base deficit	<2	2 to <10	≥10
Bicarbonate score	≥24	15 to <24	<15
Respiratory rate score	<20	20 to <40	≥40

NOTES:

1. The preferred method for calculating CAM is from GCS and base deficit. However, if base deficit is not available then either bicarbonate or respiratory rate can be used as indicators of acidosis. Respiratory rate is inferior to bicarbonate.

2. Patients with a CAM score <2 at hospital admission may be safely treated in a general ward, provided that renal function can be monitored.

Bulaquine is said to lack the haemolytic potential of primaquine, although it appears to be at least partially metabolized to primaquine in the bloodstream.

Antimalarial prophylaxis

Advice on prophylaxis against malaria presents a great problem because of the difficulty in predicting drug resistance. Chloroquine has been widely used, but its usefulness has been seriously undermined by the spread of resistance in *P. falciparum*. Moreover, it has a bitter taste and more serious side effects, such as skin photosensitization and retinal damage, may become apparent after prolonged use. Chloroquine should not be continued long term owing to chronic toxicity. In general, it is preferable to use an antifolate agent (pyrimethamine or proguanil) whenever possible, but the unpredictability of resistance has led some authorities to recommend combinations of antifolates with chloroquine in an attempt to reduce the chances of breakthrough of protection. Sulphonamide and sulphone-containing mixtures should be avoided in persons known to be hypersensitive to these compounds or to suffer from glucose-6-phosphate dehydrogenase deficiency. If antifolate agents are used during pregnancy, folic or folinic acid supplements should be given. The combination of pyrimethamine with sulfadoxine has been associated with some fatal reactions and is no longer recommended as a prophylactic agent.

Mefloquine is a reliable prophylactic drug for short-term use in areas in which chloroquine resistance is prevalent, and is widely recommended despite its neurotoxicity. Atovaquone–proguanil and doxycycline also appear effective. Doxycycline is unsuitable for pregnant women and young children.

Advice on the choice of prophylactic regimen is under constant review depending on information on drug resistance in individual travel destinations and the availability of new agents. It is therefore wise for anyone counselling a traveller to a malarious area to seek advice from a specialist, or make use of the excellent databases held nationally by travel clinics and the expert tropical medicine institutes. The choice of agent—or the decision to take any antimalarial—is a risk assessment that depends on the duration and likelihood of exposure against toxicity. Pregnant women and elderly patients on extensive medication might be well advised to travel to less exotic parts of the world if the reason for their journey is tourism.

The most important aspects of prophylaxis are regular medication and continuance of therapy after the last possible exposure in order to eradicate any residual parasites. Prophylaxis needs to continue after leaving the malarious area for one week for atovaquone-proguanil and for four weeks for all other regimens. The reason for the shorter duration with atovaquone-proguanil is that it has the ability to act on the liver and blood stage of the malaria infection whereas all other regimens only act on the blood stage. It is important for the traveler to understand that prophylaxis does not prevent infection entirely, hence the need to continue after leaving the malarious area. Although it is not essential to premedicate patients it is advisable to start a routine a week or two before travelling in order to ensure acceptability and to enable adequate drug concentrations to be achieved before exposure. Atovaquone-proguanil only needs to be started one to two days before travelling. Of great importance, but often neglected, is practical advice to keep exposed parts of the body covered, especially in the evening when mosquitoes are active, and to use insect repellants such as diethyltoluamide (DEET). Screening windows and sleeping under mosquito nets impregnated with insecticide (permethrin) is also a wise precaution. It is important to stress to all travellers that prophylaxis may not be effective, so that any fever developing within two years of visiting an endemic area should be treated with suspicion until malaria has been excluded by examination of adequate blood slides.

Amoebiasis

Entamoeba histolytica may live harmlessly in the lumen of the gut, usually in the cyst form, or may invade the gut mucosa to cause amoebic dysentery. The factors that govern the transformation from harmless commensal to invasive pathogen are poorly understood, although it is now clear that some strains of *E. histolytica* (morphologically identical forms now often classified as *E. dispar*) do not have pathogenic potential. Secondary spread from the primary intestinal focus sometimes occurs to give rise to abscess formation in various parts of the body, usually the liver.

The treatment of symptomless cyst passers, especially those living in endemic areas, is not worthwhile unless there is evidence of recurrent attacks of dysentery. Acute intestinal amoebiasis is characterized by bloody diarrhoeic stools. Motile amoebae with phagocytosed red cells are seen on direct microscopy of a freshly passed specimen. This is an indication for therapy to relieve symptoms and prevent possible complications such as local haemorrhage or invasion. Metronidazole is the agent of choice in a high initial dose, which should be continued for three to five days. This drug gives a high cure rate; if there is a relapse and cysts are seen in the stool an agent more active against them such as diloxanide furoate should be given for 10 days.

Invasion of trophozoites into tissues, especially into the liver, may occur without dysentery and the first indication of amoebiasis may be a hepatic abscess. Metronidazole therapy needs to be of longer duration than with uncomplicated disease; although most cases respond within 72 h, treatment for five to 10 days is recommended. Where there is a large abscess or one that is easily drained, surgical aspiration speeds recovery. There is no evidence of drug resistance in amoebae. Metronidazole is easy to administer and gives rise to few adverse reactions. The only drawback in the poorer countries of the world where amoebiasis is hyperendemic is cost and availability. In such situations emetine hydrochloride or chloroquine may be given.

Giardiasis

The flagellate protozoon *Giardia lamblia* is found only in the intestinal lumen. There is no invasion of the surface, the trophozoite being attached to the mucosa of the small intestine, especially the jejunum. Cysts are passed in the stools and infection is transmitted by contamination of food and water. *Giardia* is a frequent cause of chronic diarrhoea and is often underestimated as a pathogen. However, many infections are asymptomatic and, even with a heavy infection in adults, the symptoms may be mild: nausea, flatulence, and steatorrhoea. In young children the condition may give rise to malabsorption. Although worldwide in distribution this intestinal infection, like most, is more common in less hygienic communities. Giardiasis is fairly common in the UK as well as being the most frequently imported parasitic disease.

Metronidazole is the treatment of choice, administered in a similar regimen to that used to treat amoebic dysentery, although lower doses may suffice. Cases that do not respond to metronidazole require albendazole or mepacrine (quinacrine) after re-infection has been excluded.

Cryptosporidiosis

Cryptosporidium parvum is a common cause of acute diarrhoea in people who have had direct contact with animals or have drunk contaminated water. The disease is generally mild and self-limiting in otherwise healthy individuals, and fluid replacement is all that is usually required. Nitazoxanide appears to be effective if treatment is thought to be necessary. Various drugs, including the macrolide azithromycin and the aminoglycoside paromomycin, have been used (alone or in combination) with modest results against the more severe disease seen in patients with AIDS. Whether nitazoxamide therapy is effective in these patients is presently unclear. Fortunately, the incidence of the disease has declined in this group since effective antiretroviral therapy has become available.

African trypanosomiasis

Human trypanosomiasis due to *Trypanosoma brucei rhodesiense* is a sporadic disease in east and central Africa, although occasional outbreaks occur. The clinical course of the disease found in this area is more acute than that caused by *T. brucei gambiense*, which is a major health hazard in rural west Africa. Both parasites eventually infect the brain to give the clinical manifestations of 'sleeping sickness'. Before this stage a clinical diagnosis is difficult because of the non-specific nature of the symptoms. However, an early diagnosis is important as treatment is more effective and less toxic at this stage. Laboratory confirmation may be difficult to obtain except in specialized centres because the trypanosomes are often scanty in peripheral blood. Before central nervous system involvement suramin or pentamidine may be used in therapy, but when a lumbar puncture indicates meningo-encephalitis it is necessary to use an organic arsenical. Melarsoprol has replaced the more toxic tryparsamide for this purpose. All the antitrypanosomal drugs are toxic; treatment should be given in hospital and expert advice sought.

An important advance in the treatment of sleeping sickness caused by *T. brucei gambiense* has been achieved with the introduction of eflornithine. This drug is effective even in the late meningo-encephalitic stages of the disease, but unfortunately, *T. brucei rhodesiense* appears to be refractory to treatment.

Chagas' disease

This form of trypanosomiasis is widespread in South America. The causative organism, *T. cruzi*, invades heart muscle causing myocardial damage, which may eventually be fatal. The nitrofuran agent nifurtimox may succeed in eradicating parasites in the acute stage of the disease at the expense of some toxicity. Its value in established infection is more dubious. Similar considerations appear to apply to the nitroimidazole derivative benznidazole, which some specialists prefer to nifurtimox.

Leishmaniasis

Kala azar

Visceral leishmaniasis is a chronic, often fatal, condition characterized by fever, anaemia, and gross splenomegaly. Microscopy and culture of bone marrow or splenic aspirate confirm the diagnosis. Pentavalent antimonials have been traditionally used although relapse due to drug resistance or inadequate dosage and duration of treatment is not uncommon, especially in India. Sodium stibogluconate or meglumine antimonate is given by the parenteral route in high dosage for at least 30 days and preferably longer. Drug resistance may be suppressed by use of high-dose antimonials for extended periods, but toxic effects such as cardiac irregularities are inevitable. Pentamidine has been used as an alternative but patients fare little better on this toxic compound.

In an effort to reduce the toxicity of antimony derivatives, attempts have been made to package the drugs in artificial liposomes—minute fat globules that are phagocytosed by cells of the reticulo-endothelial system, where they release drug at the target site. Unfortunately, preparation of a suitable carrier that is stable in tropical conditions, and other problems, has militated against the success of this tactic. More success has been achieved with a liposome-encapsulated formulation of the antifungal agent amphotericin, which is also useful in kala azar.

Treatment of leishmaniasis continues to evolve. Miltefosine, a compound originally developed as an anticancer agent, is now in successful use in India, where kala azar is a major problem. Claims have been made for the efficacy of antifungal imidazoles, including itraconazole, ketoconazole, and fluconazole, and for the aminoglycoside antibiotic paromomycin.

Cutaneous and mucocutaneous leishmaniasis

Cutaneous leishmaniasis is usually localized and often resolves spontaneously. Topical paromomycin or injections of sodium stibogluconate into the margins of the lesion aid resolution. Mucocutaneous leishmaniasis requires systemic treatment with antimonials and may also need surgical intervention. Miltefosine is showing promise and may replace earlier therapies for these conditions.

Co-infection with HIV

In parts of the world in which both infections are common, disseminated leishmaniasis may cause a serious problem in patients with HIV. Relatively minor cutaneous lesions that would respond to topical treatment or self-heal in the immunocompetent person present as disseminated disease that is difficult to cure. Where it is available, effective antiretroviral therapy has reduced the incidence of this complication. Elsewhere, suppression is all that may be achievable in HIV-positive patients.

Toxoplasmosis

Toxoplasma gondii is a ubiquitous organism that normally passes harmlessly from rodents to cats, but can cause human infection by ingestion with contaminated food or close contact with infected cats. Toxoplasma infections may cause death or abnormalities in the fetus by transplacental spread during pregnancy. However, many infections pass unrecognized and the parasite may encyst in muscle or brain. Latent organisms then re-emerge in immunocompromised individuals to cause cerebral toxoplasmosis, which may present like a brain abscess in AIDS patients.

The antifolate combination pyrimethamine–sulfadiazine is the usual treatment except during pregnancy, when spiramycin is used. Neither of these agents is particularly efficacious in HIV-infected patients, in whom clindamycin, and macrolides such as azithromycin have been tried. Co-trimoxazole used to prevent pneumocystis pneumonia in HIV also suppresses toxoplasma.

Balantidiasis

Treatment of infection with the ciliate *Balantidium coli* has not been properly defined, but tetracyclines and metronidazole appear to be effective.

Babesiosis

Infections in splenectomized patients, usually caused by *Babesia divergens*, is life threatening and requires urgent treatment, but experience is limited. There is evidence that the combination of clindamycin and quinine is useful, but exchange transfusion may also be needed. Infection with *B. microti* in previously healthy persons is usually self-limiting, but clindamycin and quinine can be used if therapy is warranted. The combination of azithromycin and atovaquone has also been used with success.

Other protozoan infections

Treatment of infection with intestinal protozoa such as *Isospora belli*, *Cyclospora cayetanensis*, and various microsporidia is poorly defined, although co-trimoxazole (isosporiasis and cyclosporiasis) and albendazole (microsporidiosis) have been successfully used. In patients with AIDS these opportunist infections usually remit when the CD4 lymphocyte count improves on antiretroviral therapy.

Treatment of infection with the flagellate protozoon *Trichomonas vaginalis* is considered in Chapter 24.

Nematode infections

Filariasis

Well over 200 million people harbour filarial worms and in some areas of the tropics nearly the whole population is infected. Diagnosis is made by microscopical demonstration of the larval forms (microfilariae) in blood or, in the special case of *Onchocerca volvulus*, in superficial shavings of skin. Some of the blood microfilariae exhibit a curious periodicity in that they are found in peripheral blood during only the day (*Loa loa*) or the night (*Wuchereria bancrofti*). *Brugia malayi* (which is restricted to south-east Asia) usually exhibits a less complete nocturnal periodicity. *W. bancrofti* and *B. malayi* cause a clinically identical condition (lymphatic filariasis) sometimes resulting in elephantiasis owing to blockage of the lymphatics of the lower trunk. The clinical syndrome is due to a variety of factors depending on degree of exposure and host reaction to the worms, and in any area a small proportion will have gross elephantiasis. Often by this stage the disease may be 'burnt out' and an anthelminthic may do little to improve the patient's condition, for which surgical and supportive measures are all that is left. *O. volvulus*, the causative parasite of river blindness, affects large numbers of people in west Africa and central America. As with the other filariases, many infected persons exhibit only minor symptoms such as skin swelling and itching.

The introduction of ivermectin and albendazole has revolutionized the therapy of filarial infections. These relatively non-toxic drugs are now preferred for the treatment of onchocerciasis and lymphatic filariasis respectively. One of the benefits of their use is that reactions to treatment are a good deal milder than with the traditional drug, diethylcarbamazine, although ivermectin sometimes gives rise to an encephalopathy in individuals co-infected with *Loa loa*. Ivermectin is administered as a single oral dose, which is repeated annually in endemic areas. Mass treatment with ivermectin, together with vector control, has virtually eradicated onchocerciasis in some districts, and there are hopes that lymphatic filariasis will be similarly controlled with a combination of ivermectin and albendazole. The manufacturers of these drugs are providing them free for control programmes in countries where the diseases are endemic.

Toxocariasis

Infection with the dog roundworm *Toxocara canis* may cause a condition known as visceral larva migrans, which may result in serious eye infection usually presenting as a visual loss in childhood. Although not a common disease it is found worldwide and is probably under-recognized. The larvae of the worm migrate to the retina, setting up an inflammatory response. Treatment with diethylcarbamazine has been recommended but hypersensitivity reactions may require steroids to be given as well. Albendazole (or mebendazole) appears to offer an effective and less toxic alternative.

Intestinal nematode infections

Single doses of the common agents such as piperazine, levamisole, and pyrantel pamoate give acceptable cure rates. Table 35.2 shows the differential activity of these and the oral benzimidazole derivatives, which have a broader spectrum and have largely superseded them, but are more expensive. Among benzimidazoles, albendazole exhibits the best broad-spectrum anthelminthic activity. Tiabendazole (thiabendazole) is often poorly tolerated and is best avoided if possible.

In warm countries with poor water supplies and inadequate methods of sewage disposal re-infection with intestinal worms is almost inevitable, though simple health education advice on preventive measures may be valuable.

Trematode (fluke) infections

Schistosomiasis

Schistosomes (also known as bilharzia, or blood flukes) give rise to a chronic debilitating condition with hepatosplenomegaly and diarrhoea or haematuria. The adult worms adopt a more or less benign relationship with the host, and it is fibrosis and tissue damage arising from the deposition of eggs which is responsible for most of the unpleasant manifestations of schistosomiasis. In the days when trivalent antimonials were the only available agents for therapy of bilharzia, the decision to treat a specific case would depend on balancing the toxic effects of treatment with the severity of the patient's illness and the likelihood of rapid re-infection. With several effective and safer compounds now available, treatment has become more routine. One drug, praziquantel, is effective against all the major types of schistosomiasis and offers the possibility of single-dose therapy for mass treatment campaigns. Less useful alternatives include oxamniquine, which is active only against *Schistosoma mansoni*, and metrifonate (trichlorfon), which is effective against the urinary form, *S. haematobium*.

With the advent of these relatively safe and cheap antischistosomal drugs, it has become possible to use chemotherapy as a means of control of the disease, in conjunction with the use of molluscicides to control the snail host and the provision of safe means of disposal of excreta. Unless there is development of drug resistance on a wide scale, such methods offer a good hope for the control of one of the major parasitic scourges of mankind. However, an unexpected consequence of mass campaigns involving intramuscular injection has been the iatrogenic spread of blood-borne viruses, particularly hepatitis C virus (HCV) infection. There is good epidemiological evidence to support the hypothesis that the high rates of HCV carriage (roughly 20% of the population) seen in Egypt (the HCV 'capital' of the world), have arisen because of the use of inadequately sterilized needles in schistosomiasis campaigns dating back to the 1950s and continuing through to the 1980s.

Other trematode infections

Praziquantel has also transformed the treatment of most other trematode infections, including those caused by the Chinese liver fluke *Clonorchis sinensis* and the lung fluke *Paragonimus westermani*. However, the liver fluke *Fasciola hepatica* does not usually respond to praziquantel. The treatment of fascioliasis is problematic, but the veterinary anthelminthic triclabendazole may be effective.

Cestode infections

Tapeworms

In addition to its use in trematode infections, praziquantel has emerged as an important agent in the treatment of tapeworm infections, including those caused by *Taenia saginata, T. solium, Diphyllobothrium latum*, and *Hymenolepis nana*. A single oral dose is usually effective, although more prolonged therapy is needed in cerebral cysticercosis caused by *T. solium*. In intestinal tapeworm infection, niclosamide is a suitable alternative.

Hydatid disease

Surgery to remove hydatid cysts after injection of a scolicide such as hypotonic saline, formalin, or cetrimide into the cyst remains the treatment of choice in hydatid disease, but is not without risk. Therapy with benzimidazole derivatives, particularly albendazole, has been successful in some cases and may be the only option in inoperable conditions, including disease caused by *Echinococcus multilocularis*.

Ectoparasites

A variety of arthropods feed on human blood. Some, such as ticks, lice, and mosquitoes, may act as vectors of disease; others, including most mites and fleas, are more of a nuisance. These parasites of the ectoderm are often visible and may produce skin lesions and itching after biting. In hygienic surroundings they are very emotive, even though it is estimated that over half the children in UK schools have head lice at some time and scabies is common in the elderly in institutions.

Scabies

The mite, *Sarcoptes scabiei*, causes scabies in man and is spread by close contact. The commonest sites of infection are the hands, wrists, forearm, and axillae, or the genitalia after sexual contact. The mite burrows into the skin to form tunnels, which are diagnostic of the condition. There is often a more generalized hypersensitivity rash away from the area of penetration. All areas are itchy and scratching can lead to secondary bacterial infections, including impetigo.

Benzyl benzoate is effective, but is unpleasant to use, frequently causes irritation, and is not recommended for children. This has led to the use of the pyrethroid, permethrin, and the organophosphorus compound, malathion. Malathion should not be used repeatedly over a short period. Lindane (hexachlorocyclohexane; now discontinued in the UK) is strongly suspected to be carcinogenic and should not be used.

The key to treatment of scabies is careful, complete application of the lotion and reapplication if hands have been washed during the period the insecticide is in contact with the skin. The whole body should be covered, with particular attention to hands, fingers, and nails, and left to act overnight, or preferably 24 h.

Immunocompromised patients, such as those with HIV and old people, may develop a very heavy infestation that may crust over—so-called Norwegian scabies. Oral treatment with ivermectin has been tried with some success.

Lice

The most common infestation in the developed world is due to head lice (*Pediculus capitis*). The adult lice pass from person to person during close contact and attach their eggs (nits) to hair. The infestation may spread in schools and the community and total eradication is probably impossible, though most people develop resistance to re-infection.

There is no ideal insecticide for treatment of head lice. Among agents that are used, resistance to permethrin, phenothrin, and malathion occurs; carbaryl is usually effective, but there are fears about possible toxicity. 'Wet combing', by passing a fine-tooth comb through hair that has just been washed with conditioner, is useful, but should be repeated two to three times a week for several weeks to remove all the lice. Various herbal shampoos, such as tea tree oil, have advocates, but there is little evidence that they are effective. Shaving the head is a drastic measure, which is not recommended.

Pubic lice (*Phthirus pubis*; 'crab' lice) hold tenaciously to pubic hair, but can also be found on the head and eyelashes. Aqueous preparations of insecticides, such as malathion, should be applied overnight to all parts of the body. They are generally easier to treat than head lice, but it is important to find and treat sexual contacts and to remember that other sexually transmitted infections may be present.

Key points

- Parasites (protozoa, helminths, and arthropods) have an obligatory relationship to human beings or other animals. They tend to cause chronic disease and many individuals, once infected, remain so for long periods.

- Parasitic infections are particularly common in tropical countries. However, some parasites such as *Trichomonas vaginalis* and threadworm are at least as common in developed countries. Moreover, the speed and extent of international travel ensures that infections acquired in the tropics may present therapeutic challenges to medical practitioners everywhere.

- Malaria is the most important of all parasitic diseases in terms of mortality. Although indigenous malaria is now virtually restricted to the tropics and subtropics, it is commonly imported into many temperate countries because of the rapid increase in international business travel and tourism.

- Artemesun is now recommended as the treatment of choice for malaria and is more effective than quinine for severe malaria. However, because of concerns about development of resistance artemesun should be combined with another antimalarial.

- The most important aspects of prophylaxis are regular medication and continuance of therapy after the last possible exposure in order to eradicate any residual parasites. Prophylaxis needs to continue after leaving the malarious area for one week for atovaquone-proguanil and for four weeks for all other regimens.

Further reading

World Health Organization (2010), *Guidelines for the treatment of malaria, second edition*. Geneva: WHO. Available at http://www.who.int/malaria/publications/atoz/9789241547925/en/index.html.

World Health Organization (2010), *World Malaria Report 2010*. Geneva: WHO. Available at: http://www.who.int/malaria/world_malaria_report_2010/en/index.html.

Chapter 36

The development and marketing of antimicrobial drugs

Until the 1990s, most effort towards the discovery and development of new antimicrobial agents was expended on compounds active against bacteria, but the demands of the market place have caused the emphasis to shift. Of 67 new antimicrobial agents released on to the UK market between 1990 and 2004 (Table 36.1), only 26 (39%) were antibacterial agents; in the subsequent six years, only four of 18 (22%) new antimicrobial agents were antibacterials. Antiviral agents now represent the largest single group of newly marketed compounds. Moreover, nearly all new antibacterial agents are chemically modified variants of existing compounds, although entirely new classes of antiviral and antifungal agents have emerged. Fourteen classes of antibiotics were introduced for human use between 1935 and 1968; since then, only six have been developed (Fig. 36.1). There is a particular lack of new agents with novel targets or mechanisms of action against multidrug-resistant Gram-negative bacteria.

The cost of development of a new antimicrobial, risk of failure to gain regulatory approval (especially considering the number of current agents), and perceived profit margin (unlike drugs prescribed for chronic diseases, antibiotics are typically given for only a few days to each patient) has led to many pharmaceutical companies ceasing development of antibiotics. Only five major pharmaceutical companies (GlaxoSmithKline, Novartis, AstraZeneca, Merck, and Pfizer) still had active antibacterial discovery programmes in 2008. In the same year, an investigation of the development pipeline of both small and large pharmaceutical companies, found that only 15 of 167 antimicrobial agents had a new mechanism of action with the potential to meet the challenge of multidrug resistance. Most of those were in the early phases of development, and thus the chance of these successfully navigating the clinical investigation pathway required for new drugs is slim (Fig. 36.2).

When a new antimicrobial drug is discovered or invented, the first indications of its activity and spectrum are usually gleaned from fairly simple *in vitro* inhibition tests against a few common representative organisms. Organisms with special growth requirements, such as chlamydiae, mycobacteria, and mycoplasmas are usually excluded from such primary screening. *In vitro* screening tests will not detect potentially useful activity if *in vivo* metabolism of the compound is a prerequisite for the antimicrobial effect (e.g. Prontosil; see Historical introduction); nor will such tests reveal agents that might modify microbial cells sufficiently to render them non-virulent or susceptible to host defences, without actually preventing their growth. Furthermore, conventional laboratory culture media occasionally contain substances that interfere with the activity of certain antimicrobial compounds, which may consequently go undetected.

Despite these difficulties, *in vitro* screening offers an extremely simple and generally effective way of detecting antimicrobial activity, which has yielded a rich harvest of therapeutically useful compounds over the years. In contrast, the rational design of antimicrobial agents that can disable vulnerable stages of microbial development has not been very fruitful so far, although the use of newer approaches such as genomics, molecular modeling, and combinatorial chemistry offer the

Table 36.1 Newly marketed antimicrobial agents in three year periods 1990–2004 (UK)

Period	Antibacterial agents	Antiviral agents	Antifungal agents	Antiparasitic agents
1990–1992	10	1	2	2
1993–1995	7	4	1	1
1996–1998	3	9	1	1
1999–2001	3	8	0	1
2002–2004	3	8	2	0
2005–2007	3	7	1	0
2008–2010	1	4	2	0

prospect that this might change in the future. Indeed, some of the new antiviral agents have been developed by targeting specific viral processes.

Development of new compounds

Compounds that pass the initial screening tests must be made available in sufficient quantities and in sufficiently pure form to enable preliminary tests of toxicity and efficacy to be carried out in laboratory animals, and more extensive and precise *in vitro* tests to be performed. Pilot-stage production usually presents little problem, although considerable difficulties may be experienced in scaling up production at a later date, when relatively large quantities of highly purified drug are needed for clinical trials and subsequent marketing.

Animal tests of toxicity, pharmacology, and efficacy are an indispensable part of the development of any new drug, but they also have certain limitations. Idiosyncratic reactions may suggest toxicity in a compound that would be safe for human use or, more importantly, adverse reactions peculiar to the human subject may go undetected. The pharmacological handling of the drug may be vastly different from that encountered in the human subject. As regards efficacy testing, animals have important limitations in that experimental infections seldom correspond to the

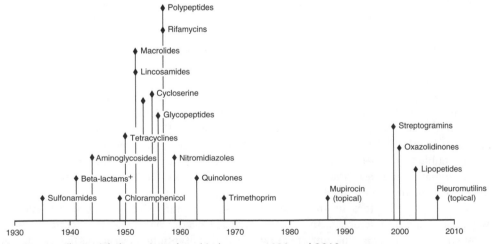

Fig. 36.1 Antibacterial classes introduced in between 1930 and 2010.

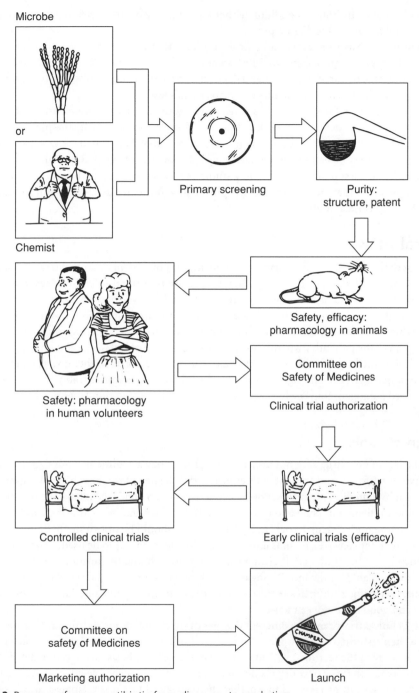

Microbe

or

Chemist

Primary screening

Purity: structure, patent

Safety, efficacy: pharmacology in animals

Safety: pharmacology in human volunteers

Committee on Safety of Medicines

Clinical trial authorization

Controlled clinical trials

Early clinical trials (efficacy)

Committee on safety of Medicines

Marketing authorization

Launch

Fig. 36.2 Progress of a new antibiotic from discovery to marketing.

supposedly analogous human condition, either anatomically or in the relationship of treatment to the natural history of the disease process.

If preliminary tests of toxicity and efficacy indicate that the compound is worth advancing further, full-scale acute and chronic toxicity tests are carried out in animals. These include long-term tests of mutagenic or carcinogenic potential, effects on fertility, and teratogenicity. Mutagenicity tests may also be performed in microbial systems (Ames test).

Provided the animal toxicity studies reveal no serious toxicity problems, the first tentative (Phase 1) trials are undertaken in healthy human volunteers to investigate the pharmacokinetic properties and safety of the new drug in man. Although animal data provide only a crude estimate of how the drug may be handled in human beings, if properly interpreted they allow an estimate to be made for the first human dose-ranging studies. Once these tests have been successfully completed, application may be made to the drug-licensing authority for permission to undertake (Phase 2 and 3) clinical trials.

Clinical trials

The proof of the pudding is in the eating, and no amount of *in vitro* or animal testing can replace the ultimate test of safety and efficacy: therapeutic use in human infection. Nevertheless, the clinical trial stage remains, in many ways, the least satisfactory aspect of the testing of any new antimicrobial drug. The reasons for this are not difficult to find: 'infection' is not a static condition in which therapeutic intervention produces an all-or-none effect. Many factors, such as mobilization of the patient's own immune response, drainage of pus, or treatment of an underlying surgical or medical condition, may crucially affect the response to therapy. The patient may improve subjectively, even though the antimicrobial therapy has demonstrably failed to eradicate the supposed pathogen; conversely, the patient's condition may deteriorate despite bacteriological 'success'.

Design of trials

Clinical trials of new drugs are not undertaken lightly. They are difficult to design, tedious and expensive to perform, and fraught with ethical pitfalls. The conduct of the trial requires close supervision by a medical practitioner dedicated to the task, who needs to have the full support of reliable and motivated nursing and laboratory staff, together with well-informed and compliant patients. Before undertaking a trial, a detailed protocol should be drawn up, defining the conditions for which the new treatment is intended, the dosage regimens to be used, and the treatment with which it is to be compared. Participating laboratories should be consulted to ensure that full facilities are available for the monitoring of microbiological progress and the detection of adverse reactions. Licensing authorities require studies to conform to strict standards of good clinical practice and good laboratory practice.

Phase 2 clinical trials examine different dosages of the investigational drug, and the 'optimum' dosage is then restudied in larger phase 3 studies. In both settings a comparator (established) drug is used for some of the recruited patients, and there is a key emphasis on collecting detailed information to assure that the new drug is not associated with unacceptable adverse events. Careful consideration should be given as to whether the trial should be open, single-blind (treatment known to the prescriber only), or double-blind (treatment randomly allocated in a fashion unknown to prescriber or recipient). In general, uncontrolled, open trials are unsatisfactory, except as preliminary indicators of safety and efficacy. They may also be used to gain information on the most appropriate dose of an agent. Controlled, double-blind trials are the most desirable scientifically, but are subject to ethical difficulties in that the prescribing doctor does not have full control over the patient's treatment. Placebo-controlled studies are normally acceptable only if adequate treatment is unavailable or controversial.

Ethical requirements

Ethical considerations need to be taken fully into account. The basic principles that should govern all research involving human subjects are embodied in the Declaration of Helsinki, which was adopted by the 18th World Medical Assembly in 1964, with subsequent revisions. In many countries, health authorities have ethical committees that monitor clinical trial protocols. The committee will need assurance that the safety of the new compound has been satisfactorily established and will wish to ensure that written informed patient consent is obtained from trial participants. It will also require adequate safeguards for the detection of unexpected adverse reactions and may have views as to whether a double-blind format, or a placebo control, is acceptable.

Statistical considerations

Ambitious trials can fail because insufficient numbers of patients are found to fulfil the criteria required for the study. Alternatively, the condition may be one (acute cystitis is a good example) in which the natural cure rate is so high, and the efficacy of standard treatment so good, that huge numbers would have to be examined to establish the superiority of a new agent, although it may be possible to determine efficacy. It is essential to be reasonably sure, before the trial starts, that sufficient patients can be recruited to satisfy statistical requirements. During the conduct of the trial, regular checks of relevant microbiological, haematological, chemical, and radiological parameters should be made. All findings should be fully documented as soon as the information is available, rather than attempting to glean information from the patients' notes retrospectively, after the trial is completed.

Concerns about the proliferation of similar antibiotics for the same types of infections has recently led the FDA to review its guidance on how new drugs are assessed. Two issues have been highlighted in particular. Firstly, a need to demonstrate that a new drug achieves early demonstrable clinical benefit; for example, fever resolution and lack of progression of skin lesions by the third day of therapy in patients with acute bacterial skin and skin structure infection. Secondly, controversial discussions are still ongoing over whether companies will be required to demonstrate that a new drug is superior to established treatment rather than simply similar or equivalent (i.e. statistically non-inferior to comparator). This may seem desirable but, in reality could set the bar so high that it is a further disincentive to drug development.

Drug licensing

Most countries have enacted some sort of legislation aimed at controlling the marketing of pharmaceutical products. In the US, federal regulations are administered by the Food and Drug Administration (FDA). Within the European Union, a Committee on Proprietary Medicinal Products issues guidelines for harmonizing regulatory requirements among member nations. The European Medicines Agency, based in London, coordinates drug licensing and safety throughout the European Union, although companies can still seek registration of their products by national regulatory authorities.

In the UK, executive powers are invested in government health and agriculture ministers, who constitute the Licensing Authority. Ministers are advised directly through the Medicines and Healthcare Products Regulatory Agency of the Department of Health. The Agency, through its specialist advisory committees, reviews all pharmaceutical products intended for medical or veterinary use. The licensing, manufacture, promotion, and distribution of all medicines intended for human use are supervised by the Commission on Human Medicines, which combines the functions of the Committee on Safety of Medicines and the Medicines Commission. The Commission acts as an independent agency in relation to particular issues and concerns, including any challenge to the decisions of the Licensing Authority.

Before clinical trials can be performed on a new drug in the UK, full toxicological data must be submitted to the Medicines and Healthcare Products Regulatory Agency together with a full trial protocol and the names of the proposed investigators. Such applications are scrutinized by the Committee on Safety of Medicines, who must satisfy themselves that all reasonable criteria are met before recommending that a clinical trial authorization should be issued. If the authorization is approved, investigators must undertake to notify any adverse reaction arising during the trial, or any other matter that might reasonably cause the Licensing Authority to doubt the safety or quality of the product.

When clinical trial data have been accumulated, an application for a marketing authorization (formerly called a product licence) may be made. All valid applications are again passed to the Committee on Safety of Medicines for scrutiny. In the UK new applications are judged solely on the grounds of safety, efficacy, and quality. If marketing authorization is refused, the application may be withdrawn or the applicant may elect to answer the objections raised, either in writing or in person before the committee. Should the application still be refused, the applicant has the right of appeal to the Medicines Commission. Marketing authorizations, once issued, are valid for five years in the first instance.

Over the years, the requirements of licensing authorities worldwide (particularly for toxicological testing) have become progressively more stringent. Consequently, the cost of developing a new drug has escalated enormously. The period between the discovery and marketing of a new product is seldom less than six years and may be substantially longer, although fast-track procedures have enabled some drugs, notably those used in the treatment of HIV infection, to be licensed much more quickly. Shortening the period is important to the company marketing the new drug, since it maximizes the time during which it can recoup the cost of research and development (which may exceed £500 million) and profit from the discovery while enjoying patent protection. Attempts are being made to harmonize the drug registration requirements of Europe, the USA, and Japan, but progress so far has been modest. Similarly, there are ongoing efforts to agree on incentives for companies to remain in or return to antimicrobial drug development. Patent extension and public-private development initiatives to target areas of unmet need are two such examples. Talk is however cheap, and there is widespread agreement that new accords are required to boost antimicrobial drug development during the next decade.

Drug marketing

Data sheets

All companies marketing products provided for the use of medical practitioners in the European Union are required to produce a Summary of Product Characteristics ('data sheet') giving relevant information about the drug, including the conditions for which its use is licensed, contraindications and known side effects. Pharmaceutical firms in the UK collaborate in producing a Data Sheet Compendium, which is freely available to registered medical practitioners (online version: electronic Medicines Compendium is available at http://emc.medicines.org.uk/).

Post-marketing surveillance

Issue of a marketing authorization is no guarantee that a compound is 100% safe, nor even that all adverse reactions have been detected before marketing. Rare, serious adverse events may not be detected among the few thousand patients exposed to the new drug in the phase 2 and 3 studies. Marketing authorization for a new drug may only be granted on the condition that the company initiates a surveillance scheme to check on aspects of drug usage, including safety and/or the detection of resistance emergence. Also, the Committee on Safety of Medicines in the UK issues postage-paid 'yellow cards' for the notification of adverse reactions. Although the scheme is voluntary, it is important that prescribers and pharmacists collaborate fully with it. Such notifications are particularly important in the first few years in which a new compound is marketed. Copies of the notification form are routinely included with each issue of the *British National Formulary*, and compounds under particular scrutiny are flagged with a black triangle.

Relationship with the medical profession

In the UK, the conduct of pharmaceutical companies in marketing their products is regulated by the Medicines and Healthcare Products Regulatory Agency. There is also a voluntary Code of Practice drawn up by the Prescription Medicines Code of Practice Authority established by the Association of the British Pharmaceutical Industry in 1993 and re-issued in revised form in 2011 (available at: http://www.abpi.org). It covers, among many other things: the content and distribution of advertisements and other promotional literature; hospitality, gifts, and inducements to the medical and allied professions; marketing research; and relationships with the general public and lay communications media.

Advertisements

The subject of advertising is a perennial bone of contention between healthcare professionals and the pharmaceutical industry. The former complain that the industry tries to cloud their professional judgement under a deluge of irrelevant, mendacious, and uninterpretable gobbledegook; the latter claim their commercial right to exploit their products to their best advantage in the market place, and point to the factual data sheets and other information services that they place at the disposal of the medical professions.

The truth, as usual, inhabits the middle ground. Advertisements are subject to the usual advertising regulations and may not tell overt lies. Nonetheless, they are intended to sway the prescriber in favour of a particular product. They are clearly cost-effective and there is ample evidence of their influence on prescribing habits.

Doctors and other healthcare workers should not delude themselves by claiming that they are uninfluenced by advertisements or other promotional activities. They should make a conscious effort to separate fact from fantasy in advertisements and cultivate a critical attitude, especially towards claims for new products. In particular, prescribers should learn to distinguish between genuine advances and new products, which, though effective, are no better than older, well-tried, and cheaper remedies. They should also be wary of impressive claims ostensibly based on published independent assessments which turn out, in the small print, to refer to unverifiable 'data on file' or papers published by, or on behalf of, the company involved.

Sources of independent advice

Within the UK the National Institute for Health and Clinical Excellence and the Scottish Medicines Consortium offer expert independent guidance on the status of medical products. In addition, the *British National Formulary* (BNF, updated at six monthly intervals), eBNF, and the *Drug and Therapeutics Bulletin* (published by the Consumers' Association), offer reliable sources of objective information to the prescriber. In the USA, the *National Formulary* and the *Medical Letter* provide a similar service. Many health authorities now produce therapeutic guides for use by medical staff in hospital or the community (see Chapter 20). Pharmacies often offer a drug information service to which medical practitioners have access, and most medical microbiology laboratories are able to offer accurate up-to-date advice on antimicrobial therapy.

Although the marketing of drugs is fairly well regulated throughout the industrially developed world, the same is not true of less favoured countries; in many nations of the world the standards of advertising and marketing often appear to overstep the bounds of what would be considered ethical in more developed countries.

Drug names

When a new antibiotic is first described in the scientific literature it usually appears under a number representing the manufacturer's laboratory code for the compound. This practice is to be discouraged, since the code is forgotten once a drug is named and, in later years, source references become difficult to locate. The reason for using a code is that names proposed by the manufacturer are not always subsequently accepted by the bodies controlling drug nomenclature. These are the British Pharmacopoeia Commission in the UK, who recommend a British Approved Name (BAN) to the Medicines Commission, the United States Adopted Name (USAN) Council in the US and equivalent bodies elsewhere. International agreement is coordinated by the World Health Organization, which specifies or recommends an International Non-proprietary Name (INN; rINN). Within the European Union, the rINN is now in general use and has replaced the British Approved Name for nearly all drugs used in the UK. In the case of antimicrobial drugs, conflated names such as co-trimoxazole and co-amoxiclav are still in use in the UK for combination products, whereas the full names of both components (e.g. trimethoprim–sulfamethoxazole) are preferred elsewhere. The British convention is adopted here.

Once the Approved Name is introduced into the national pharmacopoeia of a country, it becomes the Official Name. In addition to the Approved or Official Name, the drug may have various proprietary names under which it is marketed and these trade names often differ widely throughout the world, especially if generic versions are available. Approved Names try to avoid close nomenclatural similarities, but the profusion of 'sulfa-s' 'cefa-s', '-cillins', and '-oxacins' still produces confusion; when the same compound is marketed under different proprietary names, bewilderment is often complete.

Generic prescribing

There has been a good deal of debate as to whether doctors should use proprietary names in writing prescriptions. On the one hand, it is pointed out that formulations differ so that the pharmacological properties of a drug may vary from product to product. Moreover, adverse reactions caused by a particular formulation may be more easily detected if the product is specified. On the other hand, non-proprietary names are less likely to cause confusion; they remove the necessity of pharmacies keeping a large and varied stock of similar products, and enable the pharmacist to dispense the cheapest version of a particular drug. The *British National Formulary* sensibly recommends prescribers to use non-proprietary names in all but those few instances where bioavailability problems are so important that the patient should always receive the same brand. Policies of 'generic substitution', whereby pharmacists can dispense a generic version of a medicine even if a branded product is specified on the prescription, differ widely throughout the world.

Whither antibiotics?

The number of antimicrobial drugs available to the prescriber is now enormous and, at least as far as antibacterial compounds are concerned, the undoubted value of having a wide and varied choice has been overtaken by the confusion that is caused by the conflicting claims of so many agents with similar or overlapping indications. There are justifiable fears about antimicrobial drug resistance, but the fact remains that untreatable infection (due to antimicrobial resistance alone) is thankfully a very rare phenomenon at this point. We actually currently possess multiple antibacterial drugs to treat most common infections. This in itself can present a dilemma over which is the most efficacious or cost-effective agent, remembering that an inexpensive antibiotic can translate into a very costly course of treatment if initial therapy fails.

Indeed, most general practitioners rely on a few favourite antibiotics which they use to cover most bacterial infections. The WHO includes only a handful of antibacterial agents in its list of essential medicines (Table 36.2). The availability of antimicrobial drugs varies extensively in different countries for reasons that must be commercial rather than therapeutic: for example, over 70 β-lactam antibiotics (including 40 cephalosporins) are on the market in Japan compared with 26 in the UK; the WHO's essential drugs list has only 12, eight of which of which are penicillins.

Concern about antimicrobial drug resistance still offers some impetus for continuing research into antibacterial agents and new technologies have been harnessed to the hunt for compounds that will circumvent resistance mechanisms in some common pathogens. But the harsh truth is that the declining financial rewards available in this area have led pharmaceutical companies to divert many of their resources to the more lucrative field of antiviral and, to a lesser extent, antifungal compounds. Antiparasitic drugs remain grossly neglected, except for veterinary use.

Chemotherapeutic options for the treatment of non-bacterial infection remain very unsatisfactory. Although great strides have been made in the prevention of viral infection by immunization (Chapter 18), and there have been important developments in antiviral agents, notably for the treatment of HIV infection, chemotherapy for viral disease is still extremely constrained (see Chapters 4–6). Some sort of effective chemotherapy is available for most fungal, protozoal, and helminth infections, but the choice is very limited and, in many ways, unsatisfactory (see Chapters 7 and 8). On a global scale these conditions are responsible for much of the morbidity and mortality from infectious disease that afflicts mankind. The greatest challenge for the future is to provide for these diseases the same sort of safe, effective chemotherapy that is now available for most bacterial infections, and to make effective therapy for all infections readily available for those who need it most.

Key points

- There has been a marked reduction in the number of new antibiotics and especially drugs exploiting novel targets or modes of action.
- Clinical trials of new antimicrobial agents comprise phase 1 (healthy volunteer), phase 2 (dosage investigation) and phase 3 studies.
- Post-marketing surveillance is key to check for rare and potentially serious adverse events.

Table 36.2 Antimicrobial agents (excluding topical agents) on the WHO model list of essential medicines (2010). Drugs shown in brackets are on the complementary list

Antibacterial agents	Antimycobacterial agents[a]	Antifungal agents	Antiviral agents	Antiprotozoal agents	Anthelminthic agents
Amoxicillin	Clofazimine	Clotrimazole	Antiherpes	Amoebiasis and giardiasis	Intestinal worms
Ampicillin	Dapsone	Fluconazole[d]	Acidovir	Diloxanide[d]	Albendazole
Azithromycin[b]	Ethambutol	Griseofulvin	Antiretroviral[a]	Metronidazole[d]	Levamisole
Benzathine penicillin	Isoniazid	Nystatin	Abacavir	Leishmaniasis	Mebendazole[d]
			Atazanavir		
Benzylpenicillin	Pyrazinamide	(Amphotericin)	Didanosine	Meglumine antimonate[d]	Niclosamide
Cefalexin					
Cefazolin[e]					
Cefixime[c]	Rifampicin	(Flucytosine)	Efavirenz	(Amphotericin)	Praziquantel
			Emtricitabine		
Chloramphenicol	Streptomycin	(Potassium iodide)	Indinavir	(Pentamidine)	Pyrantel
Ciprofloxacin[d]	(Amikacin)		Lamivudine	Malaria[a]	Filariasis
Cloxacillin[d]	(p-Aminosalicylic acid)		Lopinavir + ritonavir	Amodiaquine	Ivermectin
Co-amoxiclav	(Capreomycin)		Nelfinavir	Artemether + lumefantrine	(Diethylcarbamazine)
Co-trimoxazole	Cycloserine		Nevirapine	Chloroquine	(Suramin)
Doxycycline	(Ethionamide)		Saquinavir	Doxycycline	Trematodes
			Stavudine		
			Tenofovir		
Erythromycin[d]	(Kanamycin)		Zidovudine	Mefloquine	Praziquantel
Gentamicin[d]	(Levofloxacin)			Primaquine	Triclabendazole
Metronidazole[d]	(Ofloxacin)		Influenza	Proguanil	(Oxamniquine)
Nitrofurantoin			Oseltamivir	Quinine	

Phenoxymethylpenicillin	
Procaine penicillin	
Spectinomycin	
Sulfamethoxazole + Trimethoprim	
(Ceftazidime)	
(Clindamycin)	
(Ceftriaxone[c])	
(Imipenem + cilastatin)	
(Vancomycin)	
	(Artemether)
Viral Haemorrhagic Fevers	(Artesunate)
Ribivarin	(Sulfadoxine + pyrimethamine)
Trypanosomiasis	
Benznidazole	
Melarsoprol	
Nifurtimox	
Suramin	
(Eflornithine)	
(Pentamidine)	

Data from the World Health Organization website (March 2010 update): http://www.who.int/medicines/publications/essentialmedicines/Updated_sixteenth_adult_list_en.pdf.

[a] Most of the antimycobacterial, antiretroviral and antimalarial drugs are used in combination and many are available in fixed-dose combination preparations.

[b] For genital and ocular chlamydial infections only.

[c] For single-dose treatment of uncomplicated ano-genital gonorrhoea only.

[d] Examples of a therapeutic group for which acceptable alternatives exist.

[e] For surgical prophylaxis.

Further reading

Infectious Diseases Society of America (IDSA) (2004), Bad bugs, no drugs. As antibiotic discovery stagnates . . . a public health crisis brews. Available from: http://www.idsociety.org/WorkArea/linkit.aspx?LinkIdentifier= id&ItemID=5554.

Talbot GH, Bradley J, Edwards JE Jr, Gilbert D, Scheld M, Bartlett JG, Antimicrobial Availability Task Force of the Infectious Diseases Society of America (2006), 'Bad bugs need drugs: an update on the development pipeline from the Antimicrobial Availability Task Force of the Infectious Diseases Society of America', *Clinical Infectious Diseases* **42**:657–68.

ECDC/EMEA Joint Technical Report (2009), The bacterial challenge: time to react. Available at: http://www.ecdc.europa.eu/en/publications/Publications/0909_TER_The_Bacterial_Challenge_Time_to_ React.pdf.

Recommendations for further reading

General texts

Since the availability and use of antimicrobial agents vary widely in different countries, no one book has universal applicability. Among the most authoritative general texts in the English language are:

Bryskier A. (2005), *Antimicrobial agents—antibacterial and antifungals*. Washington DC: ASM Press.

Finch RG, Greenwood D, Norrby SR, Whitley RJ. (2010), *Antibiotic and chemotherapy: anti-infective agents and their use in therapy* (9th edn). London: Saunders, Elsevier.

Greenwood D. (2008), *Antimicrobial Drugs*. Oxford: Oxford University Press.

Kucers A, Grayson ML, Crowe SM, McCarthy JS, Mills J, Mouton JW, Norrby SR, Paterson DL, Pfaller MA. (2010), *The use of antibiotics: a clinical review of antibacterial, antifungal, antiparasitic and antiviral drugs* (6th edn). London: Hodder Arnold.

An indispensable guide to the use of all therapeutic drugs for practitioners in the UK is provided by: *British National Formulary*. British Medical Association and the Royal Pharmaceutical Society of Great Britain (revised twice yearly). Also available as an electronic version at http://bnf.org/bnf.

Comprehensive monographs on antimicrobial agents are to be found in large reference texts on drugs including:

Dollery C (ed.) (1999), *Therapeutic drugs* (2nd edn). Edinburgh: Churchill Livingstone.

Sweetman SC (ed.) (2011), *Martindale: the complete drug reference* (37th edn). London: Pharmaceutical Press. (Also available online.)

Other useful texts on specific topics

Antiviral agents and the chemotherapy of viral infections

Butera ST (ed.) (2005), *HIV Chemotherapy: a critical review*. Norwich: Horizon Bioscience.

Driscoll JS. (2005), *Antiviral Drugs*. Chichester: John Wiley & Sons.

Zuckerman AJ, Banatvala JE, Schoub BD, Griffiths PD, Mortmier P (eds) (2009), *Principles and Practice of Clinical Virology* (6th edn). Oxford: Wiley-Blackwell.

Richman DD, Whitley RJ, Hayden FG. (eds) (2009), *Clinical Virology* (3rd edn) Washington DC: ASM Press 2009.

Diseases caused by protozoa and helminths (see also WHO publications below)

Aden Abdi Y, Gustafsson LL, Ericsson O, Hellgren U (eds.) (1996), *Handbook of Drugs for Tropical Parasitic Infection* (2nd edn). London: Taylor and Francis, London.

Rosenthal PJ. (2010), *Antimalarial Chemotherapy: mechanisms of action, resistance, and new directions in drug discovery*. Totowa, NJ: Humana Press, Totowa, NJ.

Mode of action of antimicrobial agents and mechanisms of resistance

European Commission: Key documents on antimicrobial resistance. Available at http://ec.europa.eu/health/antimicrobial_resistance/key_documents/index_en.htm (24th February 2011 data last accessed).

Franklin TJ, Snow GA. (2005), *Biochemistry and Molecular Biology of Antimicrobial Drug Action*, (6th edn). New York: Springer-Verlag.

Richman DD (ed.) (1996), *Antiviral Drug Resistance*. Chichester: Wiley, Chichester.

Salyers AA, Whitt DD. (2005), *Revenge of the Microbes: how bacterial resistance is undermining the antibiotic miracle*. Washington DC: ASM Press.

Scholar EM, Pratt WB.(2000), *The Antimicrobial Drugs* (2nd edn). New York: Oxford University Press, New York.

Standing Medical Advisory Committee Report (1998), *The Path of Least Resistance*. London: Department of Health/Public Health Laboratory Service.

Walsh C. (2003), *Antibiotics: Actions, origins, resistance*. Washington DC: ASM Press, Washington.

White DG, Alekshun MN, McDermott PF. (2005), *Frontiers in Antimicrobial Resistance. A tribute to Stuart B Levy*. Washington DC: ASM Press.

Laboratory methods

Lorian V. (ed.) (2005), *Antibiotics in Laboratory Medicine* (5th edn). Baltimore, MD: Lippincott Williams & Wilkins.

Versalovic J, Carroll KC, Kunke G, Jorgensen JH, Landry ML, Warnock DW. (eds.) (2011), *Manual of Clinical Microbiology* (10th edn). Washington DC: American Society for Microbiology.

Jerome KR. (ed.) (2010), *Lennette's Laboratory Diagnosis of Viral Infections* (4th edn). London: Informa Healthcare, London.

Antibiotic resistance monitoring

Centers for Disease Control and Prevention, Atlanta, GA. Antibiotic/antimicrobial resistance. http://www.cdc.gov/drugresistance/index.htm.

European Union: European Antimicrobial Resistance Surveillance Network (EARS-Net) http://www.ecdc.europa.eu/en/activities/surveillance/EARS-Net/Pages/index.aspx The website has links to various national and international networks.

UK and Ireland: British Society for Antimicrobial Chemotherapy resistance surveillance. http://www.bsacsurv.org.

Surveillance of antibiotic prescribing

European Surveillance of Antimicrobial Consumption (ESAC). http://app.esac.ua.ac.be/public/. The website has publications from the project, which has collected and published data about community and hospital use of antibiotics across Europe from 1997. There are links to various national and international networks.

Antibiotic policies and guidelines

British Society for Antimicrobial Chemotherapy (BSAC). This site has guidelines and recommended standards from BSAC Working Parties and links to other educational resources: http://www.bsac.org.uk/Standards.

European Society for Clinical Microbiology and Infectious Diseases (ESCMID). This site has links to guidelines in the fields of clinical microbiology and infectious diseases endorsed by ESCMID and to guidelines from other organisations and societies: http://www.escmid.org/escmid_library/medical_guidelines/.

Health Protection Agency. Management of infection guidance for primary care for consultation & local adaptation http://www.hpa.org.uk/servlet/Satellite?c=Page&cid=1197637041219&pagename=HPAweb%2FPage%2FHPAwebAutoListName (26th February 2011, date last accessed).

Health Protection Agency & Department of Health. *Clostridium difficile* infection: How to deal with the problem. http://www.dh.gov.uk/prod_consum_dh/groups/dh_digitalassets/documents/digitalasset/dh_093218.pdf.

NICE (National Institute for Health and Clinical Excellence) has guidelines on treatment of specific infections and information about implementation http://guidance.nice.org.uk/.

Scottish Antimicrobial Prescribing Group: Policies and guidance also has information about results of quality improvement interventions. Available at http://www.scottishmedicines.org.uk/SAPG/Policies_and_Guidance (24th February 2011 data last accessed).

Scottish Intercollegiate Guidelines Network (www.sign.ac.uk) has guidelines on antibiotic prophylaxis in surgery and treatment of specific infections.

Learning resources about antimicrobial chemotherapy

The PAUSE Project: Prudent Antibiotic User.

http://www.pause-online.org.uk/.

The website has learning resources (clinical problems and prescribing exercises) created by medical schools in the UK with the aim of teaching prudent use of antibiotics in all clinical contexts. A list of PAUSE resources linked to Antimicrobial Chemotherapy chapters is provided at the end of this chapter.

Outpatient Parenteral Antibiotic Therapy database and business case: http://www.e-opat.com/.

Pagani L, Gyssens IC, Huttner B et al. (2009), Navigating the Web in search of resources on antimicrobial stewardship in health care institutions. *Clinical Infectious Diseases* **48**: 626–32.

WHO publications

The World Health Organization issues a wide variety of publications many of which are available on-line through the website http://www.who.int/. Of particular relevance to antimicrobial chemotherapy are:

Crompton DWT, Montresor A, Nesheim MC, Savioli L. (2004), *Controlling Disease due to Helminth Infections*. Geneva: World Health Organization.

Frieden T. *Toman's Tuberculosis. Case Detection, Treatment and Monitoring*, (2nd edn), 2004. http://whqlibdoc.who.int/publications/2004/9241546034.pdf.

Mehta DK, Ryan RSM, Hogerzeil H. (2004), *WHO Model formulary*. Geneva: World Health Organization. http://mednet3.who.int/EMLib/wmf.aspx.

WHO Essential Drug Monitor. http://www.who.int/medicines/publications/monitor/en.

WHO Global malaria programme. http://malaria.who.int.

WHO Global strategy for containment of antimicrobial resistance. http://www.who.int/drugresistance/en/.

WHO Guidelines for the treatment of malaria. http://www.who.int/malaria/docs/TreatmentGuidelines2006.pdf.

WHO Model Prescribing Information (2005), *Drugs used in parasitic diseases* (2nd edn). Geneva: World Health Organization.

WHO (2004), TB/HIV: *a clinical manual* (2nd edn). Geneva: World Health Organization. http://www.who.int/tb/publications/who_htm_tb_2004_329/en/index.html.

Journals

Papers dealing with aspects of the use of antimicrobial drugs appear in numerous journals. English language journals specifically devoted to antibiotics and antimicrobial therapy include:

Antibiotics and Chemotherapy

Antimicrobial Agents and Chemotherapy

Antiviral Chemistry and Chemotherapy

Antiviral Research

Chemotherapy

Clinical Microbiology and Infection

International Journal of Antimicrobial Agents

Journal of Antibiotics

Journal of Antimicrobial Chemotherapy

Journal of Chemotherapy

Prudent Antibiotic User (PAUSE) learning resources linked to Antimicrobial Chemotherapy Chapters

http://www.pause-online.org.uk/.

Antimicrobial Chemotherapy Chapter	PAUSE Vignette or Learning Resource
9 The problem of resistance	012 - Sarah Moss
	018 - Catheter-related MRSA in a hospital setting
	019 - UTI in the community setting
11 Control of the spread of resistance	018 - Catheter-related MRSA in a hospital setting
	019 - UTI in the community setting
16 Outpatient Parenteral Antibiotic Therapy	021 - Outpatient Parenteral Antibiotic Therapy
19 Guidelines, formularies & policies	Prescribing exercises
	IVOST (IV to oral switch) protocol and exercises
21 Respiratory tract infections	001 - Pneumonia, 015 - Sore Throat
23 Urinary tract infections	005 - UTI Pyelonephritis, 006 - UTI in Pregnancy, 007 - UTI in the Elderly, 008 - Pyelonephritis, 009 - Catheter Associated Infection, 019 - UTI in the community setting
25 Gastrointestinal infections	020 - Clostridium difficile associated disease
26 Serious blood stream infections	002 - Septic Shock, 004 - Infective Endocarditis, 011 - Pancreatitis
27 Infections of the bones and joints	013 - Foot Infection in Diabetic Ulcer, 014 - Septic Arthritis
28 Infections of the central nervous system	002 - Septic Shock
29 Infections of the skin and soft tissues	003 - Cellulitis, 013 - Foot Infection in Diabetic Ulcer
30 Tuberculosis and other mycobacterial diseases	010 - Tuberculosis, 016 - Tuberculosis
33 HIV infections	017 - Needlestick Injuries
35 Viral hepatitis	017 - Needlestick Injuries

Index

abacavir 63, 179, 184
absorption 149, 155–6
　children 164
Acanthamoeba spp. 83
acedapsone 47
acetyltransferases 112
aciclovir 6, 52–3
　adverse reactions 183
　analogues 53–6
　chemoprophylaxis 339
　herpesvirus infections 334, 335, 336, 337, 338
　mode of action 52–3
　resistance 53, 122
　sexually transmitted infections 257
　structure 54
　topical use 237, 238, 257, 335
Acinetobacter spp. 96, 99, 109, 233
acne 239
acquired resistance 95–6
　mechanisms 107–19
　types of 96
actimoycetes 5
actinomycin 5
active immunization 59
acyclovir see aciclovir
adefovir 55, 70, 71
　resistance 71
adenoviruses 50, 225, 264
adicillin 4
adsorbents 262–4
adverse reactions 151, 175
　antiviral drugs 183–5
　determinants of toxicity 175–7
　elderly patients 169
　hypersensitivity 178–9
　outpatient parenteral antimicrobial therapy
　　(OPAT) 173
　prevention 185
　tissue- and organ-specific toxicity 180–2
　see also specific drugs
advertisements 200, 373
African trypanosomiasis 1–2, 361
agar diffusion tests 141
age-related infection 164, 168
AIDS 6, 61, 324, 331–3, 343
　see also antiretroviral agents; HIV
albendazole 6
　anthelminthic effects 87, 89, 90, 363–4, 365
　protozoan infections 85, 361, 363
alisporivir 74
allylamines 77, 80
amantadine 53, 57–8, 194, 341
　adverse effects 57
　combination therapy 58
　structure 57

amdinocillin (mecillinam) 14
American wormseed 1
amikacin 28, 29–30
　adverse reactions 182, 318
　immunocompromised patients 329
　tuberculosis 100, 318, 321
aminoglycosides 25–30, 31
　adverse reactions 176, 181–2, 185, 240–1
　antimicrobial spectrum 94
　assay 27, 281
　bacteraemia 275
　classification 25–6
　dosing 150
　elderly patients 168
　endocarditis 281, 282
　general properties 26
　immunocompromised patients 329
　mode of action 27–9
　placental passage 167
　resistance 97, 111–13, 118
　see also specific drugs
aminopenicillin 179, 232
amodiaquine 85, 358
amoebae 82–3
amoebiasis 82–3, 360
amoebic dysentery 6, 82, 360
amorolfine 81, 240
amoxicillin 14
　adverse reactions 179
　antibacterial properties 16
　endocarditis 282
　gastrointestinal infections 265, 266, 268
　respiratory tract infections 225, 226, 227, 230, 232
　sexually transmitted infections 253, 255
amphotericin 6, 76–8
　adverse effects 76–8, 182
　antiprotozoal effects 83, 84
　bacteraemia 275
　combination therapy 79
　endocarditis 285
　immunocompromised patients 330
　leishmaniasis 84, 362
　meningitis 304
　structure 78
　topical use 238, 240
ampicillin 14
　adverse reactions 179, 180, 183
　antibacterial properties 16
　children 167
　endocarditis 282, 284, 285
　gastrointestinal infections 267, 268
　meningitis 300
　resistance 93, 95–6, 244, 246
　sore throat 225
　urinary infections 244, 246

anaphylaxis 178
Anatomical Therapeutic Chemical (ATC)
   classification 216
Ancylostoma duodenale 87
anidulafungin 79–80
animals, antibiotic use in 123
animal testing 368
antagonistic effects 151–2
anthelminthics 6, 87–90, 364–5
   herbal 1
antibiotic esters 156
antibiotics 3–5
   absorption 149, 155–6
   animal use 123
   appropriate use 125–7
   availability 121–2
   bacterial cell wall synthesis inhibition 11–24
   community and hospital prescribing 123–5
   from soil microorganisms 5
   historical perspective 3–5
   inappropriate use 122–3
   policies 127, 128–30
   rotation 128
   surgical prophylaxis 186–92
   susceptibility testing 140–4
   topical use 235–41
   see also specific drugs and infections
antibiotic stewardship 205–6
   antimicrobial management team 217
   critical gaps in 218
   measurement of antimicrobial use 214–17
   medical prescribers 209–11
   non-medical prescribers 211–14
antifolates 85, 359
antifungal agents 6, 76–81
   allylamines 77, 80
   azoles 77, 78–9
   echinocandins 77, 79–80
   polyenes 76–8
   topical use 81
   see also specific drugs and infections
antihelminthic agents see anthelminthics
anti-HIV agents see antiretroviral agents
antimalarial agents 3, 6, 85–6
   resistance 86
   see also malaria
antimicrobial management teams 198–9,
   202–3, 217
antimicrobial policies 198
   content 200–2
   effectiveness 203–5
   implementation 202–3
   national policies and laws 199–200
   persuasive 198
   primary and secondary care 202
   prudent prescribing 200
   research and practice implications 206–7
   restrictive 198
   standardization benefits 200
antimicrobial use 214–17
   estimating the number treated 214–16
   estimating population size 216–17
   point prevalence surveys 217

antimonials 2, 89, 362
antimycobacterial agents 46–7
   see also mycobacteria
antiparasitic agents 6
antiprotozoal agents 6
antiretroviral agents 61–6, 344–5
   adverse reactions 63, 64, 184, 345, 346
   CCR5 binding inhibitors 65
   chemoprophylaxis 194
   combination therapy 66, 344–5
   in development 66
   fusion inhibitors 64–5
   integrase inhibitors 65
   pregnancy 347
   resistance 65–6
   targets for 62
   see also HIV; specific drugs
antiseptics 1, 235
antituberculosis therapy see tuberculosis
antiviral agents 6, 48–59
   adverse reactions 183–5
   directly acting antivirals (DAA) 73, 74
   limitations of 52
   prevention of virus infections 59
   targets for 48–50
   see also antiretroviral agents; specific drugs and
      infections
arbekacin 29
arenaviruses 49
arsenicals 2, 83–4, 256, 361
arsphenamine (Salvarsan) 2
artemether 86, 357, 358
Artemisia cina (wormseed) 1
artemisinin 6, 86, 357–8
artemotil 86, 357
artemusan 357
artesunate 86, 357
artesunic acid 357
arthritis, septic 287–9
Ascaris lumbricoides 87
aspergillosis 6, 328
Aspergillus spp. 328, 330
assessment see infection assessment
asthmatic reactions 180
astroviruses 264
atebrin (mepacrine, quinacrine) 3
atovaquone 85, 332, 359, 360, 363
atoxyl 2
avoparcin 22–3, 123
azidocillin 13
azidothymidine (AZT) 61–3
azithromycin 35
   babesiosis 363
   chemoprophylaxis 195
   cryptosporidiosis 361
   gastrointestinal infections 264
   immunocompromised patients 332, 333
   sexually transmitted infections 253, 255, 256, 258
   toxoplasmosis 332, 362
azlocillin 14
azoles 77, 78–9
azomycin 6
aztreonam 19, 21, 178

Babesia spp. 86
babesiosis 86, 363
Bacillus cereus 263
bacitracin 23, 236
bacteraemia 272
 antibiotic therapy 274–6
 immunocompromised patients 275
 laboratory investigation 274
 neonatal 275
bacterial cell wall synthesis inhibitors 11–24
 cell wall construction 11–12
 see also specific inhibitors
bacterial chromosomes 102
 mutations to antibiotic resistance 103
bacterial protein synthesis inhibitors 25–38
 see also specific inhibitors
bacterial vaginosis 257–8
bactericidal agents 148–9
bacteriophages 104
bacteristatic agents 148–9
bacteriuria 242–4, 245–6
Bacteroides fragilis 44, 273
Balamuthia mandrillaris 82–3
balantidiasis 363
Balantidium coli 86, 363
BCG vaccine 316
bed sores 239–40
benflumetol (lumefantrine) 86
benzathine penicillin 13–14, 256
benzimidazoles 364, 365
benznidazole 84, 361
benzoic acid 81, 240
benzoxazinorifamycin 319
benzyl benzoate 364
benzylpenicillin 12–13
 antibacterial properties 16
 bacteraemia 275, 276
 brain abscess 305
 endocarditis 281–2, 283, 284
 meningitis 299, 300
 plasma half-life 158
 pneumonia 232
 resistance 13
 septic arthritis 288
 sexually transmitted infections 256
 skin and soft tissue infections 309, 313
 structure 12
Bertheim, Alfred 2
bilharzia 2, 364
bioavailability 156
bites 309, 310
bithionol 89
blood fluke 364
boceprevir 73
boils 309
bone infections 170
 osteomyelitis 170, 289–91
 septic arthritis 287–9
Bordetella pertussis 193, 230
boric acid 258
brain abscess 304–5
breast milk, excretion of antimicrobial agents 167
British Approved Name (BAN) 374

British National Formulary 153, 373, 374
British Pharmacopoeia Commission 374
brodimoprim 41
bronchiolitis 340
bronchitis 203, 230
bronchopneumonia 228
Brooke, Blyth 4
Brotzu, Giuseppe 4
Brown, Rachel 6
Bruce, David 2
Brucella spp. 280
Brugia malayi 363
bulaquine 85, 358–9
Burkholderia cepacia 231
burns 239

caliciviruses 49, 264
Campylobacter jejuni 263, 264–5
Candida albicans 135, 226, 240, 257, 307
candidiasis 6, 257
 immunocompromised patients 327, 330
 topical therapy 240
capreomycin 47, 100, 318, 321
carbacephem 18
carbapenems 19, 21
 resistance 96, 111, 118
carbaryl 366
carbenicillin 14
carbuncles 309, 310
carfecillin 14
carindacillin 14
caspofungin 6, 79–80, 330
catheterized patients, urinary infections 249
CCR5 binding inhibitors 65
cefaclor 18, 20
cefadroxil 18, 20
cefalexin 15, 18, 19, 20, 21
cefaloridine 15
cefalotin 15
cefamandole 15, 17, 183
cefazolin 17
cefcapene pivoxil 18
cefdinir 18
cefditoren pivoxil 18
cefepime 15, 18
cefetamet 18
cefetamet pivoxil 18
cefixime 18, 20
 gastrointestinal infections 266
 sexually transmitted infections 253
cefmenoxime 15, 18
cefmetazole 18
cefminox 18
cefodizime 18
cefoperazone 15, 18, 183
cefotaxime 15, 18, 20, 331
 bacteraemia 275
 brain abscess 305
 endocarditis 285
 meningitis 100, 297, 299, 300, 304
 respiratory tract infections 233
 septic arthritis 289
 sexually transmitted infections 255

cefotetan 15, 18, 183
cefotiam hexetil 18
cefoxitin 15, 17–18
cefpimizole 18
cefpiramide 18
cefpirome 15, 18, 20
cefpodoxime 18, 20
cefpodoxime proxetil 18
cefprozil 18, 20
cefradine 18, 20
cefsulodin 18
ceftaroline 17, 20
ceftazidime 15, 18, 20
  bacteraemia 275
  brain abscess 305
  endocarditis 285
  immunocompromised patients 329
  meningitis 300
cefteram 18
ceftibuten 18
ceftiofur 123, 124
ceftobiprole 17
ceftrazidime 18
ceftriaxone 18, 20, 157, 171
  brain abscess 305
  gastrointestinal infections 266
  meningitis 100, 297, 298, 299, 300, 304
  sexually transmitted infections 253, 255,
    256, 258
cefuroxime 15, 17–18, 20
  respiratory tract infections 233
cefuroxime axetil 18, 156
cellulitis 309, 310, 312
central nervous system (CNS)
  adverse reactions 181
  infections 293–306
  see also specific infections
cephalosporins 4–5, 15–19
  adverse reactions 176, 178, 179, 181, 183
  antimicrobial spectrum 94
  antipseudomonal 18
  bacteraemia 275
  brain abscess 305
  categorization 17
  cephalosporin C 4–5, 12, 15
  cephalosporin N 4
  cephalosporin P 4
  endocarditis 281
  excretion in breast milk 167
  gastrointestinal infections 266, 268
  immunocompromised patients 329
  meningitis 297
  placental passage 167
  renal elimination 162
  resistance 96, 99, 110–11, 117–18
  sexually transmitted infections 253, 254, 255
  structure 12, 21
  urinary infections 247
cephamycins 18
cephem 21
cerebrospinal fluid (CSF) examination 295–6
cervicitis 254–5, 336
cestodes 90

Chagas' disease 84, 361
Chain, Ernst 4
chancroid 258
chaulmoogra oil 1
chemoprophylaxis 186
  cytomegalovirus 339
  endocarditis 192
  HIV 194, 195–6
  influenza 194
  malaria 192, 359–60
  neonatal Group B streptococcal infection 193
  pneumonia 192–3
  post-exposure prophylaxis 193–4
  primary 186–94
  recurrent bacterial infections 194
  resistance and 195
  secondary 194
  selective decontamination of the gastrointestinal
    tract 192–3
  tertiary 194–6
  travellers 192
  tuberculosis 323
  urinary infections 194, 248–9
  viral infections 194
chenopodium oil 1
chickenpox 336–7
  immunocompromised patients 337
  neonatal 337
children 164
  acute otitis media 226
  bacteraemia 276
  bone and joint infections 287, 290
  central nervous system infections 297–9, 304
  chickenpox 336–7
  gastrointestinal infections 260, 262, 264, 267
  impetigo 307
  respiratory infections 56, 226, 340
  urinary infections 245, 248
  see also paediatric prescribing
Chinese liver fluke 365
chlamydial infection 194, 251
  neonatal 255–6
Chlamydia psittaci 230, 280, 283
Chlamydia trachomatis 139, 251–2, 254–5, 258
Chlamydophila (Chlamydia) pneumoniae 230
chloramphenicol 30–2
  adverse reactions 32, 175, 176, 181, 183
  antimicrobial spectrum 94
  gastrointestinal infections 266
  meningitis 297, 300
  neonates 166
  resistance 30, 113, 116, 118
  structure 30
  topical use 237, 238
chlorhexidine 235, 239
chloroquine 3, 6
  amoebic infection 82
  malaria 85, 357, 359
  resistance 86, 357
chlorproguanil 85
chlortetracycline 32
cholera 264
cholestasis 181

chromosomes, bacterial 102
  mutations to antibiotic resistance 103
ciclopirox 81
cidofovir 53, 55–6, 339
  immunocompromised patients 333, 339
  polyomavirus infections 342
  structure 55
cilastatin 19, 161
cinoxacin 42
ciprofloxacin 6, 42, 43, 44
  adverse reactions 318
  chemoprophylaxis 299
  elderly people 169
  gastrointestinal infections 264, 265, 266, 267, 268
  immunocompromised patients 330
  meningitis 299
  pharmacokinetics 158
  resistance 95, 244, 247
  septic arthritis 288
  sexually transmitted infections 253
  structure 42
  tuberculosis 318, 321
  urinary infections 244, 247
Citrobacter spp. 109
clarithromycin 35
  chemoprophylaxis 195
  gastrointestinal infections 265
  immunocompromised patients 333
  leprosy 325
clavam 21
clavulanic acid 19, 21
clinafloxacin 44
clindamycin 31, 37
  adverse reactions 37, 176, 179, 180, 181
  babesiosis 363
  children 167
  gastrointestinal infections 268
  malaria 86, 357
  osteomyelitis 291
  placental passage 167
  Pneumocystis carinii 332
  septic arthritis 288
  sexually transmitted infections 255, 258
  skin and soft tissue infections 313
  structure 36
  topical use 237, 239
  toxoplasmosis 86, 332, 362
clinical assessment 146–7
clinical trials 370–1
clofazimine 47, 325
Clonorchis sinensis 89, 365
Clostridium botulinum 263
Clostridium difficile 120, 204, 206, 207, 232, 263, 268–70
  adverse drug effects 161, 179–80
  infection control 128–30
Clostridium perfringens 263, 268, 313
clotrimazole 6, 257
cloxacillin 14, 16
co-amoxiclav 19, 374
  resistance 244
  respiratory tract infections 225, 226, 232, 233
  sexually transmitted infections 258

skin and soft tissue infections 309
  urinary infections 244, 247
coccidia 86
cold sores 307, 335
colistin 46, 99, 330
Coma Acidosis Malaria (CAM) score 358, 359
combination therapy 151–2
  HIV 344–5
  resistance and 113–14
  tuberculosis 114, 317–18
Commission on Human Medicines 372
Committee on Proprietary Medicinal Products,
    EU 371
Committee on Safety of Medicines 372, 373
compliance issues
  children 167–8
  elderly patients 169
  HIV 345–6
  tuberculosis 100, 317–18, 322
condylomata acuminata 258
conjugation 104
control of resistance 128–30, 152
  antibiotic availability 121–2
  antibiotic policies 127, 128–30
  antibiotic rotation 128
  antibiotic use in animals 123
  appropriate antibiotic use 125–7
  community and hospital prescribing 123–5
  inappropriate antibiotic use 122–3
  surveillance 127–8
coronaviruses 49
cost issues 152–3
co-trifamole 41
co-trimazine 41
co-trimoxazole 41, 374
  adverse reactions 176, 178, 179, 182, 183
  chemoprophylaxis 193, 195
  elderly patients 169
  gastrointestinal infections 264, 266, 267, 268
  immunocompromised patients 330, 332, 362
  meningitis 300
  Pneumocystis jivoreci(P. carinii) 80, 332
  protozoan infections 86, 363
  resistance 95–6
  sexually transmitted infections 258
  urinary infections 246
cough 227
Coxiella burnetii 230
  endocarditis 280, 283
cross-resistance 97
croup 225–6
cryptococcal meningitis 304
Cryptococcus neoformans 304, 327, 330
cryptogenic abscess 305
cryptosporidiosis 361
Cryptosporidium parvum 86, 361
culture-negative pyogenic meningitis 304
CURB-65 score 202, 231–2
cutaneous leishmaniasis 84
cyclophilin antagonists 74
cycloserine 23–4, 47
  tuberculosis 23, 47, 318, 321
Cyclospora cayetanensis 86, 363

cystic fibrosis 164, 170, 231
cystitis 245
cytarabine 57
cytomegalic inclusive disease 338
cytomegalovirus (CMV) 332–3, 338–9
  immunocompromised patients 332–3, 339
  prophylaxis 339
  treatment 339
cytosine arabinoside 57

dalfopristin 37
dapsone 47
  children 167
  leprosy 47, 325
  malaria 85, 357
  Pneumocystis carinii 332
daptomycin 46, 99, 283, 284
data sheets 372
Debio-025 74
Declaration of Helsinki 371
Defined Daily Dose (DDD) 216
dehydroemetine 82
demeclocycline 32, 180, 182
dental staining 180
deoxyguanosine 54
deoxystreptamine 26
Department of Health (UK) 371
development of antimicrobial drugs 367–72
  clinical trials 370–1
  drug licensing 371–2
  drug names 374
dexamethasone 297–8
diabetic foot infections 309–10
diaminopyrimidines 40–2
diarrhoea
  antibiotic-associated 180, 185, 268
  multidrug resistant pathogens 99
  traveller's 192, 260
  see also gastrointestinal infections
dicloxacillin 14
didanosine 184
diethylcarbamazine 87, 89, 363, 364
diethyltoluamide (DEET) 360
digestive tract see gastrointestinal tract
dihydroartemisinin 86
diloxanide furoate 82
diphenoxylate 262, 264
diphtheria 226
Diphyllobothrium latum 90, 365
dirithromycin 36
dissociated resistance 116
distribution of drugs 157–61
  children 165
Domagk, Gerhard 3
doramectin 87
doripenem 19
dosing 149–50
doxycycline 32, 33, 182
  endocarditis 285
  gastrointestinal infections 264
  malaria 357, 359
  sexually transmitted infections 255, 256
Dracunculus medinensis 87–9
drug accumulation 160–1, 175–7

drug interactions 161, 177–8, 184
drug names 374
Drug and Therapeutics Bulletin 373
Dubos, René 5
dyes 2, 3
dysentery 261
  amoebic 6, 82, 360
dysuria 244

Eagle phenomenon 21
echinocandins 6, 77, 79–80
Echinococcus spp. 90, 365
econazole 78
ectoparasites 365
eczema herpeticum 335
efavirenz 6, 64, 184
eflornithine 84, 361
Ehrlich, Paul 1–2, 95
elderly patients 168–9
  adverse reactions 169
  age-related infections 168
  Norwegian scabies 365
  pharmacokinetic and pharmacodynamic
    considerations 168
  respiratory infections 228
elephantiasis 87, 363
elimination of drugs 161–2
  in children 166
  in elderly patients 168
Elixir Sulfanilamide 3
emetine 1, 82
encephalitis 295
  herpes simplex 336
Encephalitozoon cuniculi 86
endocarditis 276–86
  aetiological agents 279–80
  antimicrobial regimens 148–9, 281–5
  chemoprophylaxis 192
  combination therapy 151, 281, 282
  culture-negative 280
  epidemiology 277
  intravenous drug use and 280
  laboratory diagnosis 280
  outpatient parental antimicrobial therapy
    (OPAT) 170
  pathogenesis 277–8
  prognosis 285–6
  surgical management 285
  therapeutic principles 280–1
enfuvirtide 64–5
Entamoeba coli 357
Entamoeba dispar 82
Entamoeba histolytica 82, 263, 357, 360
entecavir 70, 71, 352
enteric fever 266
Enterobacter spp. 109
Enterobius vermicularis 87
enterococci
  endocarditis 282
  resistance 99, 114, 115
Enterococcus faecalis 282
Enterococcus faecium 282
enteroviruses 294
enzyme induction 161, 177, 178, 181

epiglottitis 226
Epstein–Barr virus (EBV) 51, 338
ertapenem 19
erysipelas 309, 310
erythromycin 34–5
    adverse reactions 35, 176, 178, 179
    derivatives 35–6, 181
    elderly patients 169
    excretion in breast milk 167
    gastrointestinal infections 265
    neonatal infection 256
    pharmacokinetics 156
    placental passage 167
    resistance 116
    respiratory tract infections 226, 230–1
    sexually transmitted infections 255, 256, 258
    structure 34
    topical use 237, 239
Escherichia coli 19
    bacteraemia 275
    gastrointestinal infections 260, 263, 267
    joint infections 287
    meningitis 164, 293, 297, 300
    resistance 93, 95–6, 126, 247
    urinary infections 246
Etest 141
ethambutol 47, 320
    adverse reactions 181, 320
    immunocompromised patients 333
    resistance 100
    tuberculosis 317, 320, 321, 324
ethionamide 47, 318, 321
etravirine 64
European Medicines Evaluation Agency 371
European Surveillance of Antibiotic Consumption
    (ESAC) project 124–5, 206, 216–17
extracellular fluid, drug distribution in 158–9

famciclovir 53, 54, 334, 335
Fasciola hepatica 89, 365
fascioliasis 365
fenbendazole 89
filarial worms 87–9, 363
filariasis 87–9, 356, 363–4
filoviruses 49
flagellates 83–5
flaviviruses 49
Fleming, Alexander 1, 4, 120
Florey, Howard 1, 3
flucloxacillin 14, 157
    adverse reactions 181, 183
    antibacterial properties 16
    bacteraemia 275
    brain abscess 305
    endocarditis 282–3, 284
    meningitis 303
    osteomyelitis 291
    septic arthritis 288, 289
    toxic shock syndrome 313
fluconazole 6, 78–9
    immunocompromised patients 330
    kala azar 362
    meningitis 297, 304
    resistance 122

sexually transmitted infections 257
    structure 79
flucytosine (5-fluorocytosine) 77, 79
    amphotericin and 304
    combination therapy 79
    endocarditis 285
    immunocompromised patients 330
    meningitis 297, 304
fluid replacement, gastrointestinal infections 261–2
flumequine 42
fluoroquinolones 44
    animal use 123
    antimicrobial spectrum 94
    antimycobacterial effects 47
    gastrointestinal infections 265, 266, 267, 268
    immunocompromised patients 330
    resistance 44, 95–6, 126
    respiratory tract infections 232, 233
    septic arthritis 288
    sexually transmitted infections 253, 254, 255, 258
    topical use 238
    tuberculosis 321
    urinary infections 247, 249
folliculitis 308
fomivirsen 53, 56, 339
Food and Drug Administration (FDA) 371
food poisoning 261
foreign material 153
formularies 198, 373
    standardization benefits 200
foscarnet 56, 339
    adverse reactions 56, 184
    immunocompromised patients 333, 339
    structure 56
fosfomycin 24, 247
framycetin 29, 330
fungal infections 6, 76, 77
    endocarditis 279
    immunocompromised hosts 327–8
    superficial 240
    see also antifungal agents; specific infections
furuncles 309, 310
fusidic acid 31, 33–4, 157
    adverse reactions 176, 181
    resistance 116
    structure 33
    topical use 236, 237, 238
fusion inhibitors 64–5

ganciclovir 53, 54–5
    adverse reactions 54–5, 183–4
    herpesvirus infections 339, 340
    immunocompromised patients 333, 339
    resistance 55
    structure 54
    topical use 238
Gardnerella vaginalis 258
gas gangrene 313
gastrointestinal infections 260–71
    antibiotic therapy 262–4
    Campylobacter 264–5
    cholera 264
    clinical manifestations 261
    enteric fever 266

gastrointestinal infections (*cont.*)
  Escherichia coli 260, 263, 267
  fluid replacement 261–2
  Helicobacter pylori 265
  intestinal parasites 268, 356
  salmonellosis 261, 265–6
  shigellosis 261, 266–7
  transmission and acquisition 260–1
  virus infections 260, 264
  yersiniosis 268
gastrointestinal tract
  adverse reactions 180
  selective decontamination 192–3, 330–1
gatifloxacin 44, 255
generic prescribing 374
genetic determinants of toxicity 175
genetics of resistance 102–6
  antibiotic selection pressure influence 107
  bacterial chromosome 102
  bacteriophages 104
  evolution of new resistance gene
    combinations 105
  genotypic resistance 106
  phenotypic resistance 106–7
  plasmids 103–4
  transfer of genetic information 104–6
genital herpes 336
genital warts 258
genotypic resistance 106
gentamicin 26, 28, 29, 171
  adverse reactions 173
  bacteraemia 275
  brain abscess 305
  combination therapy 151
  endocarditis 281, 282, 283, 284, 285
  immunocompromised patients 329, 330
  meningitis 300, 304
  resistance 15, 241
  septic arthritis 289
  skin and soft tissue infections 313
  structure 27
  topical use 236, 237
Gentles, James 6
Germanin (suramin) 2
giant cell pneumonia 340
Giardia lamblia (intestinalis) 84–5, 263, 356, 360–1
giardiasis 6, 360–1
glandular fever 225, 338
glucose-6-phosphate dehydrogenase
  deficiency 167, 175
glycopeptides 22–3
  antimicrobial spectrum 94
  resistance 114
gonorrhoea 30, 194, 251, 253–4
gramicidin 46
Gram stain 11–12
grey baby syndrome 32, 166
griseofulvin 6, 77, 80, 240
  adverse reactions 178
  skin and soft tissue infections 311
guidelines 198
  standardazation benefits 200
gut sedatives 262–4

hachimycin (trichomycin) 76
haematological toxicity 182
haemolytic uraemic syndrome 267
Haemophilus ducreyi 258
Haemophilus influenzae 164, 230, 231, 233
  acute otitis media 226
  croup 226
  joint infections 287
  meningitis 293, 297, 299
  resistance 230
halofantrine 86, 358
haloprogin 81
Hata, Sahachiro 2
Hazen, Elizabeth 6
head lice 366
Heatley, Norman 4
Helicobacter pylori 117, 265
helminths 87–90
  cestodes 90
  nematodes 87–9
  trematodes 89, 364–5
hepadnaviruses 50
hepatitis, antimicrobial drug-induced 181
hepatitis B (HBV) 51, 68–71, 347, 349–52
  treatment 350–2
hepatitis C (HCV) 51, 71–4, 347, 352–5, 364
  laboratory detection 139–40
  monitoring of therapy 354
  treatment 352–5
hepeviruses 49
herbal anthelminthics 1
herpes simplex 195, 334–6
  encephalitis 336
  genital 257, 336
  immunocompromised patients 336
  meningitis 294–5
herpesviruses 6, 50, 51, 255, 334, 335
herpes zoster 337–8
hexamine 1
highly active antiretroviral therapy (HAART) 195,
  331–2, 344
histamine release 177
historical background 1–7
Hitchings, George 5
HIV 6, 61, 326, 331
  chemoprophylaxis 194, 195–6
  combination therapy 344–5
  compliance issues 345–6
  hepatitis and 347, 352
  herpesvirus infections 337, 338, 339
  leishmaniasis and 362
  meningitis and 295
  natural history of infections 343
  Norwegian scabies and 365
  opportunistic mycobacteria 324
  replication cycle 62
  resistance 346–7
  timing of treatment 344
  tuberculosis and 315, 322–3
  viral load measurements 139
  see also AIDS; antiretroviral agents
hookworm 87
human herpesviruses 339–40

human immunodeficiency virus *see* HIV
human papillomavirus (HPV) 258
hydatid disease 90, 365
hydroxyquinolones 236
Hymenolepis nana 90, 365
hypersensitivity 178–9
hyposplenism 333

idoxuridine 57
imidazoles 44, 78, 362
　sexually transmitted infections 257
　topical use 78, 237, 238
imipenem 19, 161
　adverse reactions 181
　immunocompromised patients 329
　resistance 99, 118
　structure 21
imiquimod 258, 341
immune globulin 59
immunization 59, 196–7
immunocompromised patients
　bacteraemia 275
　chemotherapeutic principles 328
　microbial complications 327–8
　neutropenic patients 329–33
　see also HIV
immunodeficiency 326, 327
immunosuppression 326
impetigo 307–8, 310
indinavir 182
infection assessment
　clinical assessment 146–7
　inflammatory response assessment 147, 148
　laboratory assessment 147
　sepsis assessment 148
infection control 128–30
infection risk of surgery 186–7, 188, 189
infection treatment 146–53
　adverse reactions 151
　choice of regimen 149–52
　choice of therapy 148–9, 153, 375
　combined therapy 151–2
　cost 152–3
　failure of 153
　initial therapy 151
　length of therapy 150
infectious mononucleosis syndrome 338
infective endocarditis *see* endocarditis
inflammatory response assessment 147, 148
influenza 340–1
　chemoprophylaxis 194
　resistance 341
injection 156–7
integrase inhibitors 65, 344
integrons 105–6
interferon (IFN) 58–9, 68–9
　adverse effects 72, 352–3
　combination therapy 58, 71–3, 352–3
　hepatitis treatment 68–9, 71–3, 350, 351, 352
　interferon-alpha 71
　pegylated interferon (PEG-INF) 69, 72
　respiratory tract infections 340
　warts 341

International Non-proprietary Name (INN; rINN) 374
intestinal elimination 161
intracellular fluid, drug distribution in 159–61
intramuscular injection 157
intravenous injection 156–7, 171
intrinsic resistance 93–5, 102
in-vitro incompatibilities 177
in-vivo interactions 177–8
isoniazid 5, 47, 318–19
　adverse reactions 181, 319
　chemoprophylaxis 323, 333
　excretion in breast milk 167
　immunocompromised patients 333
　length of therapy 150
　resistance 100, 318–19, 323
　tuberculosis 317, 318–19, 321, 324
Isospora belli 86, 363
isoxazolypenicillins 14
itraconazole 6, 78–9
　kala azar 362
ivermectin 6, 87, 89, 363–4, 365

Jarisch–Herxheimer reaction 257
joint infections 170
　septic arthritis 287–9

kala azar 2, 84, 362
kanamycin 26, 28, 29–30
　kanamycin A 29, 112, 113
　resistance 112–13
　tuberculosis 100, 318, 321
Kaposi's sarcoma-associated herpesvirus 340
ketoconazole 6, 78, 362
ketolides 36
kidney
　adverse reactions 182
　drug elimination 161–2
　infection 245
Klarer, Josef 3
Klebsiella spp. 98, 111, 331
　K. aerogenes 17
　K. oxytoca 268
　resistance 98, 244
Koch, Robert 1

laboratory use 135, 147
　antimicrobial susceptibility testing 140–4
　detection of difficult to culture pathogens 139–40
　importance of clinical details 135–6
　non-culture methods 139
　specimen collection 136–7
　specimen processing 137–9
　specimen transport 137
beta-lactam antibiotics 12–22
　adverse reactions 178, 180, 181, 183
　combination therapy 151
　dosage 21, 150
　immunocompromised patients 329
　mode of action 19–21
　pharmacokinetics 159, 160
　resistance 14–15, 108–11, 114, 117–18
　see also specific drugs
beta-lactamases 108–11

lactation 322
  excretion of antimicrobial agents 167
  tuberculosis and 322
lamivudine 66
  adverse reactions 184
  hepatitis 70, 352
  resistance 70
  structure 70
lapdap 85
Lassa fever 342
latamoxef (moxalactam) 18
Legionella pneumophila 230
leishmaniasis 84, 362
Leishmania spp. 84
leprosy 1, 47, 324–5
levamisole 89, 364
levofloxacin 43, 44, 321
  resistance 95
  respiratory tract infections 232
  sexually transmitted infections 255
lice 366
licensing of drugs 371–2
lincomycin 36
lincosamides 36–7
lindane 365
linezolid 31, 38, 99
  resistance 38, 117
Listeria monocytogenes 275
  meningitis 293, 294, 300
liver, adverse reactions 181
liver fluke 89, 365
Livingstone, David 2
Loa loa 87
loracarbef 18
lower respiratory tract infections 164, 227–9
  elderly patients 168
  epidemiology 227–8
  hospital management 231–3
  primary care management 229–31
  viral infections 340
lumefantrine 86, 358
lung fluke 365
lymecycline 32
lymphangitis 309
lymphogranuloma venereum 258

macrolides 31, 34–6
  antimicrobial spectrum 94
  antimycobacterial effects 47
  elderly people 169
  respiratory tract infections 225, 230, 232
  toxoplasmosis 362
  see also specific drugs
mafenide 239
malaria 1–2, 85–6, 357–60
  chemoprophylaxis 192, 359–60
  combination therapy 86
  resistance 357, 358
  see also antimalarial agents
malathion 365, 366
male fern extract 1, 90
maraviroc 65
marketing 372–3

materno-fetal prescribing 166–7
matrix-assisted laser desorption/ionization time of
    flight (MALDI/TOF) 140
measles 196
mebendazole 89, 364
mecillinam (amdinocillin) 14, 16, 19, 21
  resistance 107
Medical Letter (USA) 373
Medicines Commission 372
Medicines and Healthcare Products Registry Agency
    (UK) 185, 371, 372, 373
mefloquine 86, 158, 358, 359
meglumine antimonate 84, 362
melarsoprol (Mel B) 2, 83–4, 361
membrane function, agents affecting 46
meningitis 293
  bacterial 293–4, 301–2
  haemophilus 299
  laboratory diagnosis 295–6
  meningococcal disease 298–9
  neonatal 164, 299–300
  pneumococcal 299
  rare forms 303–4
  therapeutic considerations 296–8
  tuberculous 323–4
  viral 293, 294–5
meningococcal infection 298–9
  children 164
mepacrine 3, 84–5, 90, 361
mercury 1, 256
meropenem 19
metabolic determinants of toxicity 175–7
metabolism of drugs 161
  children 165–6
methacycline 32
meticillin 14
  resistance 14–15, 114
meticillin-resistant Staphylococcus aureus
    (MRSA) 15, 21, 38, 233
  cellulitis 309
  glycopeptides 99
  nasal carriage 238–9
  resistance 97, 99, 121
  skin and soft tissue infections 313
  topical therapy 237, 238, 239
  vancomycin 275, 305
methotrexate 42
methylene blue 3
metrifonate 89, 364
metronidazole 6, 45
  adverse reactions 178, 181
  antimicrobial spectrum 94
  balantidiasis 363
  brain abscess 305
  excretion in breast milk 167
  gastrointestinal infections 180, 265, 268
  protozoan infections 82, 84, 360, 361
  sexually transmitted infections 255, 257, 258
  skin and soft tissue infections 313
  topical use 237
micafungin 79–80
miconazole 78, 238
micro-array technology 140

microsporidia 83, 363
Mietzsch, Fritz 3
miltefosine 84, 362
minimal bactericidal concentration 93, 141, 281
minimum inhibitory concentration (MIC) 93, 141,
      150, 281
minocycline 32, 325
mitral valve prolapse 277
MMR vaccine 196
monobactams 19, 21
monoclonal antibody 59
Moraxella catarrhalis 230
moxalactam (latamoxef) 18
moxifloxacin 43, 44, 99, 255, 321
MRSA *see* meticillin-resistant
      Staphylococcus aureus (MRSA)
multidrug resistance 97
   see also resistance
mumps 294–5
mupirocin 31, 37–8, 236, 239
   structure 38
mutational resistance 96
mutations 103
mycobacteria 46–7
   atypical 324
   opportunistic 324
   see also leprosy; malaria
mycobacteriosis 333
Mycobacterium avium 195, 324, 333
Mycobacterium leprae 324
   see also leprosy
Mycobacterium tuberculosis 5, 136, 139, 315
   hospital transmission 323
   immunocompromised patients 333
   laboratory detection 139, 140, 316
   meningitis 294, 303
   resistance 93–5, 100, 317, 323
   see also tuberculosis
Mycoplasma pneumoniae 230
mycoplasmas 32, 33, 34

Naegleria fowleri 82–3
nafcillin 14
naftifine 80
nagana 2
nalidixic acid 5, 42–4
   adverse reactions 175, 176, 181
   children 167
   structure 42
   urinary infection 246–7
naming of drugs 374
nasal carriage 238–9
Naseptin 239
natamycin 76, 85
National Formulary (USA) 373
National Institute for Health and Clinical Excellence
      (NICE), UK 373
near patient tests 137
Necator americanus 87
necrotic material 153
necrotizing fasciitis 311
Neisseria gonorrhoeae 251, 253, 254
   endocarditis 276

joint infections 287
   see also gonorrhoea
Neisseria meningitidis 293–4, 297, 298–9
   bacteraemia 276
   post-exposure prophylaxis 193–4
   resistance 100
   see also meningitis
nelfinavir 185
nematodes 87–9, 363–4
neoarsphenamine (Neosalvarsan) 2
neomycin 26, 28, 29
   adverse effects 29
   antiprotozoal effects 83
   immunocompromised patients 330
   topical use 236, 239, 241
neonates
   bacteraemia 275
   chemoprophylaxis 193
   chickenpox 337
   chlamydial infection 255–6
   conjunctivitis 256
   gonococcal infection 255–6
   herpes infection 336
   meningitis 164, 299–300
   prescribing for 165–6
   thrush 226
Neosalvarsan (neoarsphenamine) 2
netilmicin 28, 29
neuraminidase inhibitors 340–1
neurological adverse effects 181–2
neutropenia 149, 329–33
nevirapine 64, 179, 184
niclosamide 90, 365
nifurtimox 45, 84, 361
nimorazole 45
nitazoxanide 86, 89, 361
nitrofurans 5, 45
nitrofurantoin 5, 45
   adverse reactions 175, 176, 179, 180, 181
   resistance 244
   urinary infection 244, 246–7, 248
nitroimidazoles 6, 44–5, 361
non-nucleoside analogue reverse
      transcriptase inhibitors (NNRTIs) 6, 62,
      63–4, 344
   adverse reactions 184
norfloxacin 6, 43
normal flora, alteration by drugs 161, 179–80
norovirus 263, 264
Norwalk virus 264
Norwegian scabies 365
nucleic acid synthesis inhibitors 40–6
nucleoside analogues 52–7, 69–71
   adverse effects 181, 184
   hepatitis 351–2
   reverse transcriptase inhibitors (NRTIs) 61–3, 344
nucleotide analogues 63, 69–71
   hepatitis 351–2
nucleotidyltransferases 112
nystatin 6, 76, 226
   immunocompromised patients 330
   sexually transmitted infections 257
   topical use 237, 238, 240

ocular herpes simplex 335
ofloxacin 43, 44, 321, 325
oleandomycin 36
omeprazole 265
Onchocerca volvulus 87, 363
onchocerciasis 2, 89
ophthalmia neonatorum 256
opportunist pathogens 135–6, 324
oral administration 149, 156
oral hairy leukoplakia 338
oral rehydration 262
ornidazole 45
orthomyxoviruses 49
oseltamivir 53, 58, 194, 340, 341
osteomyelitis 170, 289–91
otitis media
  acute 226–7
  with effusion 226, 227
outpatient parenteral antimicrobial
    therapy (OPAT) 170–3
  adverse events 173
  antibiotics for 171
  indications 170
  monitoring 172–3
  requirements for 170–1
  technology 171
oxacephem 15
oxacillin 14
oxamniquine 89, 364
oxazolidinones 38
oxolinic acid 42
oxytetracycline 32

paediatric prescribing 164–6
  compliance issues 167–8
  pharmacokinetic and pharmacodynamic
    considerations 164–6
  see also children
Paine, Cecil George 4
palivizumab 59
pamaquine (plasmochin) 3
panipenem 19
papillomaviruses 50, 341
para-aminobenzoic acid 41
para-aminosalicylic acid 5, 47, 318, 321
Paracelsus 2
paracetamol 225
Paragonimus westermani 89, 365
paramyxoviruses 49
parasitic diseases 6, 82, 356
  therapeutic difficulties 356–7
  see also specific parasites and diseases
paratyphoid 266
parenteral administration 156–7
  see also outpatient parenteral antimicrobial
    therapy (OPAT)
paromomycin 29, 82, 84, 361, 362
parvoviruses 50
passive immunization 59
Pasteurella multocida 309
Pasteur, Louis 1
Patient Group Directive (PGD) 213–14
Pediculus capitis 366
pelvic inflammatory disease 255

penam 21
penciclovir 54, 334
penicillins 3–4, 12–15, 172
  acid stability 13
  adverse reactions 173, 176, 178, 179, 181, 183, 241
  antimicrobial spectrum 94
  antipseudomonal 14
  antistaphylococcal 14–15
  bacteraemia 275
  chemoprophylaxis 193
  children 165
  combination therapy 151–2
  drug dosing 149
  endocarditis 281–2
  excretion in breast milk 167
  historical perspective 3–4
  hyposplenism 333
  intramuscular injection 157
  length of therapy 150
  plasma level prolongation 13–14
  renal elimination 162
  resistance 13–15, 95–6, 99–100, 109–11, 114,
    117–18, 120
  respiratory tract infections 225, 226, 227
  sexually transmitted infections 253, 254, 256
  skin and soft tissue infections 309
  spectrum extension 14
  structure 21
  tolerance 21
  topical use 241
pentamidine 84, 332, 361, 362
peramivir 341
peripherally inserted central catheters (PICC) 171
Perkin, William 3
permethrin 360, 365, 366
persisters 21
pertussis 230–1
pharmacodynamics 162–3
  children 164–6
  elderly patients 168
pharmacokinetics 149
  absorption 149, 155–6, 165
  children 164–6
  distribution 157–61, 165
  elderly patients 168
  elimination 161–2, 166
  infection influence 162
  metabolism 161, 165–6
phenethicillin 13
phenothrin 366
phenotypic resistance 106–7
phenoxymethylpenicillin 13, 16
phosphotransferases 112
Phthirus pubis 366
picornaviruses 49
pimaricin (natamycin) 76
pipemidic acid 42
piperacillin 14
  antibacterial properties 16
  bacteraemia 275
  immunocompromised patients 329
  respiratory tract infections 233
piperaquine 86
piperazine 89, 364

pivampicillin 14, 156
pivmecillinam 247
placental passage 166–7
plasma half-life 158
plasmids 103–4, 110, 116
plasmochin (pamaquine) 3
Plasmodium spp. 85, 357
  P. falciparum 85, 357
  P. ovale 358
  P. vivax 358
  see also malaria
pneumococcal meningitis 299
Pneumocystis jiroveci (P.carinii) 76, 80–1
  immunocompromised patients 80, 195, 196,
    328, 332
  prophylaxis 80, 195, 196, 332
pneumocystosis 328
pneumonia 160, 227, 229–30, 231–3
  chemoprophylaxis 192–3
  hospital-acquired 232–3
  infants 340
  pneumocystis 80
podophyllin 258, 341
polyenes 76–8
polymyxins 46
  children 165
  immunocompromised patients 330
  topical use 236
polyomaviruses 50, 342
polypharmacy, elderly patients 168
porins 117–18
postantibiotic effect 21–2, 163
post-exposure prophylaxis 193–4, 341
post-marketing surveillance 372–3
povidone iodine 256
poxviruses 49
praziquantel 6, 89, 90, 364, 365
pregnancy
  antiretroviral therapy 347
  Group B streptococci 193
  herpesvirus infections 336
  malaria 359
  prescribing in 166–7
  tuberculosis 322
  urinary infection 246
prescribers
  medical 209–11
  non-medical 211–14
Prescription Medicines Code of Practice Authority 373
pressure sores 239–40
primaquine 3
  adverse reactions 175, 358
  malaria 85, 358
  Pneumocystis carinii 332
pristinamycin 37
probenecid 13, 162
procaine penicillin 13, 157
proctitis 257
pro-drugs 14, 156
proguanil 42, 85, 359, 360
Prontosil 3, 40
  structure 41
Prontosil red 3
propamidine 83

prophage 104
prophylaxis *see* chemoprophylaxis
propicillin 13
prostatitis 245, 249
prosthetic device infection
  endocarditis 279–80
  outpatient parental antimicrobial
    therapy (OPAT) 170
  prosthetic joint 287, 289
protease inhibitors 6, 64, 344
  adverse reactions 184
  hepatitis 73
  HIV 64
protein binding 157, 165
Proteus spp. 45, 331
protionamide 47, 318, 321
protozoa 6, 82–6
  amoebae 82–3
  flagellates 83–5
  sporozoa 85–6
  see also specific infections
Pseudomonas aeruginosa 3, 14, 231, 233
  bacteraemia 275
  cost of antipseudomonal agents 152
  immunocompromised patients 329
  osteomyelitis 290
  resistance 93–5, 102, 109, 241
  skin infection 239, 240
Pseudomonas spp. 164
pseudomonic acid *see* mupirocin
pubic lice 366
pustular lesions 308–9, 310
PVL toxin 313
pyelonephritis 245, 246
pyocyanase 3
pyrantel pamoate 89, 364
pyrazinamide 47, 317, 318, 320, 321, 324
pyrimethamine 42
  malaria 85, 357, 358, 359
  toxoplasmosis 86, 332, 362

quinacrine 3, 85, 90
quinine 1, 3, 85, 86, 162, 357
  babesiosis 363
quinolones 5–6, 42–4
  adverse reactions 42, 176, 179, 180, 181
  chemoprophylaxis 193
  dosing 150
  elderly patients 169
  resistance 116, 118
  see also fluoroquinolones

raltegravir 65
recombinant activated Protein C 276
red man syndrome 177
renal elimination 161–2, 166
reoviruses 49
research requirements 206–7
resistance 93, 120, 375
  acquired 95–6, 107–19
  clinical significance 97–8
  control of *see* control of resistance
  cross 97
  genetics of 102–6

resistance (*cont.*)
  intrinsic 93–5, 102
  mechanisms 107–19
  multiple 97
  mutational 96
  prophylaxis and 195
  surveillance 127–8
  transmissible 96
  see also specific drugs and pathogens
respiratory syncytial virus 340
respiratory tract adverse reactions 180
respiratory tract infections 215, 223
  see also lower respiratory tract infections; upper
      respiratory tract infections
retroviruses 49
  see also antiretroviral agents
reverse transcriptase inhibitors (RTIs) 6, 61–4
  non-nucleoside analogue RTIs (NNRTIs) 62,
      63–4, 344
  nucleos(t)ide analogue RTIs (NRTIs) 61–3, 344
rhabdoviruses 49
rheumatic fever 136, 225, 287
ribavirin 53, 56, 57, 58
  adverse effects 352–3
  combination therapy 71, 72–3, 352–3
  hepatitis treatment 71, 72–3, 352
  Lassa fever 342
  respiratory infections 340
rifabutin 46, 320, 333
rifampicin (rifampin) 5, 45–6, 319
  adverse reactions 46, 176, 178, 181, 319
  brain abscess 305
  chemoprophylaxis 195, 298–9
  endocarditis 283, 284
  enzyme induction 161, 177, 178, 181
  length of therapy 150
  leprosy 325
  meningitis 298–9, 303
  resistance 100, 117, 317, 323
  tuberculosis 317, 318, 319, 321, 324
rifamycin B 45
rifapentine 46
Rifater 322
Rifinah 322
rimantadine 57, 194, 341
ritonavir 64, 182
rotavirus 263, 264
roundworm 1, 87–9
roxithromycin 36

salicylic acid 258, 341
Salmonella enterica 4, 148, 263, 265, 274
  bacteraemia 276
  carriage 266
  enteric fever 266
  resistance 123, 266
salmonellosis 261, 265–6
Salvarsan (arsphenamine) 2, 256
santonin 1
saquinavir 184
Sarcoptes scabiei 365
scabies 365
Schatz, Albert 5

Schistosoma spp. (schistosomiasis) 89, 364
Scottish Medicines Consortium 373
secnidazole 45
sepsis 211, 272
  assessment 148, 272–4
  severe 272
  skin and soft tissue infections and 307, 308, 311
  see also bacteraemia
sepsis syndrome 272, 298
septicaemia 272
  see also bacteraemia
septic arthritis 287–9
septic shock 272
  management 276
sexually transmitted infections 251–9
  genital tract infections 252–8
  laboratory diagnosis 251–2
  see also specific infections
Shigella spp. 263, 266–7
shigellosis 261
shingles 58, 337
shunt-associated meningitis 303
sialic acid 58
side effects *see* adverse reactions
silver nitrate 256
silver sulfadiazine 239
sinusitis 227
skin
  adverse reactions 179, 180
  infections 211, 237–8, 307–14
  ulcers 239–40, 310
  see also topical therapy
sleeping sickness 1–2, 83–4
sodium fusidate 283, 284
sodium stibogluconate 84, 362
soft tissue infections 211, 307–14
soil microorganisms, antibiotics from 5
sore throat 223–5
specimens
  collection 136–7
  processing 137–9
  transport 137
spectinomycin 30, 253
spheroplasts 21
spiramycin 36, 86
spirochaetes 2, 32, 251
sporozoa 85–6
staphylococci
  endocarditis 279, 282–3, 284
  nasal carriage 238–9
  resistance 14–15, 38, 96, 99, 110
  see also specific species
Staphylococcus aureus
  bacteraemia 273, 274
  brain abscess 305
  cystic fibrosis 164
  endocarditis 276, 277–8, 279, 280, 282–3
  gastrointestinal infections 261, 263, 268
  joint infection 287
  meningitis 294, 303
  osteomyelitis 290, 291
  resistance 95, 99, 114, 120
  respiratory infections 230, 231, 233

skin and soft tissue infections 209, 239, 240, 307, 310, 311, 313
  see also meticillin-resistant *Staphylococcus aureus* (MRSA)
Staphylococcus epidermidis
  bacteraemia 273, 275
  endocarditis 279, 280, 283
  meningitis 303
stavudine 184
Stenotrophomonas maltophilia 231
Stevens–Johnson syndrome 179
streptamine 26
streptidine 26
streptococci
  endocarditis 279, 281–2, 284
  Group B 164, 193, 297, 300
  neonatal infection, chemoprophylaxis 193
  resistance 38
Streptococcus agalactiae 193, 275, 287
  meningitis 293, 294
Streptococcus bovis 279, 281
Streptococcus milleri 305
Streptococcus pneumoniae 164, 230, 233
  acute otitis media 226
  bacteraemia 273, 276
  endocarditis 276
  meningitis 293, 294, 297, 299
  resistance 99
Streptococcus pyogenes 136
  bacteraemia 273
  length of therapy 150
  resistance 95
  skin and soft tissue infections 239, 307, 309, 310, 311, 313
  sore throat 225
streptogramins 31, 37
streptomycin 5, 25–9, 320
  adverse effects 320
  combination therapy 151
  resistance 100, 116
  tuberculosis 29, 317, 318, 320
Strongyloides stercoralis 358
strongyloidiasis 328
sulbactam 19, 21
sulfadiazine 41
  toxoplasmosis 332, 362
sulfadoxine 85, 359
sulfalene (sulfametopyrazine) 85
sulfamethoxazole *see* co-trimoxazole
sulfamoxole 41
sulphanilamide 3, 41
sulphonamides 3, 40
  adverse reactions 175, 176, 178, 179, 180, 182, 183
  antimicrobial spectrum 94
  excretion in breast milk 167
  malaria 357, 358, 359
  pregnancy 167
  resistance 95–6, 118
  see also specific drugs
sulphone 21
suramin (Germanin) 2, 361
surgical prophylaxis 186–92
surveillance

antimicrobial use 214–17
  resistance 127–8
susceptibility testing 140–4
  clinical relevance 141–2
  interpretation of reports 144
  laboratory reports 142–4
  purpose 140–1
  selection of antimicrobial therapy 148
  test methods 141
synergistic effects 151
syphilis 1, 2, 251, 256–7
systemic inflammatory response syndrome (SIRS) 272, 273

Taenia spp. 90, 365
tafenoquine 85
tapeworms 1, 90, 365
tartar emetic 2
tazobactam 19, 233, 275, 329
teicoplanin 22, 23, 157, 171
  bacteraemia 275
  resistance 114
telaprevir 73
telavancin 23
telithromycin 36
TEM-1 110, 111
temocillin 14, 16
tenofovir 55, 63, 70, 71, 351–2
terbinafine 80, 240
tetracyclines 31, 32–3
  adverse reactions 176, 179, 180, 181, 182
  amoebic infection 82
  anthelminthic effects 87
  antimicrobial spectrum 94
  balantidiasis 363
  elderly patients 169
  excretion in breast milk 167
  gastrointestinal infections 264, 267, 268
  neonatal infection 256
  resistance 97, 117
  respiratory tract infections 225, 230, 232
  sexually transmitted infections 255, 258
  therapeutic use 33
  topical use 236, 241
tetroxoprim 41
thiacetazone 47, 318, 320–1
thiamphenicol 30, 183
threadworm 87, 356
thrush 226
  topical therapy 240
tiabendazole 89, 364
ticarcillin 14, 16
tigecycline 31, 32–3, 99
tinidazole 45, 257
tioconazole 78, 240
tipranavir 66
tissue biopsies, drug concentrations 160
tissue distribution 157
tizoxanide 86
tobramycin 26, 28, 29
togaviruses 49
tolnaftate 81
tonsillitis 136, 150

topical therapy 235–41
  acne 239
  antiseptics 1, 235
  application methods 236
  bacterial skin infections 237–8
  burns 239
  choice of 236–7
  disadvantages 240–1
  fungal infections 240
  skin ulcers 239–40
toxicity
  determinants 175–7
  tissue- and organ-specific 180–2
  see also adverse reactions; specific drugs
toxic shock syndrome 311, 313
Toxocara canis 89, 364
toxocariasis 364
Toxoplasma gondii 86, 332, 362
toxoplasmosis 86, 362
  immunocompromised patients 86, 332
trachoma 255
transduction 104
transformation 51, 104
transposons 105
traveller's diarrhoea 192, 260
treatment *see* infection treatment
trematodes 89, 364–5
Treponema pallidum 256
triacetyloleandomycin 36
triazoles 78–9
Trichinella spiralis 87
trichlorfon (metrifonate) 89
trichloroacetic acid 258
trichomonal vaginitis 6
Trichomonas vaginalis 84–5, 251, 255, 257, 356
trichomoniasis 251, 257
trichomycin 76, 85
Trichuris trichiura 87
triclabendazole 89, 365
trifluridine 57
trimethoprim 5, 40–1
  antimicrobial spectrum 94
  combination therapy 80–1
  Pneumocystis jiroveci (carinii) 80–1
  pregnancy 167
  resistance 41, 118, 244, 247
  structure 41
  urinary infection 93, 244, 246, 248
  see also co-trimoxazole
trimetrexate 42
trovafloxacin 44
trypan blue 2
Trypanosoma brucei 83–4, 361
Trypanosoma cruzi 84, 361
trypanosomiasis
  African sleeping sickness 1–2, 83–4, 361
  Chagas' disease 84, 361
tryparsamide 2
tuberculosis 5, 47, 315–24
  chemoprophylaxis 323
  combination therapy 114, 317–18
  diagnosis 316
  extrapulmonary 323–4

HIV infection and 315, 322–3
  immune response 315
  length of therapy 150
  management principles 315–16
  pregnancy and lactation 322
  resistance 100, 317, 323
  response to therapy 318
  streptomycin 29
  therapeutic response monitoring 322
  treatment 317–24
  vaccination 316
typhoid 4, 266
tyrocidine 46
tyrothricin 5, 46

undecylenic acid 81
United States Adopted Name (USAN) Council 374
upper respiratory tract infections 223–7
  acute otitis media 226–7
  children 164
  croup 225–6
  diphtheria 226
  sinusitis 227
  sore throat 223–5
  thrush 226
  viral infections 340
urethral syndrome 245, 257
urethritis 251, 254–5
urinary tract infections 242–9
  antibiotic treatment 245–8
  bacteriuria 242–4
  catheterized patients 249
  chemoprophylaxis 194, 248–9
  children 245, 248
  elderly patients 168
  nitrofurantoin 45
  recurrent 248–9
  symptomatic 244–5
urine sampling 242, 243–4

vaginal discharge 257–8
valaciclovir 53, 156
  chemoprophylaxis 339
  herpesvirus infections 334, 335
valganciclovir 53, 55, 333, 338, 339
vancomycin 22, 23, 171
  adverse reactions 176, 177
  bacteraemia 275
  brain abscess 305
  endocarditis 281, 282, 283, 284
  gastrointestinal infections 180, 268
  immunocompromised patients 330
  meningitis 299, 303
  resistance 114
varicella-zoster virus (VZV) 334, 336–8
Vibrio cholerae 263, 264
vidarabine 57
viomycin 47
viral infections 6, 48, 49, 334
  gastrointestinal infections 260, 264
  immunocompromised hosts 327
  prevention 59, 194
  properties of viruses 48

respiratory tract infections 340–1
viral replication cycle 51
virus–cell interactions 51
see also antiviral agents; sepcific infections
virginiamycin 37
volume of distribution 159–60
voriconazole 78–9, 330

Waksman, Selman A. 1, 5
warts 258, 341–2
whipworm 87
Whitfield's ointment 81, 240
whooping cough 230–1
winter vomiting disease 260

World Health Organization (WHO) 125–6
list of essential medicines 376–7
wormseed 1
Wuchereria bancrofti 87, 363

Yersinia enterocolitica 263, 268
yersiniosis 268

zalcitabine 63
zanamivir 53, 58, 194, 340, 341
zidovudine 6, 61–3, 344
adverse effects 63, 184
resistance 65